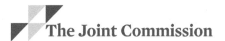
The Joint Commission

MW00846107

The APIC/JCR
Infection Prevention and Control
Workbook, 4th Edition

Edited by Patti G. Grota PhD, CNS-M-S, CIC, FAPIC
Angela H. Rupp, MT, MS, CIC, FAPIC

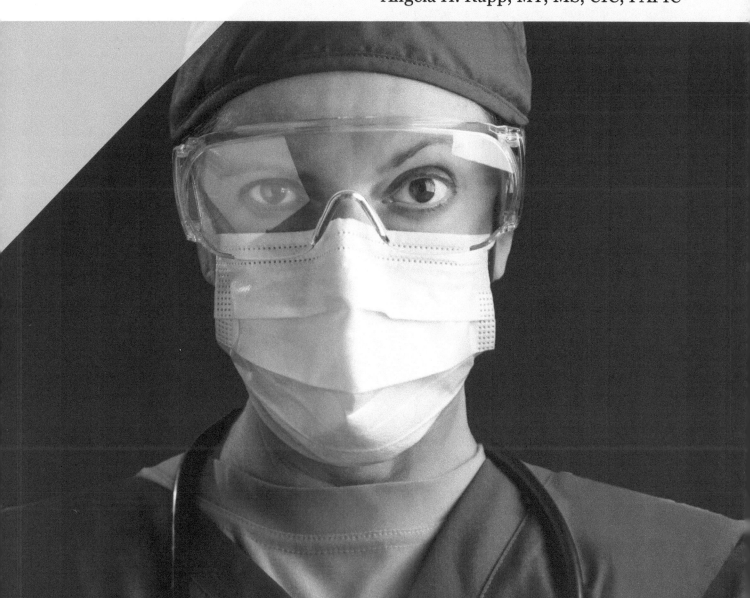

Joint Commission Resources Mission

The mission of Joint Commission Resources (JCR) is to continuously improve the safety and quality of health care in the United States and in the international community through the provision of education, publications, consultation, and evaluation services.

Disclaimers

JCR educational programs and publications support, but are separate from, the accreditation activities of The Joint Commission. Attendees at Joint Commission Resources educational programs and purchasers of JCR publications receive no special consideration or treatment in, or confidential information about, the accreditation process. The inclusion of an organization name, product, or service in a JCR publication should not be construed as an endorsement of such organization, product, or service, nor is failure to include an organization name, product, or service to be construed as disapproval.

This publication is designed to provide accurate and authoritative information regarding the subject matter covered. Every attempt has been made to ensure accuracy at the time of publication; however, please note that laws, regulations, and standards are subject to change. Please also note that some of the examples in this publication are specific to the laws and regulations of the locality of the facility. The information and examples in this publication are provided with the understanding that the publisher is not engaged in providing medical, legal, or other professional advice. If any such assistance is desired, the services of a competent professional person should be sought.

Published by Joint Commission Resources
Oak Brook, Illinois 60523 USA
https://www.jcrinc.com

Joint Commission Resources, Inc. (JCR), a not-for-profit affiliate of The Joint Commission, has been designated by The Joint Commission to publish publications and multimedia products. JCR reproduces and distributes these materials under license from The Joint Commission.

ISBN (print): 978-1-63585-205-9
ISBN (e-book): 978-1-63585-206-6

Printed in the USA

For more information about The Joint Commission, please visit https://www.jointcommission.org.

Development Team

Executive Editor: Phyllis Crittenden
Editorial Coordinator: Kristine Stejskal
Senior Project Manager: Heather Yang
Associate Director, Production: Johanna Harris
Executive Director, Global Publishing: Catherine Chopp Hinckley, MA, PhD

Reviewers

Joint Commission Division of Healthcare Improvement
Sylvia Garcia-Houchins, RN, MBA, CIC, Director, Infection Prevention and Control

Joint Commission Division of Healthcare Quality Evaluation
Helen Larios, MBA, MSN, RN, Project Director-Clinical, Department of Standards and Survey Methods

Joint Commission International
Wai Khuan Ng, PhD, RN, CIC, CPHQ, FAPIC, Principal Consultant, Asia Pacific & International Infection Prevention and Control

Table of Contents

Introduction

The Infection Prevention and Control Program—A Global Perspective

By Patti G. Grota, PhD, CNS-M-S, CIC, FAPIC, CSHE and
Barbara M. Soule, RN, MPA, CIC, FSHEA, FAPIC

Background

The twenty-first century has seen and will continue to see increasing emphasis on preventing and controlling infectious disease. Each year, millions of people in health care organizations and communities across the globe are exposed to infections from within health care settings and their communities. Globalization has led to increased transmissibility of diseases as well as to greater awareness of the social and economic effects of infectious disease. The good news is, health care providers across the globe are seeing advances in the design of medical devices, use of clinical practice techniques, faster vaccine development, and the positive effects of antimicrobial stewardship programs. These efforts and others are advancing infection prevention and control (IPC) goals in both developed and developing nations. However, health care–associated infections (HAIs)[1] and newly emerging infectious diseases, such as the ongoing global COVID-19 pandemic, have demonstrated the need for continuous efforts in mitigating and managing reemerging and evolving infectious diseases.[2]

While the *APIC/JCR Infection Prevention and Control Workbook* focuses primarily on HAIs, this new edition also underscores how infectious agents in the community can pose risks to quality care and patient safety within health care settings. Infection prevention professionals in all health care settings must plan and prepare for both HAIs and infectious disease threats from a more global perspective, including preparedness for new viruses such as SARS-CoV-2 (Novel Coronavirus 2019/COVID-19), responsible for the COVID-19 global pandemic of 2020-2021.

Global infectious disease threats are not a new health care concern. In recent years, such threats have included outbreaks such as the SARS-CoV outbreak in 2003[3]; the Middle East Respiratory Syndrome (MERS-CoV) in 2012[4]; Zika virus in tropical Africa, Southeast Asia, and the Pacific Islands, as well as transmissions in Florida and Texas in 2016[5,6]; and the West African Ebola Virus of 2014-2015, with confirmed cases in the United States.[7] Currently the world continues to battle the COVID-19 pandemic, which resulted in more than half a million deaths in the US alone and more than 2 million deaths worldwide by early 2021.[8,9] As a result, this edition of the *APIC/JCR Infection Prevention and Control Workbook* includes a global perspective on infection prevention and control by highlighting both Joint Commission domestic and Joint Commission International standards and by continuing to offer potential strategies and solutions for all health care settings.

HAIs, such as pneumonia, urinary tract infections, bloodstream infections, and surgical site infections (SSIs), can be acquired anywhere health care is delivered, including inpatient acute care and long term care facilities as well as outpatient facilities, such as ambulatory surgical and dialysis centers, to name a few. They may result in extended hospital or residential stays, additional illness and treatment, and sometimes death. In all types of facilities, HAIs increase the demands on health care for supportive leadership, trained staff, a safe environment, collaboration among staff and public health agencies, and associated medical costs. In 2011, the US Centers for Disease Control and Prevention (CDC) published a report suggesting that the annual cost of HAIs could be as high as $45 billion.[10] In a 2013 meta-analysis study, total annual costs for five major HAIs alone (central–line associated infection, ventilator-associated pneumonia, surgical site infections, *Clostridium [Clostridioides] difficile* infection, and catheter-associated urinary tract infection) were estimated to cost $9.8 billion annually (95% confidence interval, $8.3–$11.5 billion).[1] In addition, a 2019 study conducted in the Netherlands found national hospital costs attributable to SSIs following colectomy, mastectomy, and total hip arthroplasty—mainly from prolonged length of hospital stay—were estimated at €39.6 million.[11]

In the past, HAIs were thought to be inevitable and were considered a consequence of complex care delivered to increasingly ill patients. In other words, HAIs were an "expected" outcome of health care. However, there has been a shift in thinking. Many organizations are working toward achieving zero preventable infections and realizing that a proportion of HAIs are avoidable, making strides toward achieving the goal of zero preventable infections.[12,13] Eliminating HAIs is the ultimate goal of infection surveillance, prevention, and control programs. This goal makes an effective infection prevention and control program one of the most significant patient safety initiatives for any health care organization and should be a top priority for leaders and staff.

Since the third edition of this workbook was published in 2016, health care organizations have made great strides in reducing rates of several types of HAIs. In 2019, US hospitals saw 31% fewer central line–associated blood stream infections (CLABSIs) and 42% fewer *C. difficile* events compared to the 2015 national baseline. There has been a steady decline in other infections, including catheter-associated urinary tract infections and SSIs, in part due to implementation of evidence-based practices.[14] In fact, the CDC conducted a point prevalence survey and concluded that between 2011 and 2015, there was a reduction in SSIs and urinary tract infections in acute care settings that was directly attributed to evidence-based IPC practices. In general, fewer patients had HAIs in 2015 than did in 2011,[15,16] and the trend continues. During this time, antimicrobial stewardship also has become an integral part of infection prevention in many care settings, further contributing to decreasing HAIs. A greater importance also has been placed on including and educating patients and their family advocates about their role in IPC efforts, which is critical to meeting patient safety needs.[17]

Standards and Requirements for Infection Prevention and Control

The Joint Commission's philosophy and requirements are represented in its Infection Prevention and Control (IC) standards and associated elements of performance (EPs), as well as Leadership (LD), Environment of Care (EC), Human Resources (HR), and Medication Management (MM) standards. In addition, and because there is close coordination between the US Centers for Medicare & Medicaid Services (CMS) and Joint Commission domestic standards, for US organizations, CMS requirements are also discussed in this book, where applicable.

For the global community, similar requirements are addressed in JCI's Prevention and Control of Infections (PCI) standards and associated measurable elements (MEs). Other JCI standards, such as the Quality Improvement and Patient Safety (QPS), Governance and Leadership (GLD), and Staff Qualification and Education (SQE) standards, provide additional guidance.

Together these standards support infection prevention professionals in all settings to systematically develop, implement, and evaluate an effective infection surveillance, prevention, and control program. Relevant Joint Commission and Joint Commission International accreditation standards are provided in all chapters of this book.

However, please note that while relevant Joint Commission and Joint Commission International standards are included in this book, the strategies presented here may go beyond what is required by the standards. This workbook is not meant to focus strictly on compliance with standards but to show good practices.

Purpose of This Book

The *APIC/JCR Infection Prevention and Control Workbook*, 4th edition is intended to help health care organizations and their infection prevention teams identify infection risks and challenges in their designated health care settings by providing the strategies and resources to develop, implement, and evaluate a comprehensive IPC program to minimize those risks. Discussions, examples, tables, graphs, figures, case studies, and other tools are provided to support organizations and infection preventionists (IPs) achieve an effective IPC program. This book is designed to help those responsible for infection prevention and control enhance and improve all IPC practices and activities across the continuum of care to move toward safer care and healthier communities. The book discusses health care organizations other than acute care hospitals; however, it must be noted that much of the book still focuses on the hospital setting. Other types of health care organizations are encouraged to consider the good practices for hospitals and extrapolate lessons and guidance as appropriate.

Note: *The strategies, tools, and examples discussed in this book do not necessarily reflect Joint Commission and Joint Commission International accreditation requirements for all settings. Always refer to the most current TJC and JCI standards applicable to your health care setting to ensure compliance.*

Using the *APIC/JCR Infection Prevention and Control Workbook*

The chapters in this book are organized to help infection prevention professionals develop a comprehensive IPC program by first providing an overview for designing and managing an effective IPC program and then addressing in more detail the following key components of the IPC program:

- Assessing risks
- Setting goals based on those identified risks
- Developing a written IPC plan based on identified goals and risks
- Implementing the written plan
- Evaluating plan and program effectiveness

To help reduce the occurrence of infections and the likelihood of transmission of pathogenic microorganisms to patients, staff, and visitors, a systematic and proactive IPC program must be planned, implemented, and monitored and must include everyone involved in the daily operations of an organization—including top leadership and administration, clinical personnel, environmental services, sterilization and purchasing services, occupational health, and patients and their families. These topics are discussed in the following chapters:

- *Chapter 1: Designing and Managing an Effective Infection Prevention and Control Program*
- *Chapter 2: The Role of Leadership in Infection Prevention and Control*
- *Chapter 7: Maintaining a Safe Environment of Care*

- *Chapter 8: Cleaning, Disinfection, and Sterilization of Medical Devices and Equipment*
- *Chapter 10: Occupational Health Issues*

Because assessing risks, surveillance, education, and communication are such essential components for the effectiveness and success of an infection prevention program, these topics are covered in depth in the following chapters:

- *Chapter 3: A Risk-Based Approach to Infection Prevention: Performing the Risk Assessment and Creating the IPC Plan*
- *Chapter 4: Planning and Implementing an Effective Surveillance Program*
- *Chapter 5: Planning for and Managing Infectious Disease Emergencies*
- *Chapter 6: Implementing Clinical Strategies to Reduce Infection Risk*
- *Chapter 9: Communication and Education Strategies for Infection Prevention and Control Programs*

The effectiveness of an IPC program depends on vigilant assessment of the status of goals and objectives and how the program integrates with and improves patient safety and the quality of care. These chapters address these important issues:

- *Chapter 11: Evaluating the Effectiveness of an Infection Prevention and Control Program*
- *Chapter 12: Integrating Infection Prevention and Control into Patient Safety and Performance Improvement*

The figure on the next page includes the topics covered in this workbook and illustrates how they are all components of an effective IPC program.

A Collaborative Effort

This workbook continues the collaboration between the Association for Professionals in Infection Prevention and Control and Epidemiology (APIC) and Joint Commission Resources (JCR)—a division of The Joint Commission. APIC is a nonprofit professional organization whose mission is to create a safer world through the prevention and control of infections.[18] The mission of Joint Commission Resources is to continuously improve the safety and quality of health care in the US and in the international community.[19] The two organizations have joined together to create this fourth edition, which is designed to assist IPC teams in all health care settings and countries to establish comprehensive

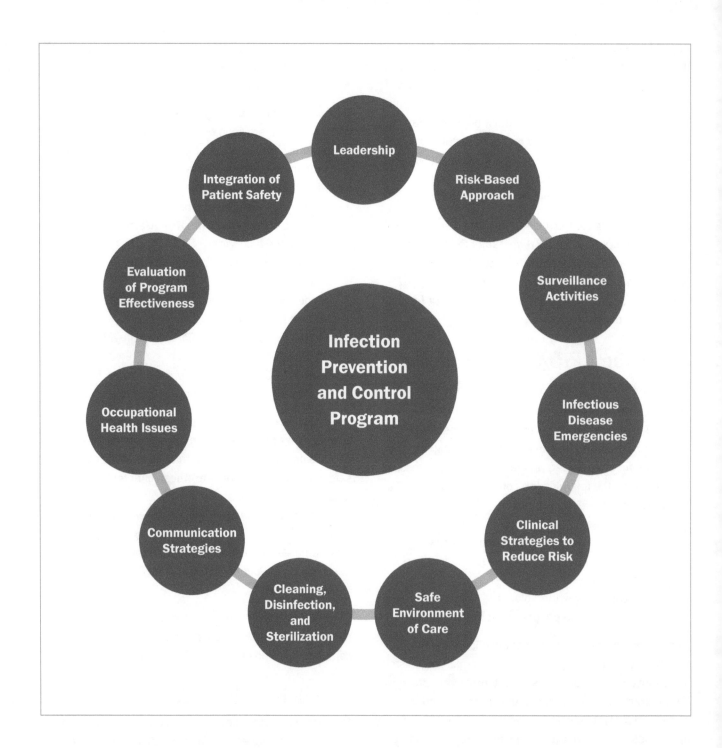

risk-based IPC programs to protect patients, staff, and families from infections acquired in the community and in health care facilities. Both APIC and JCR provide support for the development of effective IPC programs. APIC supports infection professionals through publications, education, practice guidance, policy, and advocacy. The Joint Commission[20] and Joint Commission International[21] use published standards as a structure for support. Other organizations, such as the Society for Healthcare Epidemiology of America (SHEA)[22] and CMS,[23] also support strong IPC programs with regulations, evidence-based guidelines, consensus documents, and more. All these organizations agree that IPC programs should be comprehensive, collaborative, and interprofessional and pursue HAI reduction with multi-interventional programs based on evidence-based strategies.

Finally, the *APIC/JCR Infection Prevention and Control Workbook*, 4th edition continues to incorporate the experience of the IPs who work across the US and throughout the world who have shared their expertise and knowledge of infection surveillance, prevention, and control issues.

About the Contributors

Vicki Gillie Allen, MSN, RN, CIC, FAPIC, is the Director of the Infection Prevention and Control Department at a not-for-profit community hospital in Gastonia, North Carolina. Her responsibilities include the oversight of infection prevention and control for the regional health system of CaroMont Health, including physician practices, urgent care, hospice, emergency facilities, and its anchor, a 435-bed hospital. Allen has more than 23 years of experience in infection control. In addition to her role as director, she has participated in and provided infection prevention and control consultation and education to other settings, including long term care facilities. As an RN with national board certification in infection control, Allen has been actively involved with professional organizations, including statewide programs for APIC; she was APIC North Carolina President in 2018 and Arkansas President in 2007. She also served on the national APIC Communications Committee from 2013 to 2018 and as the APIC Text Editor and Author from 2014 to 2020. Allen earned a bachelor of science degree in nursing from Kaplan University and a master of science in nursing education from the University of Texas at Tyler.

Kathleen Meehan Arias, MS, MT(ASCP), SM(AAM), CIC, FAPIC, has worked in the infection prevention and control field since 1980. She has infection prevention and control experience in a variety of health care settings, including acute care, long term care, and ambulatory health care. Arias has a bachelor of science degree in medical technology and a master of science degree in clinical microbiology. She is certified in infection control by the Certification Board of Infection Control. Arias has authored books, chapters, and articles on a variety of infection prevention and control topics. She was a coeditor and author of the first three editions of the *APIC/JCR Infection Prevention and Control Workbook* and is the author of the surveillance chapter in the *APIC Text of Infection Control and Epidemiology.*

Arias is an active APIC member and has served in many capacities at the local and national levels. She was cochair of the national APIC Education Committee from 1998 to 2000 and served as APIC President in 2006. In 2011, Arias received APIC's Carole DeMille Award in

recognition for her contributions to the field of infection prevention and control.

Ruth Carrico, PhD, DNP, FNP-C, CIC, FSHEA, FNAP, is Professor and Family Nurse Practitioner with the University of Louisville School of Medicine, Division of Infectious Diseases. She serves as Director of Epidemiological Research in the University's Center of Excellence for Research in Infectious Diseases (CERID) and as Director of the Center for Education and Training in Infection Prevention. Carrico has received training specific to health care epidemiology from the CDC in conjunction with the Rollins School of Public Health at Emory University in Atlanta and the SHEA.

Carrico served as editor for the APIC Text of Infection Control and Epidemiology from 2005 to 2012. In 2008, she was appointed to the National Biosurveillance Subcommittee (NBS) Advisory Committee to the CDC Director, and in 2010, she became a SHEA Fellow. In 2011, Carrico was appointed by Secretary Sebelius to the Healthcare Infection Control Practices Advisory Committee (HICPAC). In 2012, she was presented with the Carole DeMille Achievement Award by APIC, and she began serving as the Nurse Planner for the National Foundation for Infectious Diseases in 2013. In 2014, she became a Robert Wood Johnson Foundation Executive Nurse Fellow alumna and then served as President of the Certification Board of Infection Control and Epidemiology, Inc. (CBIC) in 2016. In 2018, Carrico served as the Editor-in-Chief for the University of Louisville's open access *Journal of Refugee and Global Health.* She became President of the Kentucky Nurses Association and in 2020 and was recognized as a Distinguished Fellow in the National Academies of Practice.

Loretta L. Fauerbach, MS, FSHEA, FAPIC, CIC, is the lead infection preventionist for Fauerbach & Associates, LLC. Fauerbach served for more than 28 years as Director of Infection Prevention and Control for Shands Hospital at the University of Florida. Her expertise encompasses the continuum of health care. Fauerbach received APIC's Carole DeMille Achievement Award in 2007 for her contributions/achievements in the field of infection prevention and control. Fauerbach is an active member of APIC, SHEA, and the American Society for Microbiology (ASM). She has served on APIC's board of directors and on a number of APIC committees. Fauerbach was also cochair of APIC's Nominating and Awards Committee. In 2002 she testified before the Institute of Medicine on

APIC's behalf related to HAI data. Fauerbach has served as APIC's liaison to the Association for the Advancement of Medical Instrumentation (AAMI), HICPAC, the US Food and Drug Administration (FDA), and the Infectious Diseases Society of America (IDSA), during times when multiple sentinel guidelines were produced by those agencies/associations. She was also APIC's leader for the SHEA/APIC/CDC Communication Network. She represented APIC on The Joint Commission's expert panels for monographs on hand hygiene, influenza vaccination, and Tdap vaccination. Fauerbach has presented at regional and national meetings and authored several books and articles for peer-reviewed journals, and she is currently a member of HICPAC.

Sylvia Garcia-Houchins, RN, MBA, CIC, Joint Commission, is the Director of Infection Control and an ambulatory care surveyor. She has provided infection prevention and control consultation in a variety of health care settings, including hospitals, health clinics, and dialysis centers, both domestically and internationally. She has trained nurses, microbiologists, and public health graduates to certification in infection control. Garcia-Houchins has been active in APIC and CBIC; most recently she chaired the Test Writing Committee. Garcia-Houchins has also conducted hospital assessments and developed educational programs responsive to the needs of the community, geographic region, and country and has authored articles and book chapters related to infection prevention and control.

Kathleen Gase, MBA, MPH, CIC, FAPIC, is the Director of Clinical Excellence at Barnes-Jewish St. Peters and Progress West Hospitals in the St. Louis area. She has previous work experience with BJC HealthCare, the New York State Department of Health, and Memorial Sloan-Kettering Cancer Center. Gase earned an undergraduate degree at Washington University in St. Louis a master's in public health at Hunter College in New York City, and an MBA at Washington University. She is certified in infection prevention and epidemiology, a Fellow of the APIC and is currently serving on the APIC Board of Directors.

Linda R. Greene, RN, MPS, CIC, FAPIC, is the Director of Infection Prevention at the University of Rochester Highland Hospital, Rochester, New York. She has extensive experience in infection prevention in acute care, long term care, and ambulatory surgery settings. She held leadership roles in her local APIC chapter before becoming a member of the APIC Board of Directors in

2010. She was Secretary of the APIC Board in 2012–2013 and served as APIC President in 2017. Greene was also President of the Board for APIC Consulting Services in 2015, and she continues to serve APIC and the infection prevention and control profession in myriad ways, including as an advisor and contributor to APIC position papers and implementation guides, as an APIC representative to the 2020 CDC Decennial Steering Committee, and as a frequent presenter at regional, national, and international conferences. The author of dozens of peer-reviewed publications, Greene is an expert on quality improvement, antimicrobial stewardship, and HAIs. She served on the *AJIC* editorial board from 2015 to 2017. In 2020, APIC awarded her with the prestigious Carole DeMille Award, which is given annually to an infection preventionist with visionary leadership and extraordinary contributions to the profession. She has also received numerous awards for leadership and nursing.

Patti G. Grota, PhD, CNS-M-S, CIC, FAPIC, CHSE, is an expert infection prevention professional with more than 30 years of experience in academia and diverse practice settings, including acute, ambulatory, and long term care. In her role as Infection Prevention Director of a Veteran's Administration health care facility for more than 15 years, Grota led the facility through successful Joint Commission accreditation cycles. She has advanced experience in developing, implementing, and evaluating infection prevention and control programs. Currently, she teaches infection prevention and control and leadership to nurses and other health care students.

Grota has served APIC both nationally and locally. She is the Clinical Editor of the 2014 edition of the *APIC Text of Infection Control and Epidemiology* and served as Chair of the *APIC Text On-line* Editorial Panel from 2014 to 2018, coordinating its transition to an electronic publication. She has served on the APIC Chapter 71, San Antonio, Board of Directors as a member and as President. Currently, she is a member of the APIC National Research Committee. She has given numerous national presentations on infection prevention, and published articles in peer-reviewed journals. Her research interests are in the impact of isolation and implementation of evidence-based practices.

Joan Ivaska, BS, MPH, CIC, is Consultant for JCR and has worked in health care for the past 17 years, with expertise in performance improvement and infection prevention and control. She currently serves as the Senior Director of Infection Prevention for Banner Health, overseeing infection prevention and control programs across 7 states, including 29 hospitals, 2 nursing care centers, a hospice, home health and ambulatory surgery organizations, and hundreds of physician clinics. Ivaska has served as the Vice President of Quality and Patient Safety for Cheyenne Regional Medical Center in Cheyenne, Wyoming, and worked in biomedical research for Oregon Health & Science University and the University of Colorado Health Sciences Center.

Ivaska holds a bachelor of science degree in biology and an MPH and is nationally board certified in infection control and epidemiology. She completed her thesis on the epidemiology of community-acquired versus health care–associated methicillin-resistant *Staphylococcus aureus* (MRSA) and has advanced training in hospital epidemiology from the CDC.

Wai Khuan Ng, PhD, RN, CIC, CPHQ, FAPIC, is Principal Consultant, Asia Pacific & International Infection Prevention and Control for Joint Commission International. She has more than 25 years of experience in health care and 18 years of experience in infection prevention and control. An expert in infection prevention and control, Ng provides consulting services for IPC in international settings and across the health care continuum, including program assessment, professional development and mentoring, education and training, and product development. Ng has broad experience practicing and teaching about infection prevention and control and has published and presented extensively in this area.

Terri Rebmann, PhD, RN, CIC, FAPIC, is a Special Assistant to the Saint Louis University President, where she assists with COVID-19 response. She also is Director of the Institute for Biosecurity, Associate Dean for Academic and Faculty Affairs, and Professor of Epidemiology at the Saint Louis University College for Public Health & Social Justice. A PhD nurse researcher with an emphasis in infectious disease emergency preparedness, Rebmann is board certified in infection prevention and epidemiology and is a Fellow of the Association for Professionals in Infection Control and Epidemiology (FAPIC). She publishes and lectures on bioterrorism, pandemic planning, emerging infectious diseases, and infection prevention practices on a national basis. Rebmann also has served on several national and international task forces and committees aimed at

minimizing morbidity and mortality related to emerging infectious diseases and bioterrorism threats, including being a member of the APIC COVID-19 Task Force, the APIC Ebola Task Force, and a former member and Chair of the APIC Emergency Preparedness Committee. She is currently a CBIC Board Member.

Chaz Rhone, MPH, CIC, FAPIC, received a master's degree of public health in epidemiology from the University of Florida in 2007 and immediately began his career as an infection preventionist. He has been certified in infection control since 2012 and has worked in both the public and private sectors, with experience in acute and long term care settings. Currently, Rhone is a Division Manager for HCA Healthcare, where he oversees the infection prevention programs for five acute care facilities in the Orlando area. Rhone is an active member with APIC, currently serving on the Professional Development Committee and the Florida Professionals in Infection Control, where he also formerly served as President and Board Member. He has published extensively in peer-reviewed journals and lectured at conferences at the state and national levels. In 2016, Rhone received the APIC Heroes of Infection Prevention Award for his work in CAUTI prevention. He also was named as one of University of Florida's College of Public Health and Health Professions Outstanding Alumni in 2018. In 2019, Rhone became an APIC Fellow. He is passionate about patient safety, leadership, and advancing the field of infection prevention.

Angela H. Rupp, MT, MS, CIC, FAPIC, began her career in infection prevention in 1998 and has served as an infection preventionist in long term care, at a community hospital, at an academic medical center, and most recently as the director at a freestanding pediatric hospital. A member of APIC, Rupp served as the 2010 and 2011 Pediatric Section Chair for APIC and, in 2017, was awarded APIC's Heroes of Infection Prevention Award for her work associated with an outbreak related to a contaminated medication. Rupp has served on the SHEA Pediatric Leadership Council Steering Committee, the Child Health Corporation of America Infection Prevention Director's Forum, and the Illinois Department of Public Health task force on hospital-acquired infections. In 2018, Rupp traveled abroad with Joint Commission International to provide infection prevention consultation in Vietnam and Egypt. She has coauthored numerous articles and presented educational topics in person and via webinars. She also served as Editor of *The Joint Commission Big Book of Checklists for Infection Prevention and Control.*

Barbara M. Soule, RN, MPA, CIC, FSHEA, FAPIC, has served as Principal Consultant in Infection Prevention and Control for Joint Commission Resources and Joint Commission International. She also served as Director of Infection Control and Epidemiology, Director of Safety, and Director of Quality Management Services at Providence St. Peter Hospital in Olympia, Washington, where she managed programs in quality and performance improvement, hospital epidemiology and infection control, risk management, utilization management, clinical research, staff education, and care management services. Soule was the Editor-in-Chief of the first APIC curriculum for infection control (now APIC Text) and served on the editorial board of the *American Journal of Infection Control* and as editor of *Best Practices in Infection Prevention and Control: An International Perspective*, which was co-published by JCI and SHEA. Soule also is member of the Editorial Board of the International Infection Control and Public Health and is former President of both APIC in 2003 and CBIC in 1988. She also was a member of the CDC's HICPAC from 2007 to 2010. Soule received the Carol DeMille Award in 1989 and the President's Distinguished Service Award in 2009 from APIC. She also was awarded the Advanced Infection Preventionist Award from SHEA in 2009.

Elizabeth E. Tremblay, MPH, CPH, CIC, is completing her third year of medical school at Florida State University College of Medicine. Prior to medical school, she was an infection control practitioner at UF Health Shands Hospital in Gainesville, Florida from 2012 to 2019. Tremblay earned a bachelor of science degree in microbiology in 2011 and a master's degree of public health in epidemiology in 2013 from the University of Florida. She has maintained certification in both public health (CPH) and infection control (CIC) since 2013. In 2020–2021, Tremblay received a research fellowship grant from the Infectious Diseases Society of America to support her work on the systematic differentiation between non-tuberculous mycobacteria (NTM) and tuberculosis when assessing the need for inpatient airborne isolation. She serves as a biostatistician for various research studies at UF Health, including laboratory diagnostics. Her infection control experience includes neurosurgical infection prevention, health informatics, gastrointestinal pathogen diagnostic testing, and research on topics such as *Pseudomonas aeruginosa* in cystic fibrosis patients, *carbapenem-resistant Enterobacterales* (CRE), and *C. diff.* Her future endeavors include further research in laboratory diagnostic testing and beginning her clinical residency in 2023.

Acknowledgments

APIC and JCR would like to thank the following individuals for their support, contributions, and technical review of chapters:

- Lorene Campbell, BSN, RN, CIC, APIC Communication Committee/Hospital Division, Director Infection Control, Kindred Healthcare
- Brenda Ehlert, BS, MT(ASCP), MBA, CIC, FAPIC, Director Infection Prevention, Ascension Wisconsin
- Patti G. Grota PhD, CNS-M-S, CIC, FAPIC, CHSE, University of Texas Health Science Center, San Antonio, Texas
- Lori Kay Groven, MSPHN, RN, CIC, Infection Preventionist, TRIA Orthopaedic Center, Bloomington, Minnesota
- Martin Levesque, MPH, MBA, CIC, FAPIC, System Director, Infection Prevention and Control, Henry Ford Health System, Detroit, Michigan
- Kathleen McMullen, MPH, CIC, FAPIC, Christian Hospital
- Sara M. Reese, PhD, MPH, CIC, FAPIC, Swedish Medical Center
- Angela H. Rupp, MT, MS, CIC, FAPIC, Cedar Lake, Indiana
- April Sutton, MSN, RN, CIC, Texas Health Resources
- Marie H. Wilson, MSN, RN, CIC, Methodist Dallas Medical Center
- Marlene Fishman Wolpert, MPH, CIC, FAPIC, Long Term Care Infection Preventionist, The Miriam Hospital, A Lifespan Partner, CITY, STATE, and Independent Consultant, Providence, Rhode Island

APIC and JCR would also like to acknowledge the contributions of the following health care professionals for use of the risk assessment tools included in Chapter 3:

- Michelle A. Barron, MD, Senior Medical Director, Infection Prevention and Control, UCHealth Metro Denver
- Cathleen Carroll, MLT, CIC, Infection Prevention Supervisor at Barnes-Jewish West County Hospital
- Amber Conrad, RN, BSN, CIC, Infection Prevention Specialist at Parkland Health Center
- Ashley Heller, MPH, CIC, Manager, Infection Prevention and Control, UCHealth Metro Denver
- Kathleen McMullen, MPH, CIC, FAPIC, Interim Director of Quality and Analytics at Christian Hospital and Northwest Healthcare

- Larissa Pisney, MD, Medical Director, Infection Prevention and Control, University of Colorado Hospital and UCHealth Metro Denver
- Rachael Snyders, MPH, BSN, RN, CIC, FAPIC, Manager, Infection Prevention Center for Clinical Excellence, BJC HealthCare
- Luke Starnes, PhD, RN, Interim Manager of Infection Prevention at Missouri Baptist Medical Center
- Cheryl Wright, MSN, RN, CIC, BC, Infection Prevention Specialist at Memorial Hospital East

TRY THIS TOOL

The tools in this book are available as downloadable, customizable resources that can be distributed internally to health care staff. To access these tools, click on the Try This Tool box in each chapter or visit https://store-jcrinc.ae-admin.com/assets/1/7/ICSA20_landingpage.pdf

References

1   Zimlichman E, Henderson D, Tamir O. Health care–associated infections: A meta-analysis of costs and financial impact on the US health care system. *JAMA Intern Med.* 2013 Dec;173(22):2039–2046.

2. Nicola M, et al. The socio-economic implications of the coronavirus pandemic (COVID-19): A review. *Int J Surg.* 2020 Jun;78:185-193. doi: 10.101.

3. Varia M, et al. Investigation of a nosocomial outbreak of Severe Acute Respiratory Syndrome (SARS) in Toronto, Canada. *CMAJ.* 2003;169(4):285–292.6/j.ijsu.2020.04.018. Epub 2020 Apr 17. PMID: 32305533; PMCID: PMC7.

4. Chan JF, et al. Middle East Respiratory Syndrome coronavirus: Another zoonotic betacoronavirus causing SARS-like disease. *Clin Microbiol Rev.* 2015;28(2):465–522. doi:10.1128/CMR.00102-14162753.

5. Chang C, et al. The Zika outbreak of the 21st century. *J Autoimmun.* 2016;68:1–13. doi:10.1016/j.jaut.2016.02.006

6. McCarthy M. First US case of Zika virus infection is identified in Texas. *BMJ.* 2016 Jan 13;352:i212. doi: 10.1136/bmj.i212. PMID: 26762624.

7. US Centers for Disease Control and Prevention. The Road to Zero: CDC's Response to the West African Ebola Epidemic, 2014-2015. Accessed Feb 2021. https://www.cdc.gov/about/ebola/index.html

8. US Centers for Disease Control and Prevention. CDC COVID Data Tracker. https://covid.cdc.gov/covid-data-tracker/#datatracker-home. Accessed Feb 28, 2021.

9. World Health Organization. WHO Coronavirus (COVID-19) Dashboard. Accessed Apr 3, 2021. https://covid19.who.int/

10. Stone, PW. Economic burden of healthcare-associated infections: An American perspective. *Expert Rev Pharmacoecon Outcomes Res.* Author manuscript; available in PMC 2010 Feb 24. Published in final edited form as: *Expert Rev Pharmacoecon Outcomes Res.* 2009 Oct;9(5):417–422. doi: 10.1586/erp.09.53. PMCID: PMC2827870 Accessed Apr 3, 2021. https://www.ncbi.nlm.nih.gov/pmc/articles/PMC2827870/

11. Koek MBG, et al. Burden of surgical site infections in the Netherlands: Cost analyses and disability-adjusted life years. *J Hosp Infect.* 2019 Nov;103(3):293–302. doi: 10.1016/j.jhin.2019.07.010. Epub 2019 Jul 19. PMID: 31330166. https://pubmed.ncbi.nlm.nih.gov/31330166/

12. Schreiber et al. The preventable proportion of healthcare–associated infections 2005-2016: Systematic review and meta-analysis. *Infect Control Hosp Epidemiol.* 2018 Nov;11:1277–1295. doi: https://doi.org/10.1017.ice.208.183.

13. Bhatt J, Collier, S. Reducing health care associated infection: getting hospitals and health systems to zero. *Ann Intern Med.* 2019 Oct;171(7 Suppl):S81–S82. https://doi.org/10.7326/M18-3441

14. Centers for Disease Control and Prevention. Current HAI Progress Report: 2019 National and State Healthcare–Associated Infections Report. Accessed Feb 11, 2021. https://www.cdc.gov/hai/data/portal/progress-report.html

15. Magill SS, et al. Emerging Infections Program Healthcare-Associated Infections and Antimicrobial Use Prevalence Survey Team. Multistate point-prevalence survey of health care–associated infections. *N Engl J Med*. 2014 Mar;370(13):1198–1208.

16. Magill SS, et al. Changes in prevalence in health care–associated Infections in U.S. hospitals. *N Engl J Med*. 2018 Nov;379:1732–1744. DOI:10.1056/NE/Moal801550.

17. Fernandes Agreli H, et al. Patient involvement in the implementation of infection prevention and control guidelines and associated interventions: A scoping review. *BMJOpen*. 2019;9:e025824. doi: 10.1136/bmjopen-2018-025824.

18. Association for Professionals in Infection Control and Epidemiology. Vision and Mission Statement. Accessed Feb 13, 2021. https://apic.org/about-apic/vision-and-mission/

19. Joint Commission Resources. Mission Statement. Accessed Apr 3, 2021. https://www.jcrinc.com/about-us/mission/

20. The Joint Commission. SAFER Dashboard. Accessed Feb 28, 2021. https://www.jointcommission.org

21. The Joint Commission International. JCI Navigator. Accessed Feb 28, 2021. https://www.jointcommissioninternational.org

22. Society for Healthcare Epidemiology of America (SHEA). Accessed Feb 28, 2021. https://www.shea-online.org/

23. Centers for Medicare & Medicaid Services (CMS). Accessed Feb 28, 2021. https://www.cms.gov

Chapter 1

Designing and Managing an Effective Infection Prevention and Control Program

By Kathleen Meehan Arias, MS, MT(ASCP), SM(AAM), CIC, FAPIC

Disclaimer: Strategies, tools, and examples discussed in this book do not necessarily reflect Joint Commission or Joint Commission International requirements for all settings. Always refer to the most current standards applicable to your health care setting to ensure compliance.

Introduction

Health care–associated infections (HAIs) result in considerable morbidity and mortality as well as increased health care costs worldwide.[1-6] An effective infection surveillance, prevention, and control program can reduce the risk of HAIs and improve health care outcomes.[7-8] Since the landmark Study on the Efficacy of Nosocomial Infection Control (SENIC) Project, conducted in the 1970s, other studies have demonstrated that organizations with intensive infection surveillance, prevention, and control programs have been able to reduce infection rates in a variety of health care settings through multidisciplinary performance improvement initiatives.[7-9]

The primary goal of an infection prevention and control (IPC) program is to prevent HAIs. This chapter discusses how to design, manage, and allocate resources for IPC programs that can effectively prevent the risk of and eliminate the occurrence of HAIs across the continuum of care, including acute, ambulatory, nursing care center, behavioral health, and home care settings.

Relevant Joint Commission Standards Addressed in This Chapter

Note: These standards were in effect at the time of publication. They refer to Joint Commission standards effective January 1, 2021. Always consult the most recent version of Joint Commission standards for the most accurate requirements for your setting.

IC.01.01.01 The [organization] identifies the individual(s) responsible for the infection prevention and control program.

EP 1 The [organization] identifies the individual(s) with clinical authority over the infection prevention and control program.

EP 2 When the individual(s) with clinical authority over the infection prevention and control program does not have expertise in infection prevention and control, he or she consults with someone who has such expertise in order to make knowledgeable decisions.

(continued)

(continued)

EP 3 The [organization] assigns responsibility for the daily management of infection prevention and control activities. (See also HR.01.01.01, EP 1; LD.03.06.01, EP 2)

Note: *Number and skill mix of the individuals(s) assigned should be determined by the goals and objectives of the infection prevention and control program.*

EP 4 For [organizations] that use Joint Commission accreditation for deemed status purposes: The individual with clinical authority over the infection prevention and control program is responsible for the following:

- Developing and implementing [organizationwide] infection surveillance, prevention, and control policies and procedures that adhere to nationally recognized guidelines
- Documenting the infection prevention and control program surveillance, prevention, and control activities
- Communicating and collaborating with the quality assessment and performance improvement program on infection prevention and control issues
- Training and educating staff, including medical staff, on the practical applications of infection prevention and control guidelines, policies, and procedures
- Preventing and controlling health care–associated infections, including auditing of adherence to infection prevention and control policies and procedures by hospital staff, including medical staff
- Communicating and collaborating with the antibiotic stewardship program

EP 5 For ambulatory surgical centers that elect to use the Joint Commission deemed status option: The infection control program is under the direction of a designated and qualified professional who has training in IPC.

EP 6 For [organizations] that use Joint Commission accreditation for deemed status purposes: An individual(s) who is qualified through education, training, experience, or certification in infection prevention and control is appointed by the governing body to be responsible for the infection prevention and control program. The appointment is based on recommendations of medical staff leadership and nursing leadership

HR.01.01.01 The [organization] defines and verifies staff qualifications.

EP 1 The [organization] defines staff qualifications specific to their job responsibilities. (See also HR.01.01.01, EP 32; IC.01.01.01, EP 3; RI.01.01.03, EP 2)

Note: *Qualifications for infection control may be met through ongoing education, training, experience, and/or certification (such as that offered by the Certification Board for Infection Control).*

LD.03.06.01 Those who work in the [organization] are focused on improving safety and quality.

EP 2 Leaders provide for a sufficient number and mix of individuals to support safe and quality care, treatment and services. (See also IC.01.01.01, EP 3)

Note: *The number and mix of individuals is appropriate to the scope and complexity of the services offered.*

Relevant Joint Commission International (JCI) Standards Addressed in This Chapter

Note: These standards were in effect at the time of publication. They refer to the *Joint Commission International Accreditation Standards for Hospitals, seventh edition,* ©2020. Always consult the most recent version of Joint Commission International standards for the most accurate requirements for your hospital or medical center setting.

PCI.1 One or more individuals oversee all infection prevention and control activities. This individual(s) is qualified in infection prevention and control practices through education, training, experience, certification, and/or clinical authority.

ME 1 One or more individuals oversee the infection prevention and control program and ensure that the program complies with local and national laws and regulations.

ME 2 The individual(s) is qualified for the hospital's size, complexity of activities, and level of risks, as well as the program's scope.

ME 3 The individual(s) fulfills program oversight responsibilities as assigned or described in a job description.

ME 4 This individual(s) coordinates with hospital leadership regarding priorities, resources, and quality improvement opportunities related to the infection prevention and control program.

PCI.3 Hospital leadership provides resources to support the infection prevention and control program.

ME 1 The infection prevention and control program is staffed according to the hospital's size, complexity of activities, and level of risks, as well as the program's scope.

ME 2 Hospital leadership approves and assigns staff required for the infection prevention and control program.

ME 3 Hospital leadership approves and allocates resources required for the infection prevention and control program.

PCI.12.2 The hospital develops, implements, and evaluates an emergency preparedness program to respond to the presentation of global communicable diseases.

ME 1 Hospital leaders, along with the individual(s) responsible for the infection prevention and control program, develop and implement an emergency preparedness program to respond to global communicable diseases that includes at least a) through f) in the intent.

SQE.2 Leaders of hospital departments and services develop and implement processes for recruiting, evaluating, and appointing staff as well as other related procedures identified by the hospital.

ME 2 The hospital establishes and implements a process to evaluate the qualifications of new staff.

GLD.7 Hospital leadership makes decisions related to the purchase or use of resources—human and technical—with an understanding of the quality and safety implications of those decisions.

ME 3 Hospital leadership uses the recommendations of professional organizations and other authoritative sources in making resource decisions.

Medical care, and subsequently HAIs, have spread beyond the walls of the acute care hospital to long term acute care settings and a variety of ambulatory care settings.[10] Patients receive diverse types of procedures, therapeutic care, and diagnostic testing in ambulatory settings such as hospital-based outpatient clinics, non-hospital-based clinics and physician offices, ambulatory surgery centers, office-based surgery settings, pain clinics, oncology centers, dental offices, urgent care centers, hemodialysis centers, and ambulatory behavioral health and substance abuse clinics. Many of these outpatient procedures and treatments were previously performed in hospitals, are invasive, and carry risks for infection.[10] Patients and residents also receive care in non-hospital settings such as nursing homes, rehabilitation facilities, and behavioral health care and human services facilities, as well as in home care. In addition to occurring in hospitals, HAIs and infection outbreaks have been reported in most of these non–acute care settings.[10-18]

IPC Program Issues That Are Unique to Non–Acute Care Settings

The Joint Commission IPC requirements apply to a variety of health care settings. However, implementing an effective IPC program in some ambulatory and non-hospital health care settings can be particularly challenging. Many of these settings are not certified by a state agency or by the US Centers for Medicare & Medicaid Services (CMS), and they are not accredited by an accreditation agency. As a result, some facilities are not being held to minimum safety standards for IPC or other aspects of patient care.[2-4] Because of this lack of oversight, increasing reports of outbreaks—and the identification of poor IPC practices in diverse non-hospital heath care settings—regulatory and accrediting agencies, public health agencies, professional organizations, and consumer groups have increased their attention to the need for evidence-based infection surveillance, prevention, and control programs in all health care settings.[3,10-15]

Some recognized barriers to implementing an effective IPC program in non-hospital settings include the following[16]:
- Inadequate staffing for patient/resident care and support services staff
- Failure to recognize and prevent infection risks for patients/residents and staff

- Lack of protocols for and noncompliance with evidence-based practices for hand hygiene; cleaning, disinfection, and sterilization of medical devices and instruments; safe injection and medication practices; and use of personal protective equipment (PPE)
- Lack of a trained, dedicated individual to oversee the IPC program
- Lack of accountability, oversight, and IPC training for all personnel
- Lack of time for staff overseeing the IPC program, particularly for individuals who are also responsible for managing other areas, such as employee health and quality assurance/performance management
- Lack of leadership support of individual(s) overseeing the IPC program
- Lack of appropriate supplies, such as hand sanitizer, PPE, and cleaning and disinfecting agents
- An aging population with multiple patient comorbidities
- The presence of patients and families (some with undiagnosed communicable diseases) in common waiting rooms
- Lack of laboratory and information technology support
- Lack of private rooms in hospitals, long term acute care facilities, and nursing care centers, which can increase the risk of exposure to infectious agents

Organizations that are aware of these barriers and other infection risks and obstacles in their setting are more likely to succeed in designing and implementing an effective IPC program that can effectively prevent HAIs in their patient/resident population.

Experience with emerging and highly infectious diseases has highlighted a critical need for effective infection surveillance, prevention, and control programs in all health care delivery systems. The pandemics of Severe Acute Respiratory Syndrome (SARS) in 2003, Middle East Respiratory Syndrome (MERS) in 2012, and, more recently, Novel Coronavirus 2019 (SARS-CoV-2/COVID-19) in 2020 spread rapidly not only within communities but also within a variety of heath care settings.

Designing an Effective Infection Surveillance, Prevention, and Control Program

Practices and protocols vary among health care settings depending on the type of organization, the populations served, and the care, treatment, and services provided. However, when designing an IPC and surveillance program, certain principles apply across the board. In all health care settings, the IPC program should be built on hierarchy that accounts for the following elements, as appropriate:

- Local, state, and federal rules and regulations
- CMS Conditions of Participation (CoPs) and Conditions for Coverage (CfCs)*
- Manufacturers' instructions for use
- Evidence-based guidelines and national standards, such as those from The Joint Commission standards, the US Centers for Disease Control and Prevention (CDC), and the World Health Organization (WHO)
- Consensus documents

An IPC program should be implemented organizationwide and designed to involve all relevant locations, programs, services, and departments. It must address IPC issues related to patient care, including licensed independent practitioners, contractors, patients, residents, students, volunteers, families, and visitors, as applicable. The IPC program must be integrated into the organization's programs for quality assurance; performance improvement; employee health, education, and training; emergency preparedness; patient safety; and environment of care, as discussed later in this book.

Initial steps for developing an IPC program in any health care setting include the following:

- Identify the organization's care, treatment, and services provided and perform a risk assessment that also accounts for the geographic location, community, and population served.
- After risks are prioritized and goals are developed based on those risks, then a written IPC plan produced based on those findings. It is helpful to include IPC personnel and staff from management, clinical and support services, and finance, as appropriate for the organization.

A thorough facility risk assessment should be the foundation for an infection surveillance, prevention, and control program in any health care organization. Conducting a risk assessment and developing an IPC plan are discussed in further detail in Chapter 3.

Health care organizations must designate an individual (or individuals) responsible for the IPC program, but it may also be helpful to identify a group with ongoing

> **TIP** Integrate the IPC program into the organization's quality assurance/ performance improvement; employee health, education, and training; emergency preparedness; patient safety; and environment of care/facility management and safety programs.

oversight of the IPC and surveillance programs. It is recommended that this oversight group be composed of representatives from a variety of disciplines, such as patient care services, administration, environmental services, microbiology, safety, and performance improvement, as appropriate for the organization.

Essential Components of an IPC Program

IPC programs must extend beyond the acute care hospital to include diverse health care settings, such as nursing care centers, ambulatory health care settings, same-day surgery centers, behavioral health care and human services facilities, rehabilitation care facilities, and home care, to meet the needs of a changing health care delivery system.[10,19] A variety of groups and organizations have defined the essential components of an effective infection surveillance, prevention, and control program for various health care settings.[10,20-32] These key components include, but are not limited to, those listed in Sidebar 1-1. These critical elements are recommended when designing or evaluating an IPC program.

Managing the Infection Prevention and Control Program

As stated previously, Joint Commission and Joint Commission International standards require that the organization's leaders assign one or more individuals responsibility for the IPC program and that leaders allocate adequate resources for the program. The following sections discuss some strategies for how organizations can accomplish this and offer guidance for identifying and managing responsibility in a variety of settings.

---

*For organizations that use Joint Commission accreditation for deemed status purposes or that are required by state regulation or directive, CoPs and/or CfCs should be reviewed for applicable mandatory requirements.

Sidebar 1-1. Components of an Effective IPC Program

- Dedicated resources for infection surveillance, prevention, and control
- Adequate number of trained personnel managing the IPC program
- Periodic facility infection risk assessment
- Written infection surveillance, prevention, and control plan based on risk assessment
- Capability to identify and investigate epidemiologically important organisms, outbreaks, and clusters of infectious disease
- Surveillance program that monitors outcomes and practices
- System for obtaining, managing, and reporting critical data and information
- Use of surveillance findings in quality assurance/performance improvement activities
- Internal and external communication systems
- Written policies and procedures based on evidence-based practices
- Compliance with applicable regulations, standards, guidelines, accreditation requirements, and other requirements
- IPC activities integrated with employee health, patient safety, quality assurance/performance improvement, engineering/construction, disinfection/sterile processing, emergency preparedness, and environment of care/facility management and safety programs
- Authority to implement IPC measures
- Education and training of health care personnel, patients, and visitors
- Monitoring of personnel compliance with IPC practices
- Competency assessments for personnel, including the infection preventionist (IP)
- Periodic evaluation of the effectiveness of the IPC program
- Integration with emergency preparedness systems in the community
- Collaboration with local, state, and federal public health departments
- Accountability for complying with IPC practices and standards

Depending on the organization, leadership may identify an individual (or individuals) who has knowledge of the clinical principles and practices used to prevent and control the transmission of infection and meets recognized core competencies. In addition to the IP, some organizations may also have a health care epidemiologist; in some cases, a physician is assigned to direct or act as a clinical consultant for the IPC program. The Society for Healthcare Epidemiology of America (SHEA) has published guidelines outlining the roles and necessary skills for a health care epidemiologist.[33]

The organization should provide those responsible for the IPC program with the authority to take quick action when steps are needed to prevent or control the spread of infectious agents. For example, when an IP responsible for the IPC program in a nursing care center discovers that carbapenem-resistant *Klebsiella pneumoniae*—an emerging multidrug-resistant nosocomial pathogen that causes several types of HAIs—has been isolated from the urine of residents on one unit, ideally, the IP should initiate contact precautions for those residents and oversee implementation of other actions, if necessary, to prevent transmission to other residents, such as instituting a cohort.

Although not required by current Joint Commission and Joint Commission International standards, many organizations have a written statement that authorizes specified personnel, such as the IP and the health care epidemiologist and/or designee, to institute appropriate control measures when there is a risk of infection to patients and health care workers. Such measures may include the following:
- Instituting transmission-based precautions for a patient or resident
- Recommending relevant cultures and other laboratory tests to licensed independent practitioners (LIPs)
- Restricting visitors and staff and movement of patients or residents from one area to another
- Recommending temporarily closing a unit or ward to further admissions in case of a suspected or actual outbreak

In addition, some states and local health agencies may require an organization to have an authority statement for the IP or responsible physician.

Many organizations have a job description for the IP and health care epidemiologist positions. The organization defines the reporting structure, job summary, qualifications, duties, and responsibilities. A sample job description for an IP is shown in Figure 1-1 on pages 18–20 and is provided as a downloadable tool (see Tool 1-1).

TRY THIS TOOL

Tool 1-1. Sample Job Description for an Infection Preventionist

Using Qualified Clinical Resources

The organization's leadership is responsible for identifying a resource who can assist the individual with clinical responsibility in making knowledgeable decisions related to infection surveillance, prevention, and control. These persons with expertise may be employees of the organization, contractual agents, outside consultants, or volunteers. Local resources may include state or local health department staff and members of professional organizations such as the Association for Professionals in Infection Control and Epidemiology (APIC), SHEA, and the International Association of Healthcare Central Service Materiel Management (IAHCSMM).

For example, the leaders of a nursing care center, a behavioral health care and human services facility, or an ambulatory surgery center may arrange for an IP from a local hospital or the epidemiologist from an academic medical center to provide consultation services, as needed, to help individuals assigned with responsibility for managing the facility's IPC program.[10]

Organizations should base their considerations on the goals and objectives of the IPC program and keep in mind the following:

- The organization's leaders should provide for a sufficient number and mix of individuals to support safe, quality care, treatment, and services.
- Organization leaders should identify competencies needed by those assigned responsibility for the IPC program and select persons that either possess these competencies or can be trained to attain them.

Staffing and competencies for IPC staff are discussed below. *See Chapter 2 for a more detailed account of leadership responsibilities.*

Staffing

In most health care settings, leaders are responsible for assigning clear responsibility for the daily management of the IPC program to at least one person who is knowledgeable about infectious diseases; IPC risks; the principles of infection surveillance, prevention, and control; and data collection, analysis, and presentation, for example.[20-22] As stated earlier, the number and types of individuals assigned should be determined by the scope, goals, and objectives of the organization's IPC and surveillance program.

Figure 1-1. Sample Job Description for an Infection Preventionist

NOTE: This job description is an example and lists job duties that may not apply to all health care settings.

Job Title:	Infection Preventionist
Date created: Date revised:	
FLSA status:	
Job summary	

Coordinates a comprehensive organizationwide infection surveillance, prevention, and control program in accordance with current requirements of regulatory, government, and accrediting/licensing agencies and organizational policies and procedures. Duties include surveillance for health care–associated infections (HAIs); collection, analysis, interpretation, and reporting of surveillance data; outbreak identification and investigation; and program evaluation. Responsible for the day-to-day administration and development of the infection surveillance, prevention, and control program.

Reporting Structure

Reports to the Vice President, Quality Improvement.

Major Duties

1. Conducts a facility infection prevention and control risk assessment annually and whenever risks significantly change
2. Develops a plan for infection surveillance, prevention, and control activities based on the facility risk assessment
3. Maintains an infection surveillance, prevention, and control program based on the organization's risk assessment and plan and in accordance with local, state, federal, and other reporting requirements
4. Collects, manages, and analyzes surveillance data using standardized methodology and defined criteria for HAIs
5. Organizes and maintains surveillance data and records
6. Reports surveillance data, findings, and analyses to the appropriate committees, patient care units, personnel, and external agencies
7. Monitors patients for the occurrence of communicable diseases, HAIs, and resistant and epidemiologically important organisms
8. Monitors infectious diseases and epidemiologically significant organisms occurring in the community via laboratory reports and public health reports
9. Identifies and evaluates clusters of infections and potential outbreaks
10. Institutes an outbreak investigation and control measures as needed
11. Recommends isolation precautions according to the organization's policies and procedures
12. Develops evidence-based infection prevention and control policies and protocols in accordance with regulatory, government, and accrediting/licensing agency requirements and recommendations of relevant professional organizations
13. Updates policies and protocols as needed to maintain compliance with regulations, standards, and evidence-based guidelines

(continued)

Figure 1-1. Sample Job Description for an Infection Preventionist (continued)

14. Assists the organization to evaluate and maintain readiness for local, state, federal, and accrediting agency surveys
15. Monitors and evaluates the efficacy of infection prevention and control strategies
16. Collaborates with other departments throughout the facility to design and implement strategies to prevent HAIs and transmission of multidrug-resistant organisms and other epidemiologically important organisms
17. Investigates exposures to communicable disease and initiates appropriate measures to prevent the transmission of disease
18. Maintains confidentiality of patients, personnel, and related information
19. Provides consultation services relating to infection prevention and control to the various departments in the organization
20. Evaluates products, devices, and equipment relating to infection prevention and control
21. Actively participates in quality assurance/performance improvement activities
22. Maintains departmental records for compliance with regulatory and accrediting agencies
23. Provides written and verbal reports to administration and relevant committees, departments, personnel, and external agencies
24. Communicates with local and state health departments
25. Participates in orientation programs and required annual education programs
26. Provides education on hand hygiene, aseptic technique, infection prevention and control strategies, antiseptics and disinfectants, specific infectious diseases, and other related health care issues
27. Develops or obtains educational materials and programs, as needed, for personnel, patients, and visitors
28. Collaborates with employee health personnel on matters such as exposure management and immunization
29. Works with facilities management and other personnel to evaluate infection risks associated with renovation and construction projects and identify control measures
30. Is an active member of the following committees: Infection Prevention and Control, Patient Care Council, Quality and Performance Improvement, and Product Standardization, as applicable to the organization
31. Assists leaders in identifying appropriate personnel as potential members of the IPC committee, as applicable
32. Either leads or participates on work groups tasked with identifying and implementing effective infection prevention and control measures
33. Collaborates with leaders and financial personnel to identify and implement evidence-based, cost-effective strategies for reducing the risk and occurrence of infections

Qualifications
- ___ years of experience in clinical/patient care services or relevant health care position
- Minimum Bachelor of Science degree in nursing, microbiology, public health, medical technology, or related field required. Related license or certification.
- CIC certification from the Certification Board of Infection Control and Epidemiology preferred. Ability to take certification examination within three years of employment required.

(continued)

Figure 1-1. Sample Job Description for an Infection Preventionist (continued)

Knowledge/Skills/Abilities

- Familiarity with relevant local, state, federal, and accrediting agency requirements
- Knowledge and experience in areas of patient care practices, microbiology, asepsis, cleaning, disinfection and sterilization, adult education, infectious diseases, epidemiology, statistics, communication, and program management
- Self-motivated, organized, and detail oriented
- Able to collect, analyze, and report data
- Computer literate, including Microsoft Office (Word, Excel, and PowerPoint) and ability to obtain, enter, and manage electronic data
- Excellent oral and written communication skills
- Able to facilitate performance improvement initiatives
- Able to organize and manage time and multiple tasks
- Participates in ongoing personal education and professional development
- Is an active member of relevant professional organizations
- Adheres to the principles and to the mission of the organization
- Able to manage and lead infection prevention and control department staff (when applicable)
- Exhibits leadership and team building skills

The above statements are intended to describe the general duties and level of work performed by those persons assigned to this position. These statements are not designed to contain or be interpreted as a comprehensive inventory of all duties, responsibilities, and qualifications required of employees assigned to the job. Management retains the discretion to add to or change the duties of the position at any time.

Note: FLSA, Fair Labor Standards Act; CIC, Certified in Infection Control.

Source: Arias Infection Control Consulting, LLC. Used with permission.

Due to transformative changes in health care, and depending on how an organization defines responsibilities, the scope and responsibilities for many IPs have grown beyond infection surveillance, prevention, and control to also include quality assurance/performance improvement, patient safety, occupational health, construction and renovation, emergency preparedness, mandatory reporting, sterile processing, and antimicrobial stewardship.[19-27] An IP in a hospital may be responsible for overseeing the IPC programs in a variety of affiliated long term care, ambulatory health care, home health, and behavioral health care and human services facilities. Regardless of an organization's type, size, or complexity, the infection, prevention, and control program must be aligned with the organization's mission and values, meet the organization's needs, comply with applicable regulations and other requirements, and incorporate standards and evidence-based guidelines, as applicable.

Successful implementation of IPC programs across the continuum of care depends on adequate numbers of trained personnel responsible for the daily management of the programs' activities. Some examples of such activities may include, but are not limited to, the following:

- Identifying and assessing actions aimed at eliminating the risks and occurrence of HAIs
- Conducting surveillance activities
- Collecting, analyzing, and presenting data

- Reporting surveillance findings to management, frontline staff and other appropriate personnel, and external agencies, as required
- Monitoring and reporting trends in antimicrobial resistance
- Educating personnel about strategies to prevent and control the spread of infections
- Leading and participating in quality assurance/performance improvement activities
- Promoting the use of evidence-based infection prevention and control practices
- Collaborating with personnel in all areas of the organization to promote implementation of effective infection prevention and control measures
- Identifying and responding to acute events such as an influx of potentially infectious patients, outbreaks, emerging infectious diseases, and pandemics (discussed in Chapter 5)
- Ensuring follow-up of US Food and Drug Administration (FDA) and local authority alerts on medical devices
- Monitoring the effectiveness of the IPC program (discussed in Chapter 11)
- Communicating with staff and leadership
- Interfacing with public health authorities on issues relating to reportable diseases, outbreaks, and pandemics

Currently, no nationally recognized standard for staffing infection surveillance, prevention, and control programs exists; however, several studies and reports have attempted to quantify the issue. The historic SENIC Project in the 1970s linked the availability of one IP per 250 occupied hospital beds with an effective hospital infection surveillance, prevention, and control program.[7] However, in 1996, a SHEA Consensus Panel noted that, for the hospital setting, "the old ratio of one ICP [infection preventionist] per 250 beds is no longer adequate, because the notion of a ratio tied to beds is insufficient to define the scope of the work of an infection preventionist."[32(p. 53)]

A similar consensus panel was established by APIC and SHEA in 1997 to develop recommendations for optimal infrastructure and essential activities of infection control and epidemiology programs in out-of-hospital settings.[20] This panel noted that the IPC program must be "the responsibility of at least one designated person. In some HCOs [health care organizations], this person may also have other responsibilities (i.e., IPC activities will be part

time). In this situation, the expected number of hours per week that are devoted to infection control should be clearly stated."[20(p. 425)]

In 2012, the Ontario Ministry of Health and Long-Term Care Public Health Division/Provincial Infectious Diseases Advisory Committee, Toronto, Canada, issued *Best Practices for Infection Prevention and Control Programs in Ontario in All Health Care Settings*, third edition.[23] This guideline discusses several reports that address IP staffing levels and concludes that "staffing levels must be appropriate to the size and complexity of care of the health care facility. Recommendations for staffing should not be based exclusively on bed numbers. The ratio of ICPs will vary according to the acuity and activity of the health care facility and the volume and complexity of the ICP's work. This includes high-risk ambulatory care centers such as oncology and dialysis."[23(p. 48)]

In some cases, particularly in ambulatory health care, nursing care, and behavioral health care and human services centers, the person who manages the IPC program may also oversee related areas, such as employee health, staff development, nursing, and quality assurance/performance improvement.[16,35] In some settings, such as office-based practices or very small hospitals, it may be cost-effective to contract out all or some IPC functions, such as staff education and training, employee health, and exposure follow-up. Some organizations have successfully used infection control liaisons in a variety of health care settings to support infection surveillance, prevention, and control activities.[36]

No matter the size and scope of an organization, its leaders and the person(s) responsible for developing, maintaining, and managing the IPC program must collaborate to identify resource capabilities and match them with the organization's needs and external requirements. They should prioritize infection surveillance, prevention, and control activities and streamline work processes to increase efficiency. This can be accomplished by the following:

- Conduct a facility infection prevention risk assessment and use the findings to develop an infection prevention, control, and surveillance plan. (See Chapter 3 for information on conducting an infection prevention risk assessment.)
- Use the IPC and surveillance plans to identify the essential activities needed to provide a safe environment and reduce the risks of infection.

Remember that the risk assessment and IPC plan should support the vision, mission, and goals of the organization.

- Conduct a time study to determine the time needed to complete each of the essential activities identified above. Use a time sheet to collect activity data.[34] From these data, the number of hours of IPC labor per week/month/year needed can be quantified, and the number of personnel needed to complete these tasks can be calculated. An example of a time sheet that can be used to document IP activities can be downloaded and customized (see Tool 1-2).

TRY THIS TOOL

Tool 1-2. IPC Staff Activity Time Study for Preparing a Business Case

---

To assist in obtaining sufficient personnel resources, the IP should consider building a business case for IPC and presenting this to the organization's leaders and appropriate decision makers.[34,37-39] Additional information on quantifying IPC activities and staffing needs can be found in an article by Bartles et al.[34] For information on building and presenting a business case for IPC, refer to the websites section in the Resources at the end of this chapter and refer to the STRIVE courses on conducting a business case, also referenced at the end of this chapter.

TIP Once essential elements of the IPC program are identified, IPC personnel can then use this information to conduct a time study to quantify the number of hours needed to complete those activities per week/month/year and calculate the number of personnel needed to complete them.

Competencies

IPs come from different professional backgrounds, such as nursing, medical technology, microbiology, medicine, public health, and other health care fields, and they have varying academic preparation and degrees.[40-42] Regardless of background or training, a good practice is

to ensure that an IP has defined competencies to manage an infection prevention and control program.

Core competencies and professional practice standards for IPs have been published by a variety of organizations, including APIC,[22,40] the Certification Board of Infection Control and Epidemiology (CBIC),[43] a task force convened by APIC and the Community and Hospital Infection Control Association of Canada (CHICA-Canada) (now Infection Prevention and Control Canada [IPAC Canada]),[21] the Infection Prevention Society,[44] the European Centre for Disease Prevention and Control,[45] and consensus panels convened by SHEA.[20,27,32] A partial list of recommended competencies, based on these publications, is presented in Sidebar 1-2 on page 24.

TIP Any infection preventionist, regardless of background or training, must meet the organization's defined competencies to effectively manage an infection surveillance, prevention, and control program.

Many of the competencies identified by organizations fit into the six IP competency domains in the 2019 APIC Core Competency Model,[40] shown in Figure 1-2 on pages 25.

Joint Commission–accredited organizations are responsible for the orientation and training of the individual(s) as required by their program-specific standards. One way a new IP can obtain infection control related training is to attend a basic training course in infection surveillance, prevention, and control, such as that provided by APIC. Another way IPs may be trained is to work closely with an experienced IP at another facility that provides similar services. Download Tool 1-3 for a sample checklist that organizations can modify and use during IP orientation.

TRY THIS TOOL

Tool 1-3. Sample Orientation Checklist for an Infection Preventionist

---

Some strategies that may be used to evaluate the competency of persons assigned to the daily management of IPC activities include the following:

- *Evaluate the ability of the individual to meet defined competencies.* Use a competency checklist or tool based on defined core competencies. APIC has published a self-assessment tool that can be used for this purpose.[46]
- *Assess the individual for the defined skills needed.* Professional organizations have defined and published particular skills that the IP should possess related to communication, collaboration, program management, critical thinking, and the ability to provide education and training.[22,40,44] Assess skills using a performance evaluation/position description tool that includes these abilities.[46]
- *Determine the ability of the individual to fulfill the organization's needs and job specifications.* The criteria in the assessment should be included among the organization's performance evaluation tools to evaluate all types of personnel. Performance evaluation and competency assessment should be an ongoing process.
- *Designate responsibility for managing infection surveillance, prevention, and control activities within the organization.* A key responsibility of the IP is to coordinate and oversee the many infection surveillance, prevention, and control activities in an organization. Many of these activities take place during direct patient care or while providing support services. It is not possible for an IP to directly observe whether all personnel adhere to appropriate infection prevention and control practices, such as performing hand hygiene, cleaning and disinfecting medical equipment and devices according to policy and manufacturer's instructions, or screening visitors who may present an infection risk to others. Therefore, IPs must work to ensure that clear policies and procedures exist that meet regulatory requirements and provide guidance on best practices required by the organization, that personnel and patients or residents are aware of these policies, and that mechanisms are in place to ensure compliance with IPC policies and practices.

To effectively coordinate IPC activities, the IP should develop partnerships and obtain the cooperation of managers, point-of-care providers, and other personnel who will accept the responsibility for implementing IPC efforts in their area. Although the IP may delegate responsibility for adhering to appropriate IPC practices, managers must hold these persons accountable to ensure that IPC efforts are carried out.[38,39] The IP can promote this collaboration by sharing information and data and encouraging communication among the IP and leaders, managers, point-of-care providers, and other personnel.

IPC efforts improve with multidisciplinary participation in the IPC program, such as when there is broad representation on an IPC committee and direct communication with nursing, patient safety, and quality assurance/performance improvement committees. For instance, the IPC committee should be composed of representatives from disciplines such as patient services, administration, environmental services, microbiology, safety, and performance improvement, as appropriate for the organization. The IP must have access to, and participate in, the work of these groups to facilitate communication and collaboration throughout the organization (see Sidebar 1-3 on page 26).

An organization can successfully reduce the risk and occurrence of health care–associated infections when it has an evidence-based IPC program supported by strong leadership that promotes a culture of safety, collaboration, communication, problem-solving, and transparency.[38]

Sidebar 1-2. Examples of Competencies for the Infection Preventionist[20,22,40,43,45]

- Meets recommended qualifications for the profession:
    - Is an experienced health care professional with health sciences background
    - Has working knowledge of the following: patient care practices; microbiology; asepsis; cleaning, disinfection, and sterilization practices; infectious disease processes; epidemiology and disease transmission, surveillance, and outbreak investigation techniques; information technology; statistical measures used in IPC; communication methods; program management and administration; adult education principles; occupational health issues; the environment of care/ facility management and safety; performance measurement and improvement principles; and the standards, regulations, and other requirements affecting IPC programs
- Participates in professional development:
    - Attends a basic training course in infection surveillance, prevention, and control within the first six months of entering the profession
    - Remains current in infection surveillance, prevention, and control practices
    - Has or strives to achieve the designation Certified in Infection Control (CIC) from the Certification Board of Infection Control and Epidemiology
    - Participates in related professional organizations
    - Holds self professionally accountable for developing, evaluating, and improving his or her own practices
- Demonstrates the following management, leadership, and communication skills:
    - Plans and develops an IPC program in accordance with standards and other requirements
    - Collaborates with others to improve practices and safety and to implement into practice pertinent regulatory requirements, accreditation standards, and guidelines
    - Systematically evaluates the effectiveness of the program and its appropriateness to the practice setting
    - Determines resource needs to accomplish the IPC program goals and objectives
    - Communicates resource needs to key stakeholders based on the goals and objectives
    - Uses information technology for data collection, management, reporting, and communication
    - Communicates with and provides feedback to appropriate individuals, committees, and departments
    - Makes decisions and performs in an ethical manner
    - Optimizes available resources and practices in a fiscally responsible and accountable manner
    - Serves as a consultant on IPC issues
    - Uses principles of influence, leadership, and change management
- Participates in educational activities to improve IPC practices in the organization
- Assesses learning needs and develops and implements education programs and opportunities
- Develops and participates in performance improvement activities

Figure 1-2. The 2019 APIC Competency Model

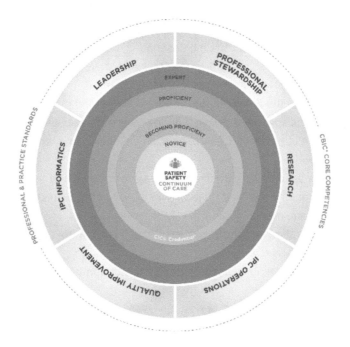

Source: Association for Professionals in Infection Control and Epidemiology. Used with permission.

During a Joint Commission survey, surveyors assess whether health care organizations that use Joint Commission accreditation for deemed status purposes meet CMS requirements. Several CMS requirements related to the individual(s) assigned responsibilities for the IPC program fall under Joint Commission Standard IC.01.01.01, EP 4; these duties are listed in the box on page 12.

An accredited organization can meet these requirements by ensuring that these duties are in the IP's job description and performance evaluation. Such duties should also be documented in the organization's written IPC and surveillance plans. Documentation that these activities are being done can be accomplished by demonstrating the availability of policies governing infections and communicable diseases and ensuring that surveillance reports are discussed in relevant committee meetings.

For an accredited ambulatory surgery center that elects the Joint Commission deemed status option, there's an additional element of performance (EP 5) under IC.01.01.01. This EP requires that oversight of the infection prevention and control program be under the direction of a designated and qualified professional who has IPC training. (See the box on pages 11–12 for details.)

An organization can meet this requirement by designating a specific individual to manage the IPC program and by providing training and competency assessments for that person, as discussed in IC.01.01.01, EP 3.

Other Related Standards

Beyond the relevant IPC standards related to designing and managing an effective IPC program, accredited organizations must also adhere to standards in the "Human Resources" (HR) and "Leadership" (LD) chapters of the Joint Commission *Comprehensive Accreditation Manuals* for their designated heath care setting. Standards HR.01.01.01, EP 1, and (for international organizations) Standard SQE.2, ME 2, require organizations to define

Sidebar 1-3. Tips for Working Effectively with Administration or Leadership to Improve Infection Prevention and Control Activities

1. Know the expectations associated with the job description.
2. Introduce yourself to the chief executive officer or president of the organization.
3. Align departmental goals with the organization's strategic plan.
4. Spend time with someone in the finance department to understand the costs of HAIs.
5. Form collaborative relationships with directors and managers of clinical support departments, particularly those who directly affect IPC activities such as laboratory, respiratory care, and sterile processing.
6. Establish close working relationships with the directors and managers of support departments such as environmental services, purchasing, and materials management to promote easy exchange of ideas for process improvements related to IPC.
7. Regularly update administration on the state of the IPC activities in the organization, including raw numbers of infection as well as rates.
8. Attend all meetings and fulfill responsibilities associated with administrative appointments to committees and task forces.
9. Negotiate for increased financial support or positions with data on cost and opportunity savings associated with infection prevention.
10. Provide a brief, easy-to-read, and understandable annual report to administration on the infection rates in the facility or organization. Be sure to include cost savings associated with a decrease in infections, including opportunity costs.
11. Establish a relationship based on mutual trust with the bedside caregivers and patient care managers because this is where the prevention and control activities take place.
12. Help remove barriers to change for managers who wish to look at new IPC products and methods to prevent and control infections.

Source: Deanie Lancaster, RN, BSN, MHSA, CIC. Used with permission.

---

staff qualifications specific to their job responsibilities. IPC personnel may be qualified through ongoing education, training, experience, and/or certification.

The organization's leadership should recognize the need for and support the IP's ongoing education and learning. The health care field and the practice of infection surveillance, prevention, and control are rapidly evolving. To ensure that the IP's knowledge remains current, leadership should make provisions that allow the IP to attend professional meetings and educational programs, access information through the Internet and other resources, purchase relevant periodicals and publications, and encourage and support the IP's efforts to successfully pass the infection prevention and control certification examination.[43]

As discussed earlier in this chapter, the number and skill mix of the persons assigned to manage the infection surveillance, prevention, and control program must be based on organizational characteristics, the types of patients or residents served, and the volume and complexity of the IP's work. Given the adverse effects due to an overwhelming influx of patients and residents during the COVID-19 pandemic, leaders should focus on providing adequate numbers of patient/resident care and support services staff as needed to support safe and quality care, treatment, and services in all health care settings. This is discussed in more detail in Chapter 5.

Responsibility and Accountability for Preventing Infections

Although the responsibility for managing the infection surveillance, prevention, and control program is assigned to a few individuals, all health care providers are responsible for using appropriate IPC practices in their daily activities. Both the "Infection Prevention and Control" and "Human Resources" standards chapters and the JCI standards address this. It is listed under Standard IC.01.05.01 for hospitals and critical access hospitals (requiring all hospital components and functions to be integrated into the IPC program) as well as ambulatory health care, behavioral health care and human services, home care, office-based surgery, and nursing care centers (giving everyone who works in the facility responsibility for preventing and controlling infections). International settings can look to JCI Standard PCI.2 for hospitals and academic medical centers.

The Joint Commission and Joint Commission International require health care organizations to integrate IPC practices throughout the organization and to educate personnel about their specific roles and responsibilities in IPC. Based on this requirement, organizations are expected to ensure that personnel are not only educated on their roles and responsibilities regarding IPC but also held accountable for adhering to appropriate IPC practices.

Summary

The goal of an infection surveillance, prevention, and control program is to prevent HAIs. Regardless of the health care setting, the infection surveillance, prevention, and control program should contain identified core elements and be managed by an individual (or individuals) who has the prescribed competencies. The types and number of personnel and other resources allocated should be based on the organization's size, type, and complexity and on an assessment of the populations served, services provided, and internal and external requirements. The organization's leaders should ensure that appropriate resources are allocated to provide an infection surveillance, prevention, and control program that effectively reduces the risk and occurrence of HAIs. In 2020, the rapid spread of COVID-19 in health care facilities worldwide called attention to the critical need for effective IPC and surveillance programs in all health care settings to prevent and control the transmission of HAIs and their resulting morbidity and mortality.

An organization's leadership is expected to ensure that personnel are both educated on their responsibilities regarding infection prevention and control and held accountable for adhering to appropriate IPC practices. Responsibilities of leadership for the IPC program are discussed in more detail in Chapter 2.

Resources

The following sections provide further information on this topic and can serve as valuable references in designing, managing, and allocating resources for an IPC program.

Tools to Try

Tool 1-1. Sample Job Description for an Infection Preventionist

Tool 1-2. IPC Staff Activity Time Study for Preparing a Business Case

Tool 1-3. Sample Orientation Checklist for an Infection Preventionist

IPC Program and Infection Preventionist Professional Practice Assessment and Evaluation Tools

Note: *Because these tools may be periodically updated, users are advised to check the provider's website to confirm they have the most recent version.*

- Centers for Disease Control and Prevention. Infection Control Tools for Healthcare Settings. This website contains assessment and infection prevention tools for a variety of health care settings including acute, long term care, and outpatient (for example, dental, orthopedic, pain management, podiatry, and hemodialysis). Accessed Dec 14, 2020. https://www.cdc.gov/infectioncontrol/tools/index.html

- Ontario Agency for Health Protection and Promotion, Provincial Infectious Diseases Advisory Committee. Summary of *Recommendations for Best Practices for IPC Programs* in Best Practices for Infection Prevention and Control Programs in Ontario in All Health Care Settings, 3rd ed. May 2012. (pp. 51–58). This summary table is intended to help with self-assessments for IPC programs. Accessed Dec 14, 2020. https://www.publichealthontario.ca/-/media/documents/b/2012/bp-ipac-hc-settings.pdf?la=en

- World Health Organization. Core Components for IPC—Implementation Tools and Resources. Accessed Dec 14, 2020. https://www.who.int/infection-prevention/tools/core-components/en/

- APIC Implementation Guide Series. APIC Implementation Guides provide practical, evidence-based strategies for surveillance and the elimination of infection. Each guide includes online tools and resources. Accessed Dec 14, 2020. https://apic.org/professional-practice/implementation-guides/

- APIC Competency Self-Assessment Activity for Novice or Becoming Proficient IPs. Accessed Dec 14, 2020. https://apic.org/wp-content/uploads/2019/05/IP_Comp_Self_Assessment-2019-Activity_5-24-19.pdf

- APIC Developmental Path of the Infection Preventionist. Accessed Dec 14, 2020. https://apic.org/professional-practice/roadmap

- APIC Sample Job Description for the Infection Preventionist, May 2019. Accessed Dec 14, 2020. https://apic.org/wp-content/uploads/2019/08/IP-Job-Description-web-version.pdf

Websites

Association for Professionals in Infection Control and Epidemiology. Accessed Dec 14, 2020. http://www.apic.org.

US Centers for Disease Control and Prevention:
- CDC Infection Control. Accessed Dec 14, 2020. https://www.cdc.gov/infectioncontrol/index.html
- CDC/STRIVE Infection Control Training. Contains courses that address the technical and foundational elements of HAI prevention. Accessed Dec 14, 2020. https://www.cdc.gov/infectioncontrol/training/strive.html
- CDC STRIVE also contains two courses on building a business case for IPC (WB-4227):
  ○ CDC STRIVE. BC 101. Creating a Business Case for Infection Prevention. Accessed Dec 14, 2020. https://www.cdc.gov/infectioncontrol/pdf/strive/BC101-508.pdf
  ○ CDC STRIVE. BC 102. Integrating the Business Case for Infection Prevention into Hospital Priorities. Accessed Dec 14, 2020. https://www.cdc.gov/infectioncontrol/pdf/strive/BC102-508.pdf

- CDC Healthcare-Associated Infections: Outbreak Investigations in Healthcare Settings. Accessed Dec 14, 2020. https://www.cdc.gov/hai/outbreaks/index.html

- CDC Healthcare–associated Infections in Outpatient Settings. Accessed Dec 14, 2020. https://www.cdc.gov/hai/settings/outpatient/outpatient-settings.html

- World Health Organization. Infection Prevention and Control. Accessed Dec 14, 2020. https://www.who.int/teams/integrated-health-services/infection-prevention-control

- Society for Healthcare Epidemiology of America. Accessed Dec 14, 2020. http://www.shea-online.org

- Infection Prevention and Control Canada (IPAC Canada). Accessed Dec 14, 2020. http://ipac-canada.org

- Certification Board of Infection Control and Epidemiology. Accessed Dec 14, 2020. http://www.cbic.org

- Ontario Agency for Health Protection and Promotion (Public Health Ontario), Provincial Infectious Diseases Advisory Committee. Best Practices for IPC. Accessed Dec 14, 2020. https://www.publichealthontario.ca/en/health-topics/infection-prevention-control/best-practices-ipac

- Infection Prevention and Control for Clinical Office Practice. 1st Revision. Toronto: Queen's Printer for Ontario; 2015. Accessed Dec 14, 2020. https://www.publichealthontario.ca/-/media/documents/B/2013/bp-clinical-office-practice.pdf?la=en

References

1. Magill SS, et al. Emerging Infections Program Hospital Prevalence Survey Team. Changes in prevalence of health care–associated infections in U.S. hospitals. *N Engl J Med*. 2018;379:1732–44.

2. Umscheid CA, et al. Estimating the proportion of healthcare-associated infections that are reasonably preventable and the related mortality and costs. *Infect Control Hosp Epidemiol*. 2011 Feb;32(2):101–114.

3. Agency for Healthcare Research and Quality. Estimating the Additional Hospital Inpatient Cost and Mortality Associated with Selected Hospital-Acquired Conditions. Accessed Dec 14, 2020. https://www.ahrq.gov/hai/pfp/haccost2017-results.html

4. Mitchell R, et al. for the Canadian Nosocomial Infection Surveillance Program. Trends in health care–associated infections in acute care hospitals in Canada: An analysis of repeated point-prevalence surveys. *CMAJ.* 2019 Sep 9;191(36):E981–E988.

5. Popovich KJ, et al. The Centers for Disease Control and Prevention STRIVE Initiative: Construction of a national Program to reduce health care–associated infections at the local level. *Ann Intern Med.* 2019;171(7 Suppl):S2–S6.

6. Zingg W, et al. Implementation research for the prevention of antimicrobial resistance and healthcare–associated infections; 2017 Geneva infection prevention and control (IPC)-think tank (part 1). *Antimicrob Resist Infect Control.* 2019;8:87 https://doi.org/10.1186/s13756-019-0527-1

7. Haley RW, et al. The efficacy of infection surveillance and control programs in preventing nosocomial infections in US hospitals. *Am J Epidemiol.* 1985 Feb;121(2):182–205.

8. Zimlichman E, et al. Health Care-Associated Infections: A meta-analysis of costs and financial impact on the US health care system. *JAMA Intern Med.* 2013;173(22):2039–2046.

9. Centers for Disease Control and Prevention. 2019 National and State Healthcare-Associated Infections Progress Report. Accessed Dec 14, 2020. https://www.cdc.gov/hai/data/portal/progress-report.html

10. Steinkuller F, et al. Outpatient infection prevention: A practical primer. *Open Forum Infect Dis.* 2018 May; 5(5). Accessed Dec 14, 2020. https://www.ncbi.nlm.nih.gov/pmc/articles/PMC5930182

11. Oppermann CM, et al. Risks of infection in health care out of the hospital setting: An integrative review. *J Epidemiol and Infect Control.* 2017;7(3):194–202.

12. Sassi HP, et al. Control of the spread of viruses in a long-term care facility using hygiene protocols. *Am J Infect Control.* 2015;43(7):702–706.

13. OYong K, et al. Health care–associated infection outbreak investigations in outpatient settings, Los Angeles County, California, USA, 2000–2012. *Emerg Infect Dis.* 2015;21(8):1317–1321. Accessed Dec 14, 2020. https://dx.doi.org/10.3201/eid2108.141251

14. Centers for Disease Control and Prevention. Outpatient Settings Policy Options for Improving Infection Prevention. Oct 2015. Accessed Dec 14, 2020. http://www.cdc.gov/hai/settings/outpatient/outpatient-settings.html

15. Centers for Disease Control and Prevention. Guide to Infection Prevention for Outpatient Settings: Minimum Expectations for Safe Care. Accessed Dec 14, 2020. http://www.cdc.gov/HAI/settings/outpatient/outpatient-settings.html

16. Pogorzelska-Maziarz M, et al. Infection prevention outside of the acute care setting: Results from the MegaSurvey of infection preventionists. *Am J Infect Control* 2017;45(6):597–602.

17. Shang J, et al. Infection in home health care: Results from national Outcome and Assessment Information Set data. *Am J Infect Control.* 2015;43(5):454–459.

18. Schaefer MK, Perkins KM, Perz JF. Patient notification events due to syringe reuse and mishandling of injectable medications by health care personnel United States, 2012–2018: Summary and recommended actions for prevention and response. *MayoClin Proc.* 2020;95(2):243–254.

19. Goldrick BA. The practice of infection control and applied epidemiology: A historical perspective. *Am J Infect Control.* 2005 Nov;33(9):493–500.

20. Friedman C, et al. Requirements for infrastructure and essential activities of infection control and epidemiology in out-of-hospital settings: A consensus panel report. *Am J Infect Control.* 1999 Oct;27(5):418–430.

21. Friedman C, et al. APIC/CHICA–Canada infection prevention, control, and epidemiology: Professional and practice standards. *Am J Infect Control.* 2008 Aug;36:385–389.

22. Bubb TN, et al. APIC professional and practice standards. *Am J Infect Control*. 2016 Jul;44(7): 745–749. Accessed Dec 14, 2020. https://apic.org/Resource_/TinyMceFileManager/PDC/PPS.pdf

23. Ontario Agency for Health Protection and Promotion. Provincial Infectious Diseases Advisory Committee. *Best Practices for Infection Prevention and Control Programs in Ontario in All Health Care Settings*, 3rd ed. Toronto: Queen's Printer for Ontario, 2012. Accessed Dec 14, 2020. https://www.publichealthontario.ca/-/media/documents/bp-ipac-hc-settings.pdf

24. Morrison J, Health Canada, Nosocomial and Occupational Infections Section. Development of a resource model for infection prevention and control programs in acute, long term, and home care settings: Conference proceedings of the Infection Prevention and Control Alliance. *Am J Infect Control*. 2004 Feb;32(1):2–6.

25. Smith PW, et al. SHEA/APIC guideline: Infection prevention and control in the long-term care facility. *Infect Control Hosp Epidemiol*. 2008 Sep;29(9):785–814.

26. US Centers for Disease Control and Prevention. Guide to Infection Prevention in Outpatient Settings: Minimum Expectations for Safe Care. 2011. Accessed Dec 14, 2020. https://www.cdc.gov/hai/settings/outpatient/outpatient-care-guidelines.html

27. Bryant KA, et al. Necessary infrastructure of infection prevention and healthcare epidemiology programs: A review. *Infect Control Hosp Epidemiol*. 2016 Apr;37(4):371–380.

28. World Health Organization. Core Components of Infection Prevention and Control Programmes in Health Care. 2011. WHO/HSE/GAR/BDP/2011.1. Accessed Dec 14, 2020. https://www.who.int/csr/resources/publications/AM_CoreCom_IPC.pdf

29. World Health Organization. Minimum Requirements for Infection Prevention and Control (IPC) Programmes. 2019. Accessed Dec 14, 2020. https://www.who.int/infection-prevention/publications/min-req-IPC-manual/en/

30. Infection Prevention and Control (IPAC) Canada. Infection Prevention and Control (IPAC) Program Standard. *Can J Infect Control*. 2016 Dec;30(Suppl):1–97. Accessed Dec 14, 2020. https://ipac-canada.org/photos/custom/CJIC/Vol31No4supplement.pdf

31. Leea GA, et al. Effectiveness and core components of infection prevention and control programmes in long-term care facilities: A systematic review. *J Hosp Infect*. 2019 Aug;102(4):377–393.

32. Scheckler WE, et al. Requirements for infrastructure and essential activities of infection control and epidemiology in hospitals: A consensus panel report. *Am J Infect Control*. 1998 Feb;26(1):47–60.

33. Kaye KS, et al. Guidance for infection prevention and healthcare epidemiology programs: Healthcare epidemiologist skills and competencies. *Infect Control Hosp Epidemiol*. 2015 Apr;36(4):369–380.

34. Bartles R, et al. A systematic approach to quantifying infection prevention staffing and coverage needs. *Am J Infect Control*. 2018;46(5):487–491.

35. Pogorzelska-Maziarz M, et al. Infection prevention staffing and resources in U.S. acute care hospitals: Results from the APIC MegaSurvey, *Am J Infect Control*. 2018 Aug;46(8):852–857.

36. Wright J, et al. Expanding the infection control team: Development of the infection control liaison position for the neonatal intensive care unit. *Am J Infect Control*. 2002 May;30(3):174–178.

37. CDC STRIVE. Building a Business Case for Infection Prevention. WB-4227. Accessed Dec 14, 2020. https://www.cdc.gov/infectioncontrol/training/strive.html

38. Perencevich EN, et al. Raising standards while watching the bottom line: Making a business case for infection control. *Infect Control Hosp Epidemiol* 2007 Oct;28(10):1121–33.

39. Stone PW, et al. The economic impact of infection control: Making the business case for increased infection control resources. *Am J Infect Control*. 2005;33(9):542–547.

40. Billings C, et al. Advancing the profession: An updated future-oriented competency model for professional development in infection prevention and control. *Am J Infect Control*. 2019 Jun;47(6):602–614. Accessed Dec 14, 2020. https://apic.org/wp-content/uploads/2019/05/June-2019-AJIC-Article-APIC-Competency-Model.pdf

41. Crist K, et al. The role of the infection preventionist in a transformed healthcare system: Meeting healthcare needs in the 21st century. *Am J Infect Control*. 2019 Apr;47(4):352–357.

42. Reese SM, Gilmartin HM. Infection prevention workforce: Potential benefits to educational diversity. *Am J Infect Control*. 2017 Jun;45(6):603–606.

43. Certification Board of Infection Control and Epidemiology. Accessed Mar 23, 2020. Home page. http://www.cbic.org

44. Denton A, Fry C, O'Connor H, Robinson. Revised Infection Prevention Society (IPS) competences 2018 *J Infect Prev*. 2019 Jan; 20(1): 18–24. Accessed Dec 14, 2020. https://www.ncbi.nlm.nih.gov/pmc/articles/PMC6346329/

45. European Centre for Disease Prevention and Control. Core Competencies for Infection Control and Hospital Hygiene Professional in the European Union. 2013. Accessed Dec 14, 2020. https://www.ecdc.europa.eu/sites/default/files/media/en/publications/Publications/infection-control-core-competencies.pdf

46. APIC Competency Self-Assessment Activity for Novice or Becoming Proficient IPs. Accessed Dec 14, 2020. https://apic.org/wp-content/uploads/2019/05/IP_Comp_Self_Assessment-2019-Activity_5-24-19.pdf

Chapter 2

The Role of Leadership in Infection Prevention and Control

By Chaz Rhone, MPH, CIC, FAPIC

Disclaimer: Strategies, tools, and examples discussed in this book do not necessarily reflect Joint Commission or Joint Commission International requirements for all settings. Always refer to the most current standards applicable to your health care setting to ensure compliance.

Introduction

When reviewing the literature for a definition of leadership, you'll find many; however, one common theme is the ability to mobilize a group or team to accomplish a specific goal. In his book *The 21 Irrefutable Laws of Leadership*, John Maxwell defines leadership simply as "influence, nothing more nothing less."[1] In terms of health care leadership, there are typically a few levels of leaders, including executive, senior, and frontline leaders.

Of course, *leader* can be a relative term; many individuals without a formal leadership title can take on a leadership role in their organization or department. The standards and best practices addressed in this chapter apply to those leaders who are directly and indirectly responsible for the infection prevention and control (IPC) program within their health care organization.

Relevant Joint Commission Standards Addressed in This Chapter

Note: These standards were in effect at the time of publication. They refer to Joint Commission standards effective January 1, 2021. Always consult the most recent version of Joint Commission standards for the most accurate requirements for your setting.

LD.01.02.01 The [organization] identifies the responsibilities of its leaders.

EP 1 Senior managers and leaders of the organized medical staff work with the governing body to define their shared and unique responsibilities and accountabilities. (*See also* NR.01.01.01, EP 3)

LD.01.03.01 The governing body is ultimately accountable for the safety and quality of care, treatment, and services.

LD.02.01.01 The mission, vision, and goals of the [organization] support the safety and quality of care, treatment, and services.

LD.03.01.01 Leaders create and maintain a culture of safety and quality throughout the [organization].

LD.03.02.01 The [organization] uses data and information to guide decisions and to understand variation in the performance of processes supporting safety and quality.

(continued)

(continued)

EP 1 Leaders set expectations for using data and information for improving the safety and quality of care, treatment, or services, decision making that supports the safety and quality of care, treatment, and services, and identifying and responding to internal and external changes in the environment.

EP 2 Leaders evaluate how effectively data and information are used throughout the [organization].

LD.03.03.01 Leaders use [organizationwide] planning to establish structures and processes that focus on safety and quality.

EP 1 Planning activities focus on improving patient safety and health care quality and adapting to changes in the environment.

EP 2 Planning is [organizationwide], systematic, and involves designated individuals and information sources.

EP 3 Leaders evaluate the effectiveness of planning activities.

LD.03.04.01 The [organization] communicates information related to safety and quality to those who need it, including staff, licensed independent practitioners, [patients], families, and external interested parties

EP 1 Communication processes are effective in fostering the safety of the patient and his or her quality of care, supporting safety and quality throughout the [organization], meeting the needs of internal and external users, and informing those who work in the [organization] of changes in the environment.

EP 2 Leaders evaluate the effectiveness of communication methods.

LD.03.05.01 Leaders manage change to improve the performance of the [organization].

EP 1 The [organization] has a systematic approach to change and performance improvement.

EP 2 Structures for managing change and performance improvement foster the safety of the patient and the quality of care, treatment, and services, support both safety and quality throughout the [organization] and adapt to changes in the environment.

EP 3 Leaders evaluate the effectiveness of processes for the management of change and performance improvement. (*See also* PI.02.01.01, EP 13)

LD.03.06.01 Those who work in the [organization] are focused on improving safety and quality.

EP 2 Leaders provide for a sufficient number and mix of individuals to support safe, quality care, treatment, and services. (*See also* IC.01.01.01, EP 3)

Note: *The number and mix of individuals is appropriate to the scope and complexity of the services offered.*

EP 3 Those who work in the [organization] are competent to complete their assigned responsibilities

LD.04.01.11 The [organization] makes space and equipment available as needed for the provision of care, treatment, and services.

IC.01.02.01 [Organization] leaders allocate needed resources for the infection prevention and control program.

EP 1 The [organization] provides access to information needed to support the infection prevention and control program. (*See also* IM.02.02.03, EP 2)

EP 2 The [organization] provides laboratory resources when needed to support the infection prevention and control program.

EP 3 The [organization] provides equipment and supplies to support the infection prevention and control program.

Relevant Joint Commission International (JCI) Standards Addressed in This Chapter

Note: These standards were in effect at the time of publication. They refer to the *Joint Commission International Accreditation Standards for Hospitals, seventh edition,* ©2020. Always consult the most recent version of Joint Commission International standards for the most accurate requirements for your hospital or medical center setting.

GLD.1.1 The operational responsibilities and accountabilities of the governing entity are described in a written document(s).

ME 1 The governing entity approves the hospital's strategic plans, operational plans, policies, and procedures, and approves, periodically reviews, and makes public the hospital's mission statement.

ME 2 The governing entity approves the hospital's capital and operating budget(s) and allocates other resources required to meet the hospital's mission.

ME 3 The governing entity approves the hospital's participation in health care professional education and research and in the oversight of the quality of such programs.

ME 4 The governing entity appoints, and annually evaluates, the hospital's chief executive(s), and the evaluation is documented.

GLD.1.2 The governing entity approves the hospital's program for quality and patient safety and regularly receives and acts on reports of the quality and patient safety program.

ME 1 The governing entity annually approves the hospital's program for quality and patient safety.

ME 2 The governing entity at least quarterly receives and acts on reports of the quality and patient safety program, including reports of adverse and sentinel events.

ME 3 Minutes reflect actions taken and any follow-up on those actions.

GLD.4 Hospital leadership plans, develops, and implements a quality improvement and patient safety program.

ME 1 Hospital leadership participates in developing and implementing a hospitalwide quality improvement and patient safety program.

ME 2 Hospital leadership selects and implements a hospitalwide process to measure, assess data, plan change, and sustain improvements in quality and patient safety, and provides for staff education on this quality improvement process.

ME 3 Hospital leadership determines how the program will be directed and managed on a daily basis and ensures that the program has adequate technology and other resources to be effective.

ME 4 Hospital leadership implements a structure and process for the overall monitoring and coordination of the quality improvement and patient safety program.

GLD.4.1 Hospital leadership communicates quality improvement and patient safety information to the governing entity and hospital staff on a regular basis.

ME 1 Hospital leadership reports on the quality and patient safety program at least quarterly to the governing entity.

ME 2 Hospital leadership reports to the governing entity include, at least quarterly, the number and type of sentinel events and root causes, whether the patients and families were informed of the sentinel event, actions taken to improve safety in response to sentinel events, and if the improvements were sustained.

ME 3 Hospital leadership regularly communicates information on the quality improvement and patient safety program to staff, including progress on meeting the International Patient Safety Goals.

(continued)

(continued)

GLD.5 The chief executive and hospital leadership prioritize which hospitalwide processes will be measured, which hospitalwide improvement and patient safety activities will be implemented, and how success of these hospitalwide efforts will be measured.

ME 1 The chief executive and hospital leadership use available data to set collective priorities for hospitalwide measurement and improvement activities and consider potential system improvements.

ME 2 The chief executive and hospital leadership ensure that, when present, clinical research and health professional education programs are represented in the priorities.

ME 3 The chief executive and hospital leadership set priorities for compliance with the International Patient Safety Goals.

ME 4 The chief executive and hospital leadership assess the impact of hospitalwide and departmental/service improvements on efficiency and resource use.

GLD.7 Hospital leadership makes decisions related to the purchase or use of resources—human and technical—with an understanding of the quality and safety implications of those decisions.

ME 1 Hospital leadership uses data and information on the quality and safety implications of medical equipment choices.

ME 2 Hospital leadership uses data and information on the quality and safety implications of staffing choices.

ME 3 Hospital leadership uses the recommendations of professional organizations and other authoritative sources in making resource decisions. (See also PC1.1, ME 3)

Note. *The number and mix of individuals is appropriate to the scope and complexity of the services offered.*

ME 6 Hospital leadership monitors the results of its decisions and uses the data to evaluate and improve the quality of its resource purchasing and allocation decisions.

PCI.3 Hospital leadership provides resources to support the infection prevention and control program.

ME 1 The infection prevention and control program is staffed according to the hospital's size, complexity of activities, and level of risks, as well as the program's scope.

ME 2 Hospital leadership approves and assigns staff required for the infection prevention and control program.

ME 3 Hospital leadership approves and allocates resources required for the infection prevention and control program.

ME 4 Information management systems support the infection prevention and control program. (See also MOI.1)

Within a health care organization, leaders should be knowledgeable of the IPC program and committed to its success to ensure that it is effective and contributes to an environment and culture of patient safety. This is necessary regardless of the setting in which health care is delivered. For an IPC program to be successful, leadership should be engaged in IPC activities.

To identify the characteristics of an engaged leader, Saint et al. conducted a series of 86 phone and in-person interviews with hospital leaders.[2] They found that engaged, successful leaders do the following:

- Cultivate a culture of clinical excellence and effectively communicate it to staff.
- Focus on overcoming barriers and dealing directly with resistant staff or process issues that impede prevention of health care–associated infection (HAI).
- Inspire their employees.
- Think strategically while acting locally. Examples of this include the following:
  - Campaigning for support before crucial committee votes
  - Leveraging personal prestige to move initiatives forward
  - Forming partnerships across disciplines

Another study by Knobloch et al., examined the effect of executive leadership rounds on HAIs at a large academic hospital. The researchers found that when top-level leadership engages with frontline staff in a way that acknowledges fallibility and models curiosity, staff members disclosed unit-specific problems and readily engaged in problem solving. Interactions with these leaders not only helped to foster a learning climate and increase psychologic safety but also played a role in reducing the rates of HAI within the organization.[3]

Health care organizations should have an organizationwide culture of safety. Regardless of the type of health care setting or where IPC programs reside, infection preventionists (IPs) should have authority delegated to them from the organization's leaders to perform essential activities and implement change to prevent HAIs.[4]

Leadership's Influence on IPC Performance

Although many senior leaders within hospital programs and health care systems are not directly involved in the day-to-day operations of an IPC program, their decisions and priorities may affect the program and outcomes of care. The actions of leadership have a direct and critical impact on the performance of the IPC program. Thus, it is essential that leadership approve the annual infection prevention plan and support its implementation strategies.

A comprehensive and effective IPC program is a critical component of a safety- and quality-based culture. The Joint Commission has identified the following key systems that influence an organization's performance with regard to establishing and supporting a culture of safety and quality[6]: (See Figure 2-1 on page 38.)

- Using data
- Planning
- Communicating
- Changing performance
- Staffing

These five key systems serve as pillars, rooted in the foundation set by leadership and supporting the many organizationwide processes, such as IPC, that contribute to the quality of patient care, treatment, and services. These systems are interrelated and need to work together to support safe, high-quality care. Permeating this entire structure is the culture of the organization. The effective performance of these systems results in a culture in which safety and quality are priorities.

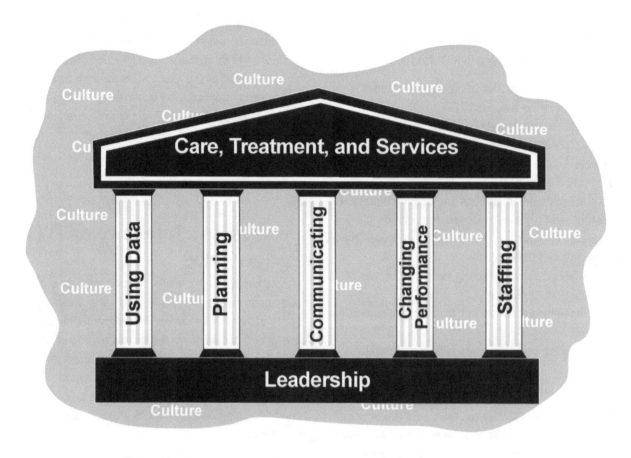

Figure 2-1. The Five Pillars of Effective Performance

Care, Treatment, and Services

Using Data

Planning

Communicating

Changing Performance

Staffing

Leadership

Culture

Source: The Joint Commission. *2020 Comprehensive Accreditation Manual for Hospitals.* Oak Brook, IL: Joint Commission Resources, 2020.

Although The Joint Commission's Leadership (LD) and Joint Commission International's (JCI's) Governance, Leadership, and Direction (GLD) standards are separate from the Infection Prevention and Control (IPC) and Prevention and Control of Infection (PCI) standards, respectively, requirements for leadership affect the entire organization, including the IPC program. It's as important for IPs to understand the role of leaders as it is for leaders to understand the work of IPs. Additionally, IPs in Joint Commission–accredited organizations should recognize their own role as leaders within the organization and how these standards can be exemplified in their work.[7] Although this chapter addresses leadership requirements relevant to the IPC program, the reader is encouraged to carefully review the entire "Leadership" (LD) chapter of The Joint Commission's *Comprehensive Accreditation Manual* for domestic organizations. For organizations outside the US, readers are encouraged to read the JCI "Governance, Leadership, and Direction" (GLD) chapter and consider how the standards relate to the IPC program in their setting.

> **TIP** **Engage leadership:** Although many executive leaders will not be directly involved in the day-to-day operations of an IPC program, the decisions they make and the initiatives they implement will affect the program and outcomes of care.

Responsibility and Accountability

In many health care organizations—particularly in hospitals—leadership is composed of three groups: the governing body, executive leadership, and medical staff leadership. It is critical that these leadership roles and responsibilities be clearly identified by the health care organization. There also should be a pathway for infection prevention to report up through the organizational chart to the chief executive, chief nurse, and chief of medical staff to ensure that IPC issues are addressed within the organization's quality and performance improvement and patient safety programs. One way to comply with this requirement is by ensuring that IPC goals are evaluated by senior leaders at least annually or when risks change and that the IPC plan is revised accordingly.

For Joint Commission–accredited hospitals, the governing body is ultimately accountable for the safety and quality of care, treatment, and services. Szekendi et al. have identified six domains of effective governance as drivers of safety and quality of care. Two of these domains directly impact IPC[8]:

1. Carefully establish and closely monitor hospital performance measures and goals through regular review of data, reports, and dashboards.
2. Intentionally create a culture that nurtures engagement, mutual trust, willingness to act, and high standards of performance.

An organization may demonstrate accountability compliance, for example, by ensuring the governing body regularly reviews HAI reports provided by the IPC program and, based on these reviews, takes the necessary decisive actions to direct and provide the internal structures and resources needed—including staff—to prevent and control HAIs. Another way for governing bodies to demonstrate compliance is to proactively invest in programs to keep patients safe from antibiotic-resistant organisms and emerging and reemerging infectious diseases.

For example, dedicating resources to preparedness efforts for high-consequence infectious disease (HCID), such as Middle East Respiratory Syndrome (MERS), Severe Acute Respiratory Syndrome (SARS), measles, Ebola virus disease (EVD), and coronavirus disease 2019 (SARS-CoV-2/COVID-19), involves standardizing a plan to include protocols for donning and doffing personal protective equipment (PPE), pertinent flow sheets and checklists, an appropriate emergency PPE cache, a defined HCID patient care area, and relevant staff education.[9]

Mission, Vision, and Goals

The organization's mission statement defines its purpose or reason for existence. Vision statements reflect the ideal image of the organization in the future and create a focal point for strategic planning. Some vision statements are bound to a specific time frame and serve to guide organizational performance to achieve desired goals. For example, most IPs are familiar with the Association for Professionals in Infection Control and Epidemiology's (APIC's) mission to "Create a safer world through prevention of infection" and its vision of "health-care without infection." This vision statement provided the focal point for APIC's strategic plan through 2020.[10] The mission and vision statements of The Joint Commission, Joint Commission Resources, and Joint Commission International—of which IPC is an unnamed subset—are not tied to specific time frames but emphasize continuous and ongoing improvements in safe, quality care. See Sidebar 2-1 for these mission statements.

Similarly, a health care organization's mission, vision, and goals guide how the organization will achieve safety and quality of care, treatment, and services—including IPC. Therefore, the IPC program's mission, vision, and goals should support those of the organization. Because the organization's goals are focused on achieving the best outcomes for all patients and residents, regardless of the setting in which care is delivered, it is important that the organization's leaders review and approve the IPC plan annually and support the IPC program's goals, objectives, and strategies for preventing HAIs. (For more information on developing goals and objectives, see Chapter 3, and for identifying specific prevention strategies, see Chapter 6.) Achieving the organization's goals requires active engagement of the governing body, executive leadership, and frontline clinicians, as well as patients and their families. Studies demonstrate that leadership support is essential to sustainable IPC practices and safe health care delivery.[11] One way an organization can demonstrate compliance with this standard is by providing evidence that organizational leaders support and promote IPC program initiatives, such as empowering patients and family members through surveys and outreach to ask, speak up, and be proactive in HAI prevention.[12]

Creating and Maintaining a Culture of Safety and Quality

The individual and aggregate beliefs, attitudes, and values of leaders and staff create the culture within an

Sidebar 2-1.
The Joint Commission Mission Statements

The mission of The Joint Commission is to continuously improve health care for the public, in collaboration with other stakeholders, by evaluating health care organizations and inspiring them to excel in providing safe and effective care of the highest quality and value. Its vision is that all people always experience the safest, highest quality, best-value health care across all settings.

Joint Commission Resources Mission

The mission of Joint Commission Resources is to continuously improve the safety and quality of health care in the United States and in the international community through the provision of education, publications, consultation, and evaluation services.

Joint Commission International

The mission of Joint Commission International is to continuously improve the safety and quality of care in the international community through education, advisory services, and international accreditation and certification.

organization and influence how effectively the organization performs. This extends to the IPC program. One of the hallmarks of a culture of safety is that all persons wish to achieve and maintain excellence and to eliminate harm to patients and staff. Personal responsibility for compliance with safe practices, such as hand hygiene and isolation precautions, is accepted and widespread. For IPC programs, this is essential to minimize infection risks and prevent infections.

Leaders can influence the culture of an organization by showing support for the IPC program. As previously mentioned in this chapter, support can be exemplified by being present and engaged in improvement efforts. For example, at one health system, an interdisciplinary clinical community that also included senior leaders was

formed to conduct a risk assessment and improve endoscopy reprocessing practices across the health system.[13] The collective effort resulted in systemwide policies and procedures and the creation of mechanisms for oversight of competency, certification, and recertification of frontline staff who perform this critical function.

In another example, nurses in a level IV neonatal intensive care unit (NICU)—with administrator and IPC program support—successfully led a quality improvement initiative to reduce central line–associated bloodstream infection (CLABSI).[14] Similarly, personnel in some nursing care centers use a team approach to prevent catheter-associated urinary tract infection (CAUTI) by joining the US Agency for Healthcare Research and Quality (AHRQ) Safety Program for Long-Term Care: HAIs/CAUTI.[15] This program focuses on reducing CAUTIs and other HAIs in nursing care centers. It promotes evidence-based methods for preventing CAUTIs and ways to incorporate these methods into a facility's regular procedures so that safety becomes the norm.

Joint Commission- and JCI-accredited organizations may demonstrate compliance with the requirement for creating and maintaining a culture of safety when leaders model safe practices and insist on teamwork and accountability to reduce the risk of adverse events, such as HAIs. IPs can support this philosophy by working with teams of caregivers to enhance best practices, such as those described in the above examples.

The safety culture promotes systems that target the elimination of HAIs, supports open communication about infections that do occur, and encourages reporting of infection issues. As IPs work collaboratively with staff or lead the implementation of performance improvement initiatives, they should note that improving care processes involves looking at system breakdowns and not blaming individuals when infections occur. To help assess your organization's culture of safety, download Tool 2-1.

TRY THIS TOOL

Tool 2-1. Organizational Assessment for Safety Culture

Using Data to Guide Informed Decisions That Support Safety and Quality

Health care organization leaders must develop the ability to deal with competing priorities. To make informed decisions, leaders should have valid and reliable data about local and national trends, clinical processes, and outcomes, as well as financial performance. They should set the expectation that data are integral to managing care and should provide the resources to obtain, analyze, and use information to maintain best practices and achieve change when necessary.

Leaders often need financial data to make decisions about overall patient care and staff safety. They may request that IPs make a business case with return on investment (ROI) for a new procedure, supplies, or equipment, or infrastructure changes.[16-18] For information on making a business case for infection prevention, see Sidebar 2-2, below, and download Tool 2-2.

TRY THIS TOOL

Tool 2-2. Steps in Developing a Business Case for HAI Prevention

An organization's leaders may not always understand the extent of the financial and personal burden of HAIs or the cost-effectiveness of IPC programs. Infection preventionists should seize every opportunity to increase leaders' understanding of the impact of HAIs as well as the current state of HAI prevention.

Sidebar 2-2. Making the Business Case for Infection Prevention and Control

An infection prevention and control (IPC) program may use limited and competing resources and requires ongoing financial commitment from the organization. Leaders often need financial data to factor IPC programs into overall patient care and staff safety investment decisions. Therefore, it is good practice for infection preventionists (IPs) to know how to develop and present an accurate, persuasive business case when seeking additional resources (for example, personnel, physical resources, or financial resources).[16]

The business case format is an important tool that provides a framework for such financial data. IPs should be trained and well positioned to create an accurate, compelling IPC business case. Proposed IPC initiatives should be expressed not only in terms of quality improvement and patient safety but also in terms of financial impact, including costs, benefits, and return on investment.[16,17] The business case should be discussed with the financial officer to ensure it is consistent with the organization's financial business plans. According to Perencevich and colleagues, a business case analysis includes the following steps[16]:

- Frame the problem and develop a hypothesis about potential solutions.
- Meet with key administrators to obtain support and identify critical costs and factors that should be included in the analysis.
- Determine the annual cost.
- Determine what costs can be avoided through reduced infection rates.
- Determine the costs associated with the infections of interest at your hospital or health care facility.
- Calculate the financial impact.
- Include the additional financial or health benefits.
- Make the case for your business case.
- Prospectively collect cost and outcome data after the program is in effect.

IPs may partner with their department of finance colleagues to determine financial returns from organizational improvement in health care–associated infections.

For example, leaders should be made aware that during the past decade, federally sponsored programs have made considerable progress in preventing some HAIs that threaten patients and that ongoing investment in comprehensive IPC programs can reduce HAIs, minimize the spread of multidrug-resistant organisms (MDROs), and address emerging pathogens (such as SARS-CoV-2), ultimately keeping patients safe.[4,19,20]

Because infection prevention resources in areas of high COVID-19 activity have had to shift to outbreak management during the pandemic, many leaders may be thinking about IPC investments differently moving forward. And while it may be too soon to know the full effect of COVID-19 on traditional HAI prevention efforts, there may be a paradigm shift in investments in IPC resources, as discussed in Sidebar 2-3.

In their organizations, IPs may demonstrate how the use of evidence-based interventions, such as care bundles and evidence-based guidelines, have reduced HAIs in a variety of health care settings. A good practice is to include an explicit section in the IPC annual report or annual evaluation to communicate changes in workloads, roles, and responsibilities and how such changes affect the overall program. For more information on data needs of an IPC program, see Sidebar 2-4 on page 42.

TIP Leaders should set the expectation that data are integral to managing care and should provide the resources to obtain, analyze, and use information to maintain best practices and achieve change when necessary.

Sidebar 2-3. Investing in HAI Prevention During a Pandemic and Beyond

Since the global COVID-19 pandemic began, infection prevention and control (IPC) resources in many health care systems, particularly in areas of high COVID-19 activity, have seen a shift away from traditional surveillance and prevention activities toward outbreak management. According to an article that appeared in *Infection Control & Hospital Epidemiology*, when the pandemic began in 2020, infection prevention and hospital epidemiology staff were asked what percentage of their time typically dedicated to infection prevention efforts had been diverted to COVID-19 response efforts. Of the respondents, 79.1% reported that greater than 75% of their time was diverted to COVID-19 response efforts. Although managing outbreaks is an understandable priority, the article also suggested that the effect of this diversion of staff away from traditional health care—associated infection (HAI) monitoring is concerning, with potential for adverse effects, such as the following:

- Reduced HAI case identification and data collection related to HAIs
- Fewer staff for process measure data collection, such as compliance with hand hygiene
- Increased rates of *Clostridium difficile* infections due to increased use of antibiotics to treat secondary bacterial infections, which affects antimicrobial stewardship efforts

The full impact of COVID-19 on traditional HAI prevention efforts remains to be seen, but leadership in health systems are encouraged to find creative ways to support their IPC programs even during a pandemic by expanding their IPC workforce with trained infection preventionists and epidemiologists at local, regional, national, and international levels.

Source: Stevens MP, et al. Impact of COVID-19 on traditional healthcare-associated infection prevention efforts. *Infect Control Hosp Epidemiol.* 2020; Aug;4(8):946–947.

Sidebar 2-4. Data and Information Needs of the Infection Prevention and Control Program

Surveillance (case finding), data collection, analysis, and reporting are critical components of a successful infection prevention and control (IPC) program. According to a study by Bartles et al., most infection preventionists (IPs) spend more than half of their working hours conducting surveillance activities.[21] It is important for leaders to support the informatics systems and networks for data collection and analysis that are increasingly critical elements of an IPC program infrastructure.

To better serve the organization and to receive accurate and timely data, leaders should evaluate and enhance the use of information technology and health informatics within the IPC program. To improve the use of such technology and to meet Joint Commission and Joint Commission International requirements, IPs should request that their organization's leaders provide the following to the IPC program staff[4,22]:

Computer workstation and internal network connectivity. These are essential for access to data needed for surveillance of health care–associated infections (HAIs), such as information on a patient's or resident's treatment, diagnostic test results, and therapy provided. Access requires connectivity to patient, pharmacy, and laboratory information systems; imaging studies; and admission/discharge/transfer information. Electronic health records (EHRs) have the potential to support IPC surveillance activities. Through the use of EHRs and an electronic surveillance program, IPs are more efficient and accurate when assessing the impact of interventions, performing algorithmic identification of HAIs, and performing syndromic surveillance related to public health concerns and identification of surgical site infections.[4,23] IPs should be involved in and provide guidance for organizational purchasing decisions related to infection surveillance systems.

Online library of resources. This is essential to allow access to infection surveillance, prevention, and control information, including guidelines, standards, best practices, online textbooks and journals, and regulatory requirements, and it is important to be able to conduct literature searches.

Computer program applications. Equally important is access to computer software applications for spreadsheet development and creation of educational materials as well as training to optimize use.

Access to computer-based systems for mandatory reporting programs and comparative databases for performance improvement. Organization leaders should support their IPC program's enrollment and use of reporting systems to submit data to federal, state, and local agencies for mandatory reporting requirements. One such reporting system is the US Centers for Disease Control and Prevention's (CDC's) National Healthcare Safety Network (NHSN). The NHSN is a secure, Internet-based application that facilitates use of HAI surveillance definitions and methods, provides a national platform for estimating magnitude and trends of HAIs, offers risk-adjusted data for intra- and interfacility comparison, and serves as a collaborative performance improvement network.[24] The US Centers for Medicare & Medicaid Services—and many states—require use of the NHSN for mandatory reporting programs.[4] Other surveillance programs that use clinical document architecture standards issued by the CDC and commercial programs can be used for meeting IPC program needs and public reporting requirements.

Secure communications networks. Electronic communication networks that use e-mail, rich site summary (RSS), social media, and other systems to distribute information and electronic alerts from professional organizations, public health agencies, and other government agencies provide an IP and an organization's leaders with up-to-date information on applicable standards, guidelines, regulations, outbreaks, product recalls, emerging infectious diseases, and other events that affect patients, personnel, and the community.

Planning Structures That Support Safety and Quality

Organizationwide planning is essential to support the functions of the IPC program. With regard to the IPC program, accredited organizations may demonstrate compliance when there is evidence that leaders have included the IPC team in the planning of quality improvement and patient safety activities and goals. An IP should secure a seat at the executive planning table as part of the interprofessional team. In this role, the IP can provide pertinent information about local, regional, national, and global trends in IPC, emerging and reemerging pathogens and diseases, new regulations, infectious diseases in community populations, and other issues that affect patient care and safety.

Leadership should understand that IPs play a critical role in providing information that can guide planning activities needed to respond to changes in the environment, such as a potential influx of patients and shortages of resources and assets, such as staff, PPE, ventilators, and airborne infection isolation rooms due to a pandemic, such as COVID-19, for example. The COVID-19 pandemic has persisted for more than a year, and its adverse effects have the potential to linger for some time. The expertise of the IP is more critical today and will continue to be necessary in the future, both to deal with the aftermath of the pandemic and to navigate the challenges that lie ahead.

Responding to Changes in the Environment

During the past decade, IPC programs have been presented with an unending series of challenges that have resulted from changes in the environment. The first such challenge was the 2014–2015 Ebola crisis, which brought to light that IPC programs are generally under-resourced and have limited infection surge capacity. This was made even more clear with the current COVID-19 pandemic.

APIC surveys illustrate this.[25] In 2014, APIC conducted a survey of IPs who practice in acute care hospitals to assess member attitudes about preparedness for EVD and other lethal infectious diseases. One year later, a second survey was conducted, and results were compared. Findings indicated that 9 in 10 hospital-based APIC members believed their facilities were better prepared in 2015 than in 2014 to receive a patient with a highly infectious and deadly disease like Ebola, but more than half (55%) said their facilities had not provided

additional resources to support their IPC programs as a result of the Ebola crisis.[25] There remains much to learn from the ongoing global COVID-19 pandemic, but IPs and epidemiologists should develop their influence skills to persuade organizational decision makers to invest in IPC programs that not only ensure that the organization has the critical resources to prevent and manage infections on a daily basis but also that it is prepared to respond to the inevitable, but unpredictable, appearance of emerging and reemerging infectious diseases. (See Chapter 5 for more information on this topic.)

Communicating Safety and Quality Information

In the context of IPC, leaders should ensure that systems are in place to allow IPs to communicate information about infection issues, processes, and outcomes to those who need it. These communications should be available to staff, patients, visitors, and volunteers throughout the organization in a timely and understandable fashion. For example, internal communication for staff may include real-time notification of infection events, periodic feedback on performance measures, and dashboards that show organizational and unit-level performance.

In addition, communication efforts should include mechanisms for the IPC program to successfully and easily communicate with external groups that collect infection-related data, statistics, and events, such as the state and local health department (for reportable infections) and/or quality improvement agencies (for HAI reporting requirements).

Implementing Change to Improve Safety, Quality, and Performance

Creating change, improving performance, and sustaining improvement are more likely to be successful with strong leadership commitment, role modeling, and a proactive, systematic, and collaborative approach. Leaders should provide adequate resources for performance improvement teams and allot sufficient time for projects to ensure effective, sustained improvement. A strong, visible emphasis on the culture of safety throughout an organization will provide a foundation for adherence to effective prevention practices and continuous performance improvement.

The World Health Organization (WHO) emphasizes the importance of a multidisciplinary team approach to improving IPC practices and preventing HAIs.[26] In this context, organizational change agents should include a wide range of disciplines, including affiliated physicians. McAlearney et al. found that the presence of local clinical champions is a key contributing factor to HAI prevention efforts, with champions playing important roles as coordinators, cheerleaders, and advocates for initiatives.[27] Saint et al. published findings from a mixed-method, representative nationwide survey of hospitals' adoption of evidence-based IPC interventions, in which clinical champions—particularly those representing nursing and physicians—were found to be effective agents for change in practices that improve performance.[28] Boev and Xia examined nurse–physician collaboration in adult intensive care units and found collaboration significantly related to decreased rates of CLABSI and ventilator-associated infections.[29] The converse was also identified.

There are both personnel and organizational attributes that inhibit adoption of new evidence-based practices or changes in work practices.[30] (*See* Tool 2-3 for ways to involve physician champions in the IPC program.)

TRY THIS TOOL

Tool 2-3. Strategies for Engaging Clinicians in IPC Activities

---

Leaders have a responsibility not only to adequately staff the patient care team and the support groups to provide the highest quality of care but also to provide time for staff to focus on performance activities. Although a thorough discussion of this topic is beyond the scope of this chapter, some studies have shown a relationship between understaffing and the occurrence of HAIs. Specifically, studies have linked compromised nurse-staffing effectiveness, the skill mix of supplementary staffing, and breakdowns in culture of safety and work assignments with increased risk of HAIs and other adverse outcomes affecting patient safety.[31,32] The need to provide sufficient staff competent to manage the IPC program is discussed in detail in Chapter 1.

The Infection Preventionist as Leader

IPs have unprecedented opportunities to influence the care of patients, in a very broad context, at every level of the health care system. To do so, they should work with and through others, guiding, directing, encouraging, and inspiring individuals and groups toward the achievement of the common goal of HAI prevention.

These critical individuals control needed resources, possess required information, set priorities on important activities, and have to agree and cooperate if IPC initiatives are to be implemented and sustained.

In other words, the success of the IP and the IPC program depends on the support of others over whom the IP may have little or no direct authority—making it critical to build influence and to leverage strategic relationships at all levels in the organization. Remember: It is not just *what* you know but *who* you know. Social ties across hierarchal positions also enhance influence—the ability to indirectly affect the actions and thoughts of others.

The 2019 APIC Core Competency Model,[33] discussed in Chapter 1, notes that the IP's leadership, which often is based on influence rather than authority, is a consequence of skills in the following key areas:

Communication
Communication (verbal and written) may be the most critical element of successful organizational leadership. Effective communication requires both emotional intelligence and situational awareness, including awareness of the audience's informational needs, cultural background, and knowledge of the subject. Being concise, accurate, and timely in communicating critical information is a skill taught in conjunction with the science of safety and a much-needed competency for IPs. Understanding barriers to effective communication is just as important as the ability to communicate well. Careful audience assessment, active listening, and calibration of the message are important strategies for reducing barriers to effective transfer of information. The art of influence and persuasion is also directly linked to communication competencies.

Critical Thinking
Critical thinking entails the use of all available information to find creative solutions to a problem or situation by applying knowledge, prior experience, data, and evidence.

Critical thinking also means frequently questioning the status quo in regard to existing processes, policies, or procedures that may no longer reflect best practices. Key skills for this subdomain include recognizing that a problem exists, developing potential solutions, applying the best solution, and examining the results. At times, there may be more than one problem that requires attention, so the ability to prioritize how to proceed is important as well.

Collaboration

As team members, facilitators, or leaders of multidisciplinary improvement efforts, infection preventionists serve as champion for a safety culture in which prevention and control of HAIs is everyone's responsibility. Managing competing agendas and priorities, while encouraging integration of IPC activities into the work of every department, takes a skilled negotiator. Additionally, effective teams need leaders, and, in turn, these leaders need followers. IPs serve a supportive (follower) role when interdisciplinary teams are formed to prevent and control HAIs. This followership role allows the IP to provide expertise and exert influence in the absence of direct or traditional authority.

Behavioral Science

Most IPC interventions involve behavior change, which requires collaboration, engagement, and communication across different disciplines and hierarchical boundaries. To effectively facilitate behavioral change and develop education and training programs, IPs should be familiar with the concepts of behavioral science theory, such as socio-adaptive strategies. By employing socio-adaptive strategies in addition to relationship management skills, IPs can build the relationships necessary to sustain the efforts of the program. Socio-adaptive strategies focus on improving culture, staff engagement, and communication. According to the AHRQ Comprehensive Unit-based Safety Program, when socio-adaptive strategies are paired with technical ones, quality improvement projects are more sustainable and have greater impact.[34]

Program Management

To have an effective IPC program, IPs need to have not only technical expertise but also the ability to manage budgets, resources, and personnel. IP managers should also build their programs to be nimble and flexible to accommodate changes in order to meet outcomes and achieve established goals. Additionally, by demonstrating

management and leadership skills such as forecasting, strategic planning, analyzing scenarios, and building consensus, IPs can increase their credibility. They will more likely be included when their expertise is required for key decision making. These skills will also equip IPs to advocate for resources and make a business case for their programs to organization leaders and stakeholders.

Mentorship

Mentors can impart infection prevention knowledge to mentees by sharing personal professional experiences. This can help the mentee translate concepts and guidelines into practice. Being intentional about mentoring can also help to improve staff retention and increase professional satisfaction. Mentorship is critical not only to sustain an organization's IPC program by investing in staff and thus reducing turnover but also to build and develop the future IPC workforce as a whole.

Organizational Leaders Provide Resources to Support the IPC Program

Joint Commission and JCI standards require organizations to allocate resources and provide access to information needed to support IPC efforts. These requirements address resource allocation in general, whereas Standards IC.01.02.01 and PCI.3 discuss resource allocation specifically as it relates to IPC. (See Chapter 1 for discussion of personnel resources related to the IPC program.) The resources allocated to services provided by the organization have a direct effect on patient outcomes. Leaders should place highest priority on high-risk or problem-prone processes that can affect patient safety. A well-known IPC high-risk process is the cleaning, disinfection, and sterilization of medical equipment and devices. Adequate space designated specifically for medical device and instrument processing is essential to control quality and ensure safety.

In outpatient care, inadequate space for instrument processing is among the most frequent problems encountered.[35] For example, endoscope reprocessing is a high-risk process consisting of multiple complex steps. Organizational leaders should provide adequate space and equipment to ensure safe, standardized endoscope reprocessing and storage.[13,35] These issues and the IP's role as it relates to cleaning, disinfection, and sterilization of medical equipment are discussed more thoroughly in Chapter 8.

One of the elements of performance (EPs) for Standard IC.01.02.01 and a measurable element (ME) for PCI.3 requires the IP to have access to laboratory resources to perform their responsibilities. Access may be accomplished by generating and providing the IP with a routine laboratory information system report. The availability of data mining and other information technology tools may also help provide evidence of compliance with these requirements.

Organizations that use reference laboratories should have immediate access to the data necessary not only to diagnose and treat infections but also to allow the IP to put in place prevention and control methods as quickly as possible. Organizations should implement policies with these laboratories to require immediate notification of significant results associated with communicable diseases and epidemiologically significant organisms, such as methicillin-resistant *Staphylococcus aureus* (MRSA) or *C. difficile*.

Smaller facilities, including long term care facilities and nursing care centers, can negotiate these policies as part of the contract with the reference laboratory. Of note, many smaller acute-care and long term care facilities may contract with commercial third-party clinical laboratories. A good practice is for leaders in these facilities to ensure that IPs have full access to laboratory information system reports and periodic analysis of microbiologic data, such as susceptibility profiles, from these third-party laboratories.

Leaders can also demonstrate their support by making available other supplies and equipment needed to sustain an effective IPC program. These may include the following:
- Hand hygiene products
- Personal protective equipment
- Sharps devices with engineered safety features
- Cleaning/disinfection/sterilization products and equipment
- Device trays/kits containing materials to promote aseptic technique
- Vaccines for patients, residents, and personnel

TIP Leaders should ensure that infection preventionists provide input when new or updated laboratory systems are being considered, particularly in microbiology. This will provide an opportunity to shape the data generation and reports that are most helpful to the organization.

Summary

An organization's administrative, patient care, and clinical leadership play an essential role in supporting the activities of the IPC program. Several concepts regarding organization leadership involvement are reviewed in this chapter, including the following:
- Leadership should provide adequate resources to support patient safety and quality in the IPC program. Gaps continue to exist between ideal resource levels for the IPC program and the current state.
- During the past decade, IPC programs have been presented with an unending series of challenges and expectations that have resulted in additional responsibilities, functions, and workload. Organizational leaders and decision makers should provide IPC resources in terms of people, technology, and funding based on these increasing expectations and demands.
- Leadership should ensure that IPC programs have the critical resources to prevent and control infections on a day-to-day basis and be prepared to respond to emerging (and reemerging) infectious diseases.
- Key leadership strategies directly influence IPC practices. Such strategies include promoting a culture of safety and quality, using data and information to make patient care decisions, engaging in organizationwide planning for care, communicating about IPC issues, managing change and performance improvement to prevent and control HAIs, and providing adequate staffing to keep patients safe and to support the IPC program.
- Clinical champions from a variety of disciplines, such as nurses, physicians, and pharmacists, are essential to realizing changes in work practices and improving the culture of safety. Organization leaders can facilitate engagement by identifying these champions and encouraging their support.

Resources

The following sections provide further information on this topic and can serve as valuable references in improving leadership involvement in IPC efforts.

Tools to Try

Tool 2-1. Organizational Assessment for Safety Culture

Tool 2-2. Steps in Developing a Business Case for HAI Prevention

Tool 2-3. Strategies for Engaging Clinicians in IPC Activities

References

1. Maxwell JC. *The 21 Irrefutable Laws of Leadership: Follow Them and People Will Follow You*. New York: HarperCollins Leadership, 2007.

2. Saint S, et al. The importance of leadership in preventing healthcare–associated infection: Results of a multisite qualitative study. *Infect Control Hosp Epidemiol*. 2010 Sep;31(9):901–907.

3. Knobloch M, et al. Leadership rounds to reduce health care–associated infections. *Am J Infect Control*. 2018 Mar;46(3):303–310.

4. Bryant KA, et al. Necessary infrastructure of infection prevention and healthcare epidemiology programs: A review. *Infect Control Hosp Epidemiol*. 2016 Apr;37(4):371–380.

5. Pogorzelska-Maziarz M, Gilmartin H., Reese S. Infection prevention staffing and resources in U.S. acute care hospitals: Results from the APIC MegaSurvey. *Am J Infect Control*. 2018 Aug;46(8):852–857.

6. The Joint Commission. *2020 Comprehensive Accreditation Manual for Hospitals*. Oak Brook, IL: Joint Commission Resources, 2020.

7. Bubb TN, et al. APIC professional and practice standards. *Am J Infect Control*. 2016 Jul;44(7):745–749.

8. Szekendi M, et al. Governance practices and performance in US academic medical centers. *Am J Med Qual*. 2015 Nov–Dec;30(6):520–525.

9. Russo N, et al. Beyond Ebola: Standardizing the approach to high consequence infection preparation. *Am J Infect Control*. 2018 Jun;46(6):S110–S111.

10. Association for Professionals in Infection Control and Epidemiology. Vision and Mission. Accessed Aug 1, 2020. http://www.apic.org/About-APIC/Vision-and-Mission

11. Carrico RM, et al. Infection prevention and control core practices: A roadmap for nursing practice. Nursing. 2018 Aug;48(8):28–29. Gould DJ, Gallagher R, Allen D. Leadership and management for infection prevention and control: What do we have and what do we need? *J Hosp Infect*. 2016;94:165–168.

12. Seale H, et al. Ask, speak up, and be proactive: Empowering patient infection control to prevent health care–acquired infections. *Am J Infect Control*. 2015 May;43(5):447–453.

13. Teter J, et al. Assessment of endoscope reprocessing using peer-to-peer assessment through a clinical community. *Jt Comm J Qual Pat Saf*. 2016 Jun;42(6):265–270.

14. Wilder KA, et al. CLABSI reduction strategy: A systematic central line quality improvement initiative integrating line-rounding principles and a team approach. *Adv Neonatal Care*. 2016 Jun;16(3):170–177.

15. US Agency for Healthcare Research and Quality (AHRQ). Toolkit to Reduce CAUTI and Other HAIs in Long-Term Care Facilities. May 2017. Accessed Apr 12, 2021. http://www.ahrq.gov/professionals/quality-patient-safety/quality-resources/tools/cauti-ltc/index.html

16. Perencevich EN, et al. Raising standards while watching the bottom line: Making a business case for infection control. *Infect Control Hosp Epidemiol*. 2007 Oct;28(10):1121–1133.

17. Swensen SJ, et al. The business case for health-care quality improvement. *J Patient Saf*. 2013 Mar;9(1):44–52.

18. The Joint Commission. Steps in Developing a Business Case Analysis. In CLABSI Toolkit and Monograph—Preventing Central Line–Associated Bloodstream Infections: Useful Tools, an International Perspective. Nov 20, 2013. Accessed Apr 12, 2021. https://www.jointcommission.org/assets/1/6/CLABSI_Toolkit_Tool_6-4_Steps_in_Developing_a_Business_Case_Analysis.pdf

19. US Centers for Disease Control and Prevention. Press Release: Progress Being Made in Infection Control in U.S. Hospitals; Continued Improvements Needed. Jan 14, 2015. Accessed Apr 12, 2021. http://www.cdc.gov/media/releases/2015/p0114-mrsa-hospitals-report.html

20. Dick AW, et al. A decade of investment in infection prevention: A cost-effectiveness analysis. *Am J Infect Control.* 2015 Jan;43(1):4–9.

21. Bartles R, Dickson A., Babade O. A systematic approach to quantifying infection prevention staffing and coverage needs, *Am J Infect Control.* 2018;46:487–491.

22. Scheckler WE, et al. Requirements for infrastructure and essential activities of infection control and epidemiology in hospitals: A consensus panel report. *Am J Infect Control.* 1998 Feb;26(1):47–60.

23. Cato KD, Cohen B, Larson E. Data elements and validation methods used for electronic surveillance of health care–associated infections: A systematic review. *Am J Infect Control.* 2015 Jun;43(6):600–605.

24. US Centers for Disease Control and Prevention: National Healthcare Safety Network (NHSN). (Updated: Apr 1, 2021.) Accessed May 20, 2021. http://www.cdc.gov/nhsn/index.html

25. Association for Professional in Infection Control and Epidemiology. Ebola Preparedness One Year Later: A Poll of APIC Members. 2015. Accessed Sep 30, 2020. http://www.apic.org/Resource_/TinyMceFileManager/Topic-specific/APIC_Ebola_Survey_Results_November_2015.pdf

26. World Health Organization. Improving Infection Prevention and Control at the Health Facility. Accessed Sept 21, 2020. https://www.who.int/infection-prevention/tools/core-components/facility-manual.pdf

27. McAlearney AS, et al. The role of leadership in eliminating health care–associated infections: A qualitative study of eight hospitals. *Adv Health Care Manag.* 2013;14:69–94.

28. Saint S, et al. A multicenter qualitative study on preventing hospital-acquired urinary tract infection in US hospitals. *Infect Control Hosp Epidemiol.* 2008 Apr;29(4):333–341.

29. Boev C, Xia Y. Nurse–physician collaboration and hospital-acquired infections in critical care. *Crit Care Nurs Q.* 2015 Apr;35(2):66–72.

30. Saint S, et al. How active resisters and organizational constipators affect health care–acquired infection prevention efforts. *Jt Comm J Qual Patient Saf.* 2009 May;35(5):239–246.

31. Stone PW, et al. Hospital staffing and health care–associated infections: A systematic review of the literature. *Clin Infect Dis.* 2008 Oct;47(7):937–944.

32. Virtanen M, et al. Work hours, work stress, and collaboration among ward staff in relation to risk of hospital-associated infection among patients. *Med Care.* 2009 Mar;47(3):310–318.

33. Billings C, et al. Advancing the profession: An updated future-oriented competency model for professional development in infection prevention and control. *Am J Infect Control.* 2019 Jun;47(6):602–614.

34. Agency for Healthcare Quality and Research. Comprehensive Unit-based Safety Program. Accessed Dec 10, 2020. https://www.ahrq.gov/hai/cusp/index.html

35. Bringhurst J. Special problems associated with reprocessing instruments in outpatient care facilities. *Am J Infect Control.* 2016 May;44(5 Suppl):e63–e67.

Chapter 3

A Risk-Based Approach to Infection Prevention: Performing the Risk Assessment and Creating the IPC Plan

By Barbara M. Soule, RN, MPA, CIC, FSHEA, FAPIC

Disclaimer: Strategies, tools, and examples discussed in this book do not necessarily reflect Joint Commission or Joint Commission International requirements for all settings. Always refer to the most current standards applicable to your health care setting to ensure compliance.

Introduction

The Joint Commission's "Infection Prevention and Control" (IC) chapter and Joint Commission International's (JCI's) "Prevention and Control of Infection" (PCI) chapter require accredited organizations to evaluate infection risks for the organization and identify, document, and prioritize risks. Accredited organizations must also establish goals and objectives based on these risks and develop an infection prevention and control (IPC) plan to achieve goals and to accomplish the best outcomes for patients and staff. A proactive risk assessment and subsequent risk-reduction strategies are intended to prevent harm before it reaches the patient. Infection preventionists (IPs) have long assessed risk—primarily based on populations served, services provided, surveillance data, outbreaks, and gaps in desired practices. The standards stipulate that assessing risk and setting goals should be a purposeful, proactive, and systematic process used to direct a well-designed, thoughtful, and practical approach to IPC activities. The primary focus of this chapter is risk assessment in acute care settings. Also addressed are other settings such as long term care, ambulatory health care, and the clinical laboratory. See the boxes on the following pages for relevant requirements for domestic and international settings.

Identifying Risks

Infection risks take many forms. Regardless of the health care setting, some infection risks are common to patients or residents (such as device-related infections) or to staff (such as sharps injuries or infection exposure). Other risks are less common but are potentially severe, such as those related to an influx of infectious patients or an emerging infectious disease or pathogen, such as Ebola virus disease (EVD), Middle East Respiratory Syndrome (MERS]), or Novel Coronavirus 2019 (SARS CoV-2/COVID-19). Risks that are shared among many health care organizations, geographic regions, and countries may have similar causes or solutions, but risk assessments and reduction activities must be tailored to each organization's specific populations, geography, and organizational environments and based on the availability of resources and the organization's unique challenges. At any time, risks that seem under control may suddenly change and require new direction for the IPC program, such as in infectious disease outbreaks. Because of the evolving nature of infection risks, they must be assessed periodically and as often as needed. Using a risk-based approach to prevent and control infections is an *ongoing process* that forms the cornerstone for an effective IPC program and safety for health care workers and the community.

The "Leadership" (LD) chapter of the Joint Commission's *Comprehensive Accreditation Manual for Hospitals* for 2021 examines risk assessment at length. Several

Relevant Joint Commission Standards Addressed in This Chapter

Note: These standards were in effect at the time of publication. They refer to Joint Commission standards effective January 1, 2021. Always consult the most recent version of Joint Commission standards for the most accurate requirements for your setting.

IC.01.03.01 The [organization] identifies risk for acquiring and transmitting infections.

EP 1 The [organization] identifies risks for acquiring and transmitting infections based on the following:

- Its geographic location, community, and population served
- The care, treatment, and services it provides
- The analysis of surveillance activities and other infection control data (*See also* IC.02.05.01, EP 2)

EP 2 The [organization] reviews and identifies its risks at least annually and whenever significant changes occur with input from, at a minimum, infection control staff, medical staff, nursing, and leadership. (*See also* IC.02.05.01, EP 2)

EP 3 The [organization] prioritizes the identified risks for acquiring and transmitting infections. These prioritized risks are documented. (*See also* IC.02.05.01, EP 2)

IC.01.04.01 Based on the identified risks, the [organization] sets goals to minimize the possibility of transmitting infections. **Note:** See NPSG.07.01.01 for hand hygiene guidelines.

EP 1 The [organization's] written infection prevention and control goals include the following:
- Addressing its prioritized risks
- Limiting unprotected exposure to pathogens

- Limiting the transmission of infections associated with procedures
- Limiting the transmission of infections associated with the use of medical equipment, devices, and supplies
- Improving compliance with hand hygiene guidelines (*See also* NPSG.07.01.01, EP 1)

IC.01.05.01 The [organization] has an infection prevention and control plan.

EP 1 When developing infection prevention and control activities, the [organization] uses evidence-based national guidelines or, in the absence of such guidelines, expert consensus.

EP 2 The [organization's] infection prevention and control plan includes a written description of the activities, including surveillance, to minimize, reduce, or eliminate the risk of infection.

"Leadership" (LD) chapter: Proactive Risk Assessment

NPSG.07.01.01 Comply with either the current Centers for Disease Control and Prevention (CDC) hand hygiene guidelines and/or the current World Health Organization (WHO) hand hygiene guidelines.

Relevant Joint Commission International (JCI) Standards Addressed in This Chapter

Note: These standards were in effect at the time of publication. They refer to the *Joint Commission International Accreditation Standards for Hospitals, seventh edition,* ©2020. Always consult the most recent version of Joint Commission International standards for the most accurate requirements for your hospital or medical center setting.

PCI.4. The hospital designs and implements a comprehensive infection prevention and control program that identifies the procedures and processes associated with the risk of infection and implements strategies to reduce infection risk.

ME 1 The infection prevention and control program is comprehensive and crosses all levels of the hospital, to reduce the risk of health care–associated infections in patients.

ME 2 The infection prevention and control program is comprehensive and crosses all levels of the hospital to reduce the risk of health care–associated infections in hospital staff.

ME 3 The hospital identifies those processes associated with infection risk.

ME 4 The hospital implements strategies, education, and evidence-based activities to reduce infection risk in those processes.

PCI.5 The hospital uses a risk-based data-driven approach in establishing the focus of the health care–associated infection prevention and control program.

ME 1 The hospital establishes the focus of the program through the collection and tracking of data related to respiratory tract, urinary tract, intravascular invasive devices, surgical sites, epidemiologically significant diseases and organisms, and emerging or reemerging infections with the community.

ME 2 The data collected in respiratory tract, urinary tract, intravascular invasive devices, surgical sites,

epidemiologically significant diseases and organisms, and emerging or reemerging infections with the community are analyzed to identify priorities for reducing rates of infection.

PCI.5.1 The hospital identifies areas at high risk for infections by conducting a risk assessment, develops interventions to address these risks, and monitors the effectiveness.

ME 1 The hospital completes and documents a risk assessment, at least annually, to identify and prioritize areas at high risk for infections.

ME 2 The hospital identifies and implements interventions to address infection risks identified through the risk assessment.

IPSG.5 The hospital adopts and implements evidence-based hand-hygiene guidelines to reduce the risk of health care–associated infections.

ME 1 The hospital has adopted current evidence-based hand-hygiene guidelines.

ME 2 The hospital implements a hand-hygiene program throughout the hospital.

ME 3 Hand-washing and hand-disinfection procedures are used in accordance with hand-hygiene guidelines throughout the hospital.

QPS.10 An ongoing program of risk management is used to identify and to proactively reduce unanticipated adverse events and other safety risks to patients and staff.

chapters of the *Joint Commission International Accreditation (JCIA) Standards for Hospitals, Seventh Edition, 2021 (for example,* "Quality and Patient Systems") lay out considerations for risk assessment. These discussions note that by undertaking a proactive risk assessment, an organization can evaluate processes to see how they could fail, evaluate the failures, and identify how to improve them, thereby reducing the likelihood of adverse events. The term *process* applies widely to include clinical procedures such as surgery, isolation, support services, management of specific pathogens, and policies and procedures for the environment. These standards require that those risks with the greatest potential for harming patients, such as sentinel events or high-risk procedures, should be the focus of the risk assessment. In addition, a proactive risk assessment helps to increase understanding and knowledge within the organization about how a process might fail and the potential consequences of that failure. The goal of the risk assessment is to use this knowledge to improve care and to safely minimize or eliminate current and future negative outcomes.

The risk assessment process should be a thoughtful, systematic, proactive examination of infection hazards in the health care environment that could cause harm to patients, staff, families and visitors, or the facility. It should address the types of information an organization must consider when identifying risks for acquiring and transmitting infections. Organizations should assess their risk for acquiring and transmitting infection based on their geographic location, the community environment, and the characteristics and behaviors of the population served.

IPs can best understand their organization's geographic and community environment by staying in contact with state and local public health services. The public health service monitors the effects of geographic and community issues on health and illness. One way to stay in touch is to register for e-mail alerts sent by the health department to health care providers and organizations, which provide information about community illnesses and trends such as tuberculosis in the homeless population, the occurrence of seasonal influenza, and the incidence of measles, mumps, and other current and emerging communicable diseases such as EVD, Zika virus, or COVID-19.

Local health departments or ministries of health also have statistics on population characteristics and health trends that can be helpful when assessing risk. IPs

should, when possible, include them in the risk assessment process.

In addition, the IP should work with the organization's admissions staff and others who maintain statistics on the populations served in the individual organization. Some hospitals have large segments of patients treated for orthopedic procedures, cardiothoracic care, maternal care and childcare, dialysis, and other distinct areas of care. The populations of long-term acute care facilities, psychiatric or rehabilitation hospitals, and others will have special characteristics that should be considered. In addition, ambulatory health care centers may provide pain management, women's health, surgery, and other services. Each health care setting has its unique challenges.

TIP Patient populations can be assessed for risk using a stratification method such as the following, which breaks patients into several groups:

- Basically healthy
- Immunocompromised (oncology patients)
- Undergoing complex procedures (ventilators, ICU, cardiothoracic surgery)
- Implanted with invasive devices (central lines)
- Very young (premature infants)
- Elderly
- Suffering from poor nutritional status
- Residents of a long term care facility
- Transferred to acute care from long term care

The risk assessment should also consider the behaviors of the patients and staff, including adherence to hand hygiene, correct disposal of sharps, or proper use of personal protective equipment (PPE).

Care, Treatment, and Services Provided

The risk assessment process should include risks for infection related to the care, treatment, and services that the health care organization provides. Some organizations perform highly invasive and risky procedures, such as surgery, interventional radiology, and endoscopy, while others rarely perform these procedures but may perform urinary catheterizations and respiratory care treatments. The IP should carefully review the procedures in each service the organization provides to ensure that they are scientifically sound and incorporate current recommendations and guidelines regarding IPC. In addition, the IP should ensure that processes are in place to assess whether staff members are educated about these procedures and are following approved IPC practices.

A thorough inventory of all services that an organization provides is invaluable to the IP in understanding the risks to patients. For IPs new to an organization, visiting each area of the organization to become familiar with the treatments and procedures provided and their policies—and the patients served—is worthwhile. The new IP should discuss IPC practices with staff and may wish to observe procedures that carry significant risk, such as the insertion of a central line or a urinary catheter, care of a surgical wound, or preparation and handling of a parenteral medication. IPs who have worked in an organization for a while should periodically revisit various departments to maintain current knowledge about IPC practices and to determine whether any new services, equipment, or procedures are being provided that may increase risk to patients or staff. Regardless of the health care setting, the IP must bear in mind that policies and procedures should also be assessed to determine if regulatory standards, manufacturers' instructions for use, and national standards are met.

There are several factors to consider when performing a risk assessment for a policy or procedure, such as preventing catheter-associated urinary tract infection (CAUTI) or processing endoscopes to determine if practice will ensure safety and also meet Joint Commission requirements, US Centers for Medicare & Medicaid (CMS) Conditions of Participation (CoP)[1] or Conditions for Coverage (CfC) requirements, as well as applicable state or federal requirements in the United States or ministry of health requirements or international settings. The steps in Figure 3-1 on page 56 are discussed in Chapter 1 and throughout this book. They provide some guidance for developing a risk assessment that addresses key considerations. It is not enough to simply have an organizational policy; several additional factors must be considered. For CAUTI prevention, for example, the risk assessment tool should ask if the organization's policy and practices meet any established rules or regulations and any mandates from state or national agencies or ministries of health, including CMS requirements[1] or those required by the US Occupational Safety and Health Administration (OSHA).[2] The organization should also verify whether manufacturer's instructions for use (IFUs)

are being followed, where applicable. It must be determined whether the practice is designed to be in agreement with evidence-based or national guidelines and consensus documents, such as, for example, recommendations from the US Centers for Disease Control and Prevention (CDC),[3] the Association for Professionals in Infection Prevention and Epidemiology (APIC),[4] the Society for Healthcare Epidemiology of America (SHEA),[5] or the Infectious Diseases Society of America (IDSA).[6] All relevant requirements should be reflected in the organization's IPC policy.

Environmental rounds, tracers, focused visits, and frequent communication with staff are also helpful in identifying potential risks of policies and procedures. Key services and their associated policies and procedures in each department should be reviewed periodically, and potential infection risks should be identified during this time.

Analyzing Surveillance Data

One of the most valuable sources for quantitative information to guide the risk assessment process is an organization's infection surveillance data. In public health, surveillance may be defined as the ongoing and systematic collection, analysis, interpretation, and dissemination of data. One of the main purposes for IPC surveillance is to provide meaningful information that can be used to identify risks for infection so that IPC practices to reduce those risks can be identified and implemented. Outcome and process data for health care–associated infections (HAIs) should be carefully collected, analyzed, and used to identify risk factors related to acquiring and transmitting these infections.[7-11] (Chapter 4 discusses surveillance in more detail.)

IPs should use surveillance data when performing a risk assessment and, where possible, compare the organization's data with existing well-validated databases, such as the National Healthcare Safety Network (NHSN) or other databases from ambulatory care services, neonatal services, long term care or other specialties, and from ministries of health, as appropriate. For the acute care setting, the NHSN is most commonly used for comparing surveillance data. Because definitions and calculation methods are updated periodically, it is important to stay apprised of NHSN criteria by reviewing the website frequently and at least once per year.

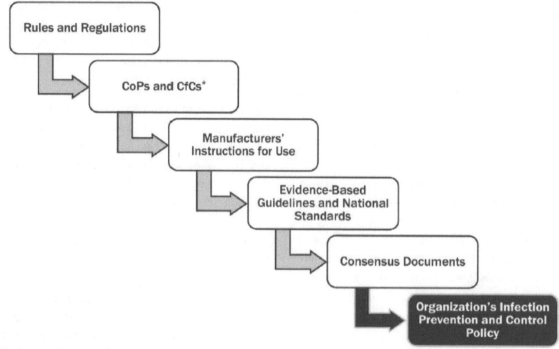

Figure 3-1. Key Considerations for Assessing Risks for Infection Prevention and Control Policies

Rules and Regulations

CoPs and CfCs*

Manufacturers' Instructions for Use

Evidence-Based Guidelines and National Standards

Consensus Documents

Organization's Infection Prevention and Control Policy

*For organizations that use Joint Commission accreditation for deemed status purposes or that are required by state regulation or directive, Conditions of Participation (CoPs) and/or Conditions for Coverage (CfCs) should be reviewed for applicable mandatory requirements.

Ongoing, Multidisciplinary Review of Identified Risks

Organizations should ensure that its IPC policies and procedures are developed by a multidisciplinary group of professionals, each of whom will bring a different perspective to the risk-evaluation process. It is also important that policies and procedures be reviewed regularly. Without input from infection control team members, medical staff, nursing staff, and leadership, the risk assessment may be incomplete, and important considerations may be missed. Those performing a risk assessment should consider at least the variables listed in Sidebar 3-1 on page 57. In addition to input from within the organization, the risk assessment should account for the key considerations illustrated in Figure 3-1.

An organization should have a continuous relationship with the risk assessment process. The written risk assessment should be a living document that is reviewed, validated, and updated at least annually. When there is a change in the organization that could affect IPC risk, the assessment should be revisited to determine whether the selected priorities are still valid.

For example, if an acute care organization acquires a new practice of neurosurgeons that perform high-risk procedures, this should be considered in the risk assessment. Likewise, a significant decrease in nurse–patient staffing ratios may require a risk reassessment, as stressed staff and lower ratios may ultimately affect IPC risks for patients, residents, or staff. Likewise, if there is an influx of infectious patients, as with a community infectious disease outbreak, an epidemic, or a pandemic, such as COVID-19, the organization's selected risks may need to

Sidebar 3-1. Variables to Consider When Performing a Risk Assessment

- Organizational mission
- IC program mission and priorities
- Rates of health care–associated infections
- Gaps in desired practices; sentinel events
- Established and new procedures and policies
- New technologies
- Medications such as antibiotics, vaccines, and chemotherapy agents
- High-risk invasive procedures
- Antimicrobial stewardship
- Populations served and services provided
- Environmental issues
- Training and education for staff
- Community characteristics
- Specific characteristics of each care setting, (for example inpatient, outpatient, office-based care)
- Outbreaks, epidemics, pandemics
- Available IPC resources

be reprioritized. The risk assessment process can be used to determine the revised priorities and precise issues that arise in a setting that has to manage a high-consequence infectious disease (HCID), such as EVD or COVID-19.

There can be several challenges with current risk assessment practices in health care organizations. These challenges include:

- Lack of consultation with a sufficiently wide multidisciplinary group of disciplines
- Lack of a usable construct for determining risk and interventions
- Lack of consistency and transparency in the process
- Insufficient risk assessment guidance for those performing scoring or analyzing the data

When such challenges exist, the risk assessment process may not be effective enough to ensure patient safety,[12] and those designing the risk assessment process should consider these challenges and address them. A framework to operationalize the risk assessment process and to train participants to be more effective in the

process is provided in Figure 3-2 on page 58. Although the framework was developed to support risk assessment in a hospital, it consists of a series of questions for each step in the assessment process that could be used in other health care settings.

The case study on page 59 provides a methodology and construct for a structured risk assessment process for patients with highly infectious diseases (for example, COVID-19, Marburg virus, Ebola virus), which warrants having care delivered in a special unit, such as a dedicated intensive care unit (ICU) or a high-level containment care (HLCC) unit devoted to these patients. Because there is often lack of adequate dedicated special units and beds when these diseases are encountered, it is imperative to have a systematic method to determine how the special units and beds are assigned.

Sometimes, a situation arises in which there is some ambiguity about risks. For example, if clinicians are concerned about whether invasive procedures can be performed at the bedside in a neonatal intensive care unit (NICU) rather than in a distant surgical suite because of the frailty of neonates, this would be an appropriate time to use a risk assessment process to analyze and assess the situation. If a new piece of equipment is purchased for use with an invasive intervention, this would also present an opportunity to perform a risk assessment to determine if the equipment is safe for use for patients. When *Clostridioides difficile* risk must be determined to guide antimicrobial efforts, a type of risk assessment—such as a risk score—can be used to assess patients. Sidebar 3-2, on page 60 describes a risk prediction model for *Clostridium (Clostridoides) difficile* infection (CDI).[13] Tools that might be helpful in determining this type of risk are described later in this chapter.

Because of differences in patient populations, services, the physical environment, and associated risks, organizations should perform a risk assessment for

---

TIP The written risk assessment should be a living document that is reviewed and updated at least annually. When there is a change in the organization that could affect risk, the assessment should be revisited to determine whether the selected priorities are still appropriate.

Figure 3-2

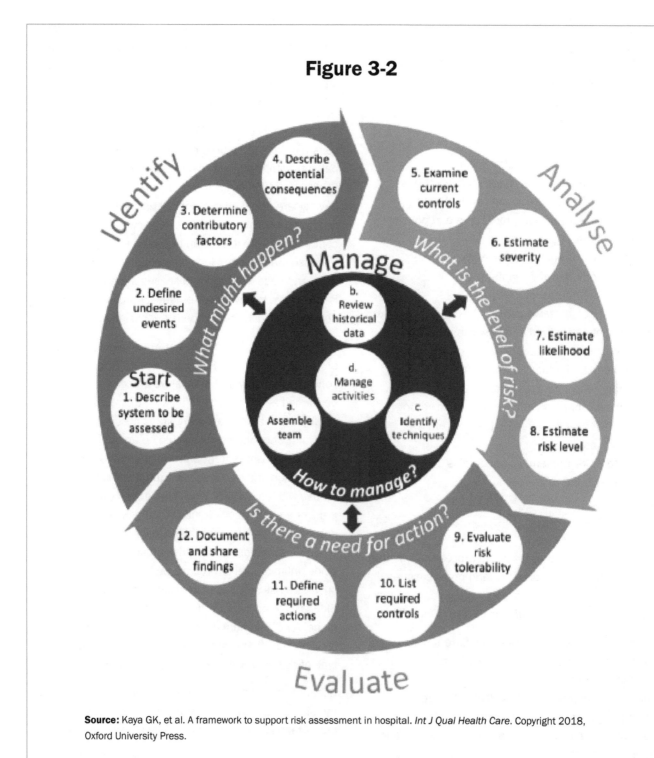

Source: Kaya GK, et al. A framework to support risk assessment in hospital. *Int J Qual Health Care*. Copyright 2018, Oxford University Press.

each care setting under its license. These various risk assessments can be presented separately or combined in one document as long as specificity for the diverse organizational setting is clearly delineated and addressed.

Part of the assessment process is to examine and prioritize the IPC risks of greatest importance and urgency to patients, staff, the patient care environment, and the organization. The analysis should incorporate a method to determine priorities from among all risks identified and analyzed. Some simple methods for establishing priorities are described later in the chapter and are illustrated in the associated tools.

A Methodology for Determining Which Infectious Diseases Warrant Care in a High-Level Containment Care Unit

The concept of high-level containment care (HLCC) in infection prevention and control dates back decades. During the 2014–2016 Ebola virus disease (EVD) outbreak in the United States, the use of HLCC units, or biocontainment units, gained increased credibility for preventing secondary infection in frontline health care workers providing care for infected patients. Such care units helped to significantly decrease mortality compared to traditional management of infectious disease and perhaps served as a lesson learned in early 2020 with the global emergence of Novel Coronavirus 2019 (SARS-CoV-2)/COVID-19. Initially, with an emerging zoonotic virus, such as EVD or COVID-19, there is limited information on virus dissemination, the level or route of infection transmissibility, viral release in bodily fluids or secretions, and the virus's ability to survive on surfaces. While it became clear that patients with viral hemorrhagic diseases such as Ebola, Lassa, and Marburg viruses require HLCC, there was no consistent construct for determining what infections require such a unit. The research team of Cieslak et al. performed a risk assessment to help medical staff determine what other infections might require this type of biocontainment care unit.

The team developed a framework for determining which infectious diseases warrant care in HLCCs that addresses existing and emerging infections. Components of the framework examine infectivity, communicability, and hazard, as shown in the figure above.

Infectivity is measured by the infectious dose needed to infect 50% of a given population. Communicability, or contagiousness, is measured by the reproductive number, which indicates the number of secondary cases resulting from a single

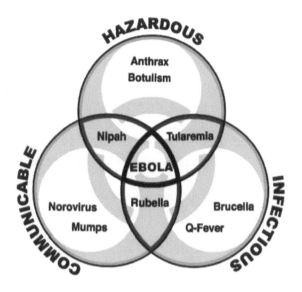

case in the absence of an intervention, such as a vaccine. Hazard is a measure of morbidity and mortality. Some infections may fulfill one or two of these criteria, in which case an HLCC may not be necessary. However, infectious diseases, such as EVD and COVID-19, which fulfill all three criteria, highly infectious, communicable, and highly hazardous—warrant HLCC management, especially if they also meet a fourth criterion: They have no known effective, available, or licensed treatment.

Through this construct, health care professionals may assess the risk of individual pathogens to determine whether an HLCC unit is required for care and to minimize the risk of transmission to other caregivers and the community.

Source: Cieslak TJ, et al. A methodology for determining which diseases warrant care in a high-level containment care unit. *Viruses.* 2019 Aug;11(9):773. Accessed Jan 29, 2021. https://www.ncbi.nlm.nih.gov/pmc/articles/PMC6784089/

After the analysis is complete, the most significant risks should be selected and documented. The results can appear in a standalone document, but the findings and selected highest risks must be integrated and evident in the IPC plan. The selected risks should be used to guide development of the goals for the IPC program. The identified risks will also provide the organization's administrative and quality and patient safety leadership, the infection prevention and control team, nursing, medicine, and support staff with information to understand the basis for the goals, objectives, activities, and resource allocation for the IC/IPC plan. Questions to ask about a risk assessment are outlined in Sidebar 3-3 on page 61, and the following section outlines the critical steps in performing a risk assessment.

Critical Steps in Performing a Risk Assessment

Performing a risk assessment involves several steps. After selecting the multidisciplinary risk assessment team members and establishing a timeline, the team must determine the method to be used for the risk assessment. The following steps are recommended when performing an IPC risk assessment:

1. **Create a Team or Advisory Group**
   Form partnerships with the following:
   - Key staff and stakeholders (for example, nursing, medicine, patient safety/quality, pharmacy, laboratory, support services, risk management, employee health, environmental and facility services, others)
   - Opinion leaders in the organization
   - Top management, including finance
   - Administrative and clinical leadership for support and endorsement

2. **Establish a Timeline**
   - Consider strategic planning and budget cycles.
   - Allow time for team/group meetings and data collection, analysis, and scoring.
   - Set time(s) for review and updating risk assessments, at least annually and if situations change.
   - Review priority risks more frequently to ensure steady progress.

3. **Gather Data and Information**
   Organizational Data
   - Gain access to key reports in the organization, for example, services provided; populations served, including their characteristics and volumes; special

environmental issues; microbiological reports; and
antibiotic use data and resistance patterns.
- Review IPC program surveillance data of HAIs in
  the organization.
- Review external databases of infections such as
  the NHSN, National Surgical Quality Improvement
  Program (NSQIP), or World Health Organization
  (WHO) reports.
- Review processes of care to prevent HAIs;
  consider medical invasive devices, multidrug-
  resistant organisms (MDROs), and antimicrobial
  stewardship, among others.
- Tap into organizational data (medical records, lab
  records, admission and discharge numbers, bed
  utilization numbers), as appropriate.

- Review sentinel event reports, risk reports, and
  mortality data.
- Review internal training programs and competency
  data.
- Review institutional costs of HAIs and MDROs.

Scientific and Professional Data

- Review the literature for new trends—for example,
  *Journal of the American Medical Association,
  The New England Journal of Medicine, Clinical
  Infectious Diseases, Pediatrics, Infection Control
  and Hospital Epidemiology, American Journal of
  Infection Control, International Journal of Infection
  Control,* and *International Journal of Infection
  Prevention.*
- Link to key websites, for example, those for the
  CDC, WHO, APIC, SHEA, The Joint Commission and
  Joint Commission International (JCI), and IDSA.
- Review statements, recommendations, and
  guidelines from professional organizations such as
  the Association of periOperative Registered Nurses
  (AORN), Association for the Advancement of
  Medical Instrumentation (AAMI), Facility Guidelines
  Institute (FGI), SHEA, APIC, IDSA, American Society
  of Health-System Pharmacists (ASHP), US Agency
  for Healthcare Research and Quality (AHRQ),
  National Quality Forum (NQF), and patient safety
  organizations.
- Review guidance from governmental agencies
  such as the CDC, National Institutes of Health
  (NIH), Centers for Medicare & Medicaid Services
  (CMS), and ministries of health.

Community Data

- Connect with the local health department to
  identify trends that may affect infection risk in the
  facility, such as emerging and reemerging
  pathogens, and infectious diseases in the
  community that could affect risk to patents and
  staff in the organization.
- Review information concerning special high-risk,
  homeless, and non-immunized community
  populations.

4. **Develop Systematic Methods and Templates**
   - Develop a systematic way of collecting and
     analyzing risk assessment data.
   - Turn qualitative data into quantitative information,
     when possible.
   - Select or design a template that is easy to use and
     understand.

- Develop a ranking scheme to determine highest priorities.
- Convene a multidisciplinary team to rank data to determine priorities.

5. **Engage and Educate Others to Assist in the Assessment**
   - Provide support and guidance for others to assess risk.
   - Provide educational sessions, as needed, to targeted audiences for how to perform a risk assessment.
   - Share collected data from surveillance, outbreaks, morbidity, and mortality incident reports and sentinel events and highlight incidence and consequences of infections and other data from the literature and the community.
   - Encourage team members to bring data they have collected from their services.
   - Present and agree on the template and assure understanding.
   - Establish rules and definitions for the risk assessment process.

6. **Perform the Risk Assessment**
   - Assemble the team.
   - Provide education and ground rules as needed.
   - Provide data and information.
   - Engage the team in dialogue.
   - Guide discussion and debate.
   - Complete the template with scoring.
   - Reach consensus on the highest priorities.
   - Present the priorities to the appropriate committee and leadership for support and approval.

7. **Use the Priorities to Develop the IPC Program Goals, Objectives, and Activities**
   - Use the highest priorities to develop the IPC plan goals.
   - Use "maintenance," or ongoing, priorities to develop goals.
   - Develop a goal and at least one measurable objective for each selected priority.
   - Create an action plan and evaluation process for each goal or measurable objective.
   - Seek approval for the IPC plan to ensure support from the IPC committee, other committees such as quality or patient safety, and the chief executive team.

8. **Disseminate the Information**
   - Market the importance of the risk assessment and share results throughout the organization as appropriate.
   - Develop a concise, clear report with key points highlighted.
   - Acknowledge those who participated in the process.

Selecting the Appropriate Method and Tools

The risk assessment begins with the selection of the method and tools to support the process. These tools may be quantitative or qualitative or a combination of the two. Some methods and tools for assessing IPC risks are discussed below.

Using a Quantitative Approach

A quantitative risk assessment uses a numeric scoring system based on definitions or criteria. Each risk event is scored with a number. Two key parameters for assessing each risk are the probability and the potential severity.

The probability of an event can be ranked in a number of ways—either on a scale such as "high," "medium," or "low" or with corresponding numbers selected by the organization such as 5, 3, 1 or 9, 5, 3. An organization may also use a five-point Likert scale that ranks the probability of occurrence from "extremely likely" to "extremely unlikely," with assigned numbers such as 5 (extremely likely) to 1 (extremely unlikely) or another numerical scale selected by the organization. If organizations or services are comparing their results, they should use the same numbers and method for analysis.

The *potential severity* of the event then should be ranked. This ranking could be from "extremely severe" to "not severe at all" or an assigned number. Depending on the method, numeric values for each variable can be *added* or *multiplied* to obtain a total score for each risk event. These scores are ranked and evaluated to select the highest priorities for the IPC program.

Other parameters may also be included in the risk assessment methodology, such as infection risks in the environment (for example, as malfunctioning utilities), risk to employees/staff (for example, sharps injuries, exposures, financial risk from infections, and legal risks) and organizational preparedness to address and manage the risk(s). Each organization can decide what it wants to measure and what parameters to include.

For consistent ranking, each category that corresponds to a term or numeric value must be clearly defined— in other words:

- What do *high*, *medium*, and *low* mean for your assessment process?
- How are they defined?
- What considerations should direct the selection of a particular numerical score?
- How is the decision made about what score to assign, such as consensus or leadership?

A critical factor in achieving a useful, consistent, and accurate risk assessment is having precise definitions. Tool 3-1 offers a sample quantitative risk assessment grid with examples that can be used to score and prioritize risk events by category and subcategory based on the characteristics of the health care organization.

TRY THIS TOOL

Tool 3-1. Consideration for Designing a Risk Assessment

Using a Qualitative Approach

Some organizations or IPs prefer to use a qualitative method to assess specific risks to better understand infection prevention practices.[14] This involves an inductive approach that begins with the event or process being analyzed by using written descriptions of populations, descriptions of risk through interviews, focus groups questionnaires, methods of analysis, and outcome indicators. This methodology makes it possible to assess risk by providing a better understanding of the context of the problem and the factors influencing IPC risk, practice, and behaviors.[15] This context helps design effective risk-reduction plans. The qualitative assessment should indicate and describe the priority for each topic and, if desired, can assign a numerical risk score.

One example of a qualitative assessment to evaluate a patient safety infection prevention policy is presented in Sidebar 3-4, at right.

Some believe that a qualitative methodology for risk rating systems has limitations that may make it unreliable, specifically due to assigning ratings that may not correctly represent the risks.[16] Therefore, qualitative techniques and methods must be administered precisely to avoid issues such as bias. During analysis of qualitative

data, some data may be converted to quantitative information such as numbers, diagrams, or matrixes.[14] Qualitative assessments can be very useful when employed carefully for evaluating risk.

One popular qualitative approach to risk assessment is gap analysis. This method uses a priority-setting method as a tool for assessing practice. The Joint Commission and others have used this tool to assess surgical site infections.[17] For a gap analysis, the organization might ask the following questions:

- What is the risk at this time?
- Where do we want to be? or What is our desired goal?
- What is the gap?
- How can we eliminate the gap to reach the goal?

Each risk is considered and assessed. The final step is to rank each of the items described in the gap analysis to determine the highest priorities. Table 3-1 on pages 65–66 is an example of a gap analysis for several IPC issues.

Another qualitative technique is SWOT (strengths, weaknesses, opportunities, and threats) analysis.[18] This method involves selecting a particular issue or risk that needs in-depth analysis, such as inadequate high-level disinfection of duodenoscopes or reduction of the incidence of CDI infections in the environment. After the strengths, weaknesses, opportunities, and threats have been described, the organization addresses the highest-priority issues to maximize opportunities and decrease or eliminate weaknesses and incorporate results into the overall risk assessment and subsequently the IPC plan. A sample SWOT analysis for central line–associated bloodstream infection (CLABSI) is presented in Figure 3-3 on page 67.

Using Criteria to Select a Risk Assessment Method

Because there are many methods to assess risk, Larson and Aiello[19] developed a set of criteria to evaluate the risk assessment method and tools an organization selects. Primary considerations are the comfort of those who will be reviewing the risk assessment and the practicality of the method. If team members do not understand the process and tool, they may defer the assessment to others rather than be active participants, whereas having a method and a tool that are comfortable and easy to use may stimulate involvement. Therefore, it is important to gain approval for both the method and the tool before beginning the process. Larson and Aiello's criteria for assessing a risk analysis method, system, model, or particular tool include asking the following questions:

- How appropriate and sound are the underlying methodological assumptions?
- Is the method or tool comprehensive, addressing all necessary information?
- Does the method contain bias? Will the results be accurate, and will there be confidence in the results?
- How practical is the method?
- Is the method time-efficient?
- Will those using the process understand it?
- Is the risk assessment process being used correctly?
- Is there expertise to perform the analysis?
- Is the process fair and ethical?
- Will the results be useful? Will they support the objectives?

Additional Risk Assessments Used for Infection Prevention and Control

Other risk assessment methods that may be used include sentinel event analysis[20] and Delphi study.[21] Sentinel event analysis helps hospitals and other health care organizations experiencing serious adverse events—not primarily related to the natural course of the patient's illness or underlying condition—learn from those adverse events and improve patient safety. A Delphi study involves convening a diverse group of experts around a particular topic to participate in several rounds of questions and analysis on that topic with the purpose of improving care.

In addition to the risk assessment methods described above, other methodologies that are often used in public health, industry, and other areas can be adapted for use in health care organizations and specifically for infection prevention and control.

Hazard Analysis Critical Control Points

A risk assessment methodology known as Hazard Analysis Critical Control Point (HACCP)[22,23] is a systematic approach to identifying potential microbial hazards in food preparation. Health care organizations can apply these principles and questions to perform reviews of nutrition and dietetics services within the organization or with contracted services. A few of the typical questions that might be asked during a HACCP assessment include:

- Does the food contain any sensitive ingredients that might present microbiological hazards, such as Salmonella or Staphylococcus aureus?
- Does food permit survival or multiplication of pathogens or toxin formation?
- Does the processing (cooking) of food destroy potential pathogens?
- Would the microbial population of the food change during storage prior to consumption?
- Are ready-to-eat foods stored separately from raw material?
- What product safety devices (for example, filters, thermometers) are used to enhance consumer safety?

Table 3-1. Sample Gap Analysis for Infection Prevention and Control Risk Assessment

This table shows one way to conduct a gap analysis and assess IPC risks. To complete the gap analysis, identify the issue and describe the current status, the desired status, and the gap between the two. State the action plan to "close" the gap and evaluation process. Indicate priority among risk issues for the organization. Convert scores to a quantitative model, if possible.

Area/Issue/Topic/Standard	Current Status	Desired Status	Gap (Describe)	Action Plan and Evaluation	Priority: High, Medium, Low
• Incomplete implementation of CDC hand hygiene guideline (NPSG.01.07.01)	• Guideline is approved by ICC. • Required elements are not implemented throughout the organization.	• Ensure full implementation of required elements throughout the organization by December 2021, e.g., Categories IA, IB, and IC.	• Only 60% of units and services are following CDC hand hygiene guideline and organization policy.	• Develop proactive implementation plan. • Make a leadership priority. • Obtain all necessary supplies. • Evaluate existing hand hygiene compliance. • Provide feedback to staff monthly. • Ensure full implementation by June 2021 for all units and services.	High
• Systematic and proactive surveillance activity to determine endemic rates of infections (IC.01.03.01)	• Current surveillance is periodic. • There is retrospective chart review of a few selected infections. Data are not always analyzed in a timely manner.	• Attain prospective surveillance for selected infections and populations on an ongoing basis using NHSN methodology; obtained by October 2021.	• There is a lack of IPC staff and computer support to perform concurrent and ongoing surveillance. • There is an absence of a well-designed surveillance plan. • Access to laboratory data is difficult. • Multiple practice issues compete for surveillance time.	• Request funding to join NHSN and obtain computer and software to enter and analyze data. • Teach IPC staff about surveillance methodologies and how to use NHSN methodology. • Work with laboratory director or contracted service to design access system for microbiology and other reports. • Delegate practice issues to other services to free up time. • Assess program status in 6 months.	Medium to high
• Inconsistent cleaning of high-touch areas in patient care settings (IC.02.02.01)	• Data from EVS supervisor and nursing servations indicate that high-touch surfaces are being cleaned with appropriate frequency per hospital policy only 58% of the time.	• EVS or nursing staff per policy clean high-touch surfaces at least daily and when visibly soiled with the hospital-approved disinfectant using correct technique. • Attain at least 95% compliance by June 2021.	• Time for daily cleaning of patient rooms may not be adequate based on current EVS staffing ratios. • There is a lack of emphasis on potential outcomes due to pathogen transmission from contaminated high-touch areas.	• Request review of staffing of EVS staff for areas requiring frequent high-touch cleaning. • Emphasize policy and necessity for nursing staff to clean high-touch areas in patient care settings on a regular basis and when visibly soiled. • Work with EVS and nursing leaders to accomplish goals. • Request additional staff for cleaning. • Continue to monitor and provide feedback to staff.	Medium to high

(continued)

Table 3-1. Sample Gap Analysis for Infection Prevention and Control Risk Assessment (continued)

Area/Issue/Topic/ Standard	Current Status	Desired Status	Gap (Describe)	Action Plan and Evaluation	Priority: High, Medium, Low
• Increasing needlestick injuries among employees (IC.02.03.01)	• The incidence of needlesticks among EVS staff is 3%. • Analysis shows that greatest risk is during changing of needle containers.	• Reduce needlesticks in EVS staff to equal to or less than 0.2% during next 6 months by January 2021. • Maintain low rate thereafter among all EVS staff.	• Observations show that needle containers are often overflowing. • There is confusion among nursing and housekeeping staff about responsibility and timing for emptying or changing containers. • Nursing supervisors are not aware of the issue.	• Clarify policy and repeat education to staff about criteria for filling/changing needle containers. • Discuss situation with nurse managers and EVS staff and emphasize responsibility. • Display ongoing data to show number of weeks without needlesticks. • Reevaluate needlestick injuries in 3 and 6 months and report to staff and ICC. • Evaluate processes implemented for improvement.	Medium to high

CDC, US Centers for Disease Control and Prevention; **EVS**, environmental services; **ICC**, Infection Control Committee; **IPC**, infection prevention and control; **NHSN**, National Healthcare Safety Network.

Failure Mode and Effects Analysis

Another method for a proactive qualitative and quantitative risk assessment process is the failure mode and effects analysis (FMEA). This method is based on engineering principles for designing systems and processes. Following are key steps in the FMEA process[24]:

1. Select a high-risk process (for example, processing of flexible endoscopes).
2. Assemble a cross-functional team of people, services, and customers with diverse knowledge about the selected process.
3. Define the scope the of the FMEA. Determine boundaries.
4. Diagram the process for clear understanding of the process.
5. Brainstorm the potential failure modes and determine their effects (for example, inability to clean particular scopes well enough to remove all organisms).
6. Use flowcharts and other tools, as appropriate.
7. Prioritize the failure modes.
8. Identify root cause of failure modes (for example, why is there a failure to effectively clean some scopes?)
9. Redesign the process.
10. Analyze and test the new process.
11. Implement and monitor the redesigned process.

TIP — **Selected Resources for the FMEA Process**

- Li X, He M, Wang H. Application of failure mode and effect analysis in managing catheter-related blood stream infection in intensive care unit. *Medicine* (Baltimore). 2017;96(51):e9339.
- Colman N, et al. Prevent safety threats in new construction through integration of simulation and FMEA. *Pediatr Qual Saf.* 2019 Jun;4(4):e189.
- Centers for Medicare & Medicaid Services. Guidance for Performing Failure Mode and Effects Analysis with Performance Improvement Projects. Accessed Apr 6, 2020. https://www.cms.gov/Medicare/Provider-Enrollment-and-Certification/QAPI/downloads/GuidanceForFMEA.pdf
- Failure mode and effects analysis. A hands-on guide for healthcare facilities. *Health Devices.* 2004 Jul;33(7):233–243. Accessed Apr 7, 2020. https://pubmed.ncbi.nlm.nih.gov/15446368/
- Quality-One. Healthcare FMEA (HFMEA). Accessed Apr 5, 2020. https://quality-one.com/hfmea/

Figure 3-3. SWOT Analysis: Central Line–Associated Bloodstream Infection Prevention Practices During Insertion and Maintenance

STRENGTHS	OPPORTUNITIES
• Policy is evidence based and current. • Current ICU staff is competent in approved practices based on periodic assessments. • Hand hygiene compliance is at 94% and improving. • Physician leadership is interested in patient safety and improving CLABSI practices.	• Educate new staff (nurses and physicians) for all CLABSI practices; e.g., formal education and competency assessments. • Identify nurse and physician champions—empower to oversee practices and guide improvements. • Revise procedure to assure availability of supplies at all times to enhance compliance (e.g., cart or kit). • Use checklist to ensure that all tasks are carried out; report analysis to staff. • Address adherence to MSB with physicians using physician champion. • Publicly report CLABSI rates.
WEAKNESSES	THREATS
• Supplies are not consistently available in a timely manner for insertion procedures. • Some physicians do not adhere to MSB. • Nonoptimal sites sometimes chosen; (e.g., femoral site often selected). • Residents do not always feel they are well trained for safe insertion procedures and sites.	• Abuse of nurses who point out lack of adherence to CLABSI insertion protocol. • Lack of proper insertion technique and placement in subclavian vein. • Interruption of supplies from vendors.

CLABSI, central line–associated bloodstream infection; **ICU,** intensive care unit; **MSB,** maximal sterile barrier

Source: Adapted from Marschall J, et al. Strategies to prevent central line–associated bloodstream infections in acute care hospitals. *Infect Control Hosp Epidemiol.* 2008 Oct;(29 Suppl 1):S22-S30.

The Survey Analysis for Evaluating Risk® (*SAFER®*) Matrix

The Joint Commission's *SAFER®* Matrix was developed to help organizations assess the risk posed by noncompliance with Joint Commission standards cited on surveys. It provides the organization with a visual assessment of the seriousness and risk levels of various risks for their program(s). This tool can be used to evaluate what compliance issues an organization has and where it needs to focus its performance improvement activities.[25,26] Figure 3-4 on pages 68–69 shows the *SAFER* Matrix template along with an explanation of the assessment categories. The matrix can be used by staff in the organization as another tool to assess IPC risk.

Tracer Methodology

Tracers provide another way for health care organizations' staff and teams to assess internal risks and evaluations.[27] Tracers accomplish many purposes, including evaluating patient care (such as how a urinary catheter is inserted);

Figure 3-4. The *SAFER*® Matrix

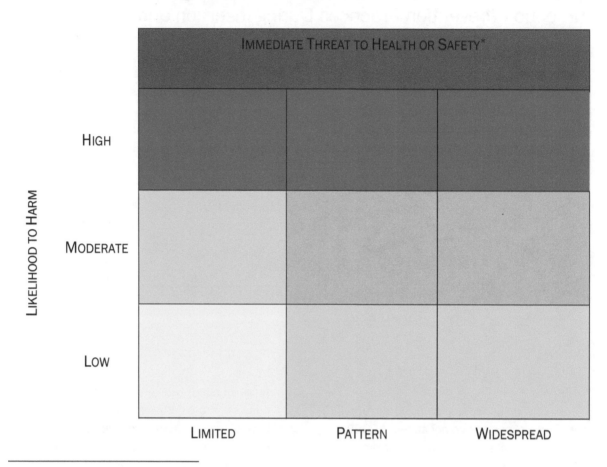

* A threat that represents immediate risk or may potentially have serious adverse effects on the health of the patient.

Category	Definition	Further Guidance
Scope		
Limited	Unique occurrence that is not representative of routine/ regular practice and has the potential to affect only one or a very limited number of patients, visitors, or staff.	An Outlier • Scope is isolated when one or a very limited number of patients are affected and/or one or a very limited number of staff are involved and/or the deficiency occurs in a very limited number of locations.

(continued)

Figure 3-4. The *SAFER*® Matrix (continued)

Category	Definition	Further Guidance
Pattern	Multiple occurrences of the deficiency or a single occurrence that has the potential to affect more than a limited number of patients, visitors, or staff.	Process Variation • Scope is a pattern when more than a very limited number of patients are affected, and/or more than a very limited number of staff are involved, and/or the situation has occurred in several locations, and/or the same patient(s) has been affected by repeated occurrences of the same deficient practice.
Widespread	Deficiency is pervasive in the facility, or represents systemic failure, or has the potential to impact most/all patients, visitors, or staff.	Process Failure • Scope is widespread when the deficiency affects most/all patients, is pervasive in the facility, or represents systemic failure. Widespread scope refers to the entire organization, not just a subset of patients or one unit.
Likelihood to Harm		
Low	Harm could happen but would be rare.	• Undermines safety/quality or contributes to an unsafe environment but very unlikely to directly contribute to harm. • It would be rare for any actual patient harm to occur as a result of the deficiency.
Moderate	Harm could happen occasionally.	• Could cause harm directly, but more likely to cause harm as a contributing factor in the presence of special circumstances or additional failures. • If the deficiency continues, it would be possible that harm could occur but only in certain situations and/or patients.
High	Harm could happen at any time.	• Could directly lead to harm without the need for other significant circumstances or failures. • If the deficiency continues, it would be likely that harm could happen at any time to any patient (or did actually happen).

assessing performance of staff providing care (such as hand hygiene or knowledge of organizational policies); and evaluating the effectiveness of established systems and processes (such as disinfection and sterilization or environmental cleaning and how improvements in care are implemented). Tracers are versatile and are ideal for identifying gaps in practice, compliance with policies, care practices, IPC goals, and other topics that present risk. Sample tracer questions for influenza vaccination are listed in Sidebar 3-5.

Sidebar 3-5. Sample Tracer Questions for an Influenza Vaccination Program

The following sample tracer questions are applicable to all Joint Commission accreditation programs/settings:

- Can you describe the organization's vaccination program?
- Who is the designated person in charge of managing the program?
- Is there an annual influenza vaccination program?
- Is vaccination offered to all licensed independent practitioners and all staff?
- How does the organization communicate information about the vaccination program?
- Does the organization provide influenza vaccination at sites accessible to licensed independent practitioners and staff?
- Does the infection control plan include the organization's goal for improving influenza vaccination rates?
- How does the organization evaluate the reasons given by staff and licensed independent practitioners for declining the influenza vaccination?
- What changes have been made as a result of the data collected?
- How do you ensure that your staff's immunizations are up-to-date?
- How do leaders, coworkers, and patients know which employees have received the influenza vaccination for the current year?

Infection Control Risk Assessment

One method familiar to many IPs is the risk assessment performed before and during construction or renovation projects, which is generally referred to as the preconstruction risk assessment (PCRA) or the infection control risk assessment (ICRA). The PCRA is completed during the documentation phase of construction, before any work begins in a health care facility. The PCRA findings that may interfere with safe construction are addressed and resolved, such as how to safely close some utilities during the construction. The ICRA is completed to determine whether IPC procedures and policies are in place and will be implemented, such as effective barriers between construction areas and non-construction areas, high-efficient particulate air (HEPA) filter exhaust systems, and traffic control. See Chapter 7 for further discussion of ICRA.

Some issues that that may be addressed during the ICRA might include the following:
- Disruptions in essential services to patients and employees during construction
- The hazards and needed protection levels for each disruption
- Location of patients by susceptibility to infection and definition of risks to each population
- Effects of potential emergencies or utility outages and protection of patients during planned or unplanned outages, including movement of debris, traffic flow, cleanup, and testing and certification
- Effective barriers during construction
- Defining the internal and external construction activities and risks
- Locations of known and potentially unknown hazards

Hazard Vulnerability Analysis

Another type of assessment is the hazard vulnerability analysis (HVA), used to determine the organization's susceptibility to disasters, emergencies, and other untoward events.[28] Some organizations incorporate the IPC risk assessment into the organization's overall HVA. Results of the HVA allow for the proactive implementation of measures that improve the facility's capability to respond to infection threats, such as floods and utility disruptions, which have infection prevention and control ramifications. This methodology is also discussed in Chapter 5. Depending on the situation, the HVA may include the following:
- Geographic considerations
- Supplies and equipment risks

- Communication risks
- Emergency preparedness
- Environmental issues
- Staff education
- Staff risks
- Community consideration

Selecting Risk Categories and Topics

A key step in the risk assessment process is to designate general risk categories for evaluation, such as the following:

- Types of infections
- Organisms of epidemiological significance
- Multidrug-resistant organisms
- At-risk patient or resident populations
- Vaccine-preventable diseases and vaccines
- Staff education
- Preparedness for IPC emergency

After general risk categories are identified, more specific risk events should be identified within each category. For example, in the general category "organisms of epidemiological significance," several multidrug-resistant organisms may be listed, such as methicillin-resistant *Staphylococcus aureus* (MRSA), *Clostridioides difficile*, vancomycin-resistant *Enterococci* (VRE), carbapenem-resistant *Enterobacteriaceae* (CRE), *Candida auris*, and *Acinetobacter* species. The risks involved with each of these should be evaluated separately. Likewise, under the general category "staff risks," more specific risks may include sharps injuries, tuberculosis, meningitis, bloodborne pathogens or influenza, and lack of compliance with hand hygiene.

Classifying Infection Risks

As previously mentioned, risks related to infections can take many forms. They can be viewed as *unexpected* or *involuntary* and include such risks as a community or organizational influx of a new community population with specific infection risks, a community outbreak of measles, or the emergence of a new pathogen, such as *Elizabethkingia* bacteria or Zika virus. Risks can also be *expected* or *voluntary*, such as risks with central lines, medication preparation and handling practices, or an elective surgical procedure. Both types of risks should be considered for a comprehensive risk assessment. Risks may also be classified as *internal* or *external* to the organization. The following sections take a closer look at these two classifications.

External Risks

External risks come from outside an organization. One type of external risk relates to geographic considerations, such as the climate of different areas. For example, some coastal areas may experience periodic hurricanes or floods and may contend with more waterborne infection risks. Geographic considerations that can affect local health care facilities include very dry or very moist climates, floods,[29] and disruption of water supply[30]; tornadoes and hurricanes; and earthquakes[31] and volcanic eruptions, all of which may have associated IPC risks. In addition, health care facilities in urban areas may be more vulnerable to events related to terrorism and may become receiving centers for persons exposed to infectious agents due to a bioterrorism event. The CDC and others have issued recommendations for preparedness for floods and hurricane preparation and remediation for these external risks.[32-34]

As new resistant organisms emerge, they may first appear in one state or country and move to other states, regions, or throughout the world, and they may be brought into a country from global travel. This introduction from one country to another occurs with influenza viruses, cholera, and emerging organisms such as SARS-CoV-2/COVID-19 and resistant organisms such as *Klebsiella pneumoniae* carbapenemase (KPC).[35,36] Swine fever is another unusual pathogen that has been seen worldwide; it is related to the importing of animals.[37] Organizations with animal visitation programs should assess risk associated with the animals interacting with patients or health care staff.

Pandemics, while infrequent, do occur and can be devastating when people become ill and then make their way to a health care organization. The 1918 influenza epidemic challenged all parts of the health care delivery system and infected or killed nearly 50 million persons globally.[38] As of this writing, the COVID-19 pandemic has infected millions and has required rapidly revised IPC risk assessments and creative IPC mitigation priorities by health care organizations globally.[39,40]

External risks can take other forms. For example, some communities have populations with a high endemic incidence of a particular infection, such as tuberculosis, malaria, or viral hepatitis. The socioeconomic level of a population can affect living conditions, which may contribute to poor health practices and the transmission of infections. Families in some areas are less likely than families in other areas to immunize their children against common vaccine-preventable disease. Some families live in close contact with animals that may transmit infections that are then brought into the community and ultimately the health care facility, such as *Salmonella*, West Nile virus, plague, and Lyme disease, to name a few. The strength of its public health department influences the community's overall health and infection risks. These factors should be considered as part of the IPC risk assessment process.

Internal Risks

Internal risks—those occurring within an organization—fall into several categories, each with special challenges and characteristics. Risks associated with patients and staff are of primary concern because of these populations' potential exposure to pathogens or injury, with subsequent morbidity and mortality.

An assessment of patient or resident risks will generally be more helpful in guiding IPC activities if it is stratified by subgroups with particular characteristics and behaviors. Such subgroups might include the following patients or residents, such as those who are

- highly immunocompromised;
- in intensive care, behavioral health care, long term care, oncology, or rehabilitation settings;
- undergoing high-risk procedures, such as total joint replacements, cardiovascular surgery, or ventilator-assisted respiratory therapy; or
- very young or old, from premature infants to the elderly.

Staff-related risks are affected by the general health habits and cultural beliefs of the staff, availability and use of PPE, and the staff's awareness of disease transmission. When conducting a risk assessment, it is important to consider staff compliance with IPC policies, such as those related to the handling of sharps, availability and use of PPE, performance of appropriate hand hygiene, and social distancing, if necessary.

In addition, the risk assessment should determine whether effective organizational processes exist for screening and protecting employees, contractual staff, or licensed independent practitioners who may be or have been exposed to infectious diseases or who have an infectious or communicable disease. Staff willingness to receive influenza and other vaccinations can determine infection risk for staff and ultimately patients or residents.

Certain procedures also present increased risk. Both diagnostic and therapeutic procedures can involve risk for the patient or the care provider. Some considerations for assessing procedure-related risks may include the following:

- The invasiveness of a procedure
- The characteristics of the equipment or devices used in the procedure
- The knowledge and technical expertise of those performing the procedure
- How staff adheres to the recommended IPC methods

For example, a surgical procedure in which a surgeon performs blind stitching poses a greater sharps-injury risk than a procedure in which visual suturing is performed. Interventional radiology performs invasive procedures, as do pain clinics, dental areas, endoscopy, and many other settings.

Some noninvasive procedures and treatments that do not appear to have an infection risk have been associated with the transmission of infectious agents. For example, therapeutic modalities that use whirlpools, swimming pools, and other water sources can transmit infection if the water is not clean or the equipment is not cleaned or disinfected regularly. In one outbreak, laundry (a seemingly low-hazard material) was implicated in the infections and deaths of five pediatric patients during a fungal outbreak.[41] In a long term care brain injury ward, regular linens were replaced with biocidal copper oxide impregnated linens to reduce HAIs.[42] It is important to consider all areas of care in the risk assessment.

IPC risks are also present in certain supplies and equipment. For example, reusable supplies and equipment that are moved from patient to patient without being cleaned and disinfected between patient use can transmit pathogenic organisms. Examples include the workstations (used by nurses to record patient information) that are moved from room to room and computers and screens that remain in a room between patents. Another risk is housekeeping supplies that are not changed between cleanings per best practice recommendations. An IP should periodically monitor these practices and consider the results during the risk assessment process.

The facility itself is vulnerable to and poses risks and hazards from the breakdown of utilities during natural or human-caused emergencies, which can result in an IPC issue. For example, defective ventilation functions in the operating rooms can create the potential for contaminated air that might come into contact with an open wound.[43,44] Likewise, construction and renovation are common in many facilities and may pose danger of infection to immunocompromised and debilitated patients from organisms such as *Aspergillus*, particularly when barriers are inadequate, HEPA filters are not used, or traffic is not controlled. Unusual but significant risks may occur internally, such as floods during construction or from defective equipment. This poses a significant mitigation risk to the facility. Further discussion on the environment and its infection control risks can be found in Chapter 7. Table 3-2 lists some categories and topics for an IPC risk assessment.

Table 3-2. Selected Categories and Topics for an Infection Prevention and Control Risk Assessment

Risk Group	Risk Factors

Geographic location	• Natural disasters such as tornadoes, floods, hurricanes, and earthquakes
	• Breakdown of municipal services such as broken water main or strike by sanitation employees
	• Accidents in the community, including mass transit (airplane, train, bus)
	• Fires involving mass casualties
	• Intentional acts of:
	    ◦ Bioterrorism
	    ◦ "Dirty bombs"
	    ◦ Contamination of food and water supplies
	    ◦ Shootings
	• Prevalence of disease linked with vectors, temperature, and other environmental factors

Community	• Community outbreaks of transmissible infectious diseases, such as influenza, meningitis, tuberculosis, and COVID-19 • Diseases linked to food and water contamination, such as *Salmonella* and hepatitis A • Vaccine-preventable illness (such as measles) in unvaccinated populations • Infections associated with primary migrant populations in a geographic area • Strength and presence of a public health structure • Socioeconomic levels of population • War or displacement
Organization programs and clinical services	• Cardiac service • Orthopedic service • Neonatology • Pediatrics • Dialysis • Long term care • Rehabilitation • Ambulatory clinics • Hospice • Home care • Acute long term care • Behavioral health

(continued)

Table 3-2. Selected Categories and Topics for an Infection Prevention and Control Risk Assessment (continued)

Risk Group	Risk Factors
Special populations served	• Women and children • Behavioral health patients • Long term care patients • Very young and very elderly patients • Persons with cognitive and physical deficiencies • Migratory populations • Persons with high-risk lifestyle issues • Other special needs populations
High-risk patients	• Surgical • ICU • NICU • Oncology • Dialysis • Transplant • Patients with MDROs
Health care worker risks	• Understanding disease transmission and prevention • Degree of compliance with infection prevention techniques and policies, such as hand hygiene, aseptic technique, and use of PPE and isolation • Sharps injuries • Screening for transmissible diseases • Work restriction guidelines • Practice accountability issues • Availability and use of supplies such as PPE
Medical procedures	• Invasiveness of procedures • Equipment used for procedures • Knowledge and technical expertise of those performing procedures • Adequate preparation of patients • Adherence to recommended IPC techniques

Equipment and devices	• Cleaning, disinfection, transport, and storage for IV pumps, suction equipment, and other equipment, such as wheelchairs, gurneys, and toys
	• Sterilization or disinfection process for the following:
	  ◦ Scopes
	  ◦ Surgical instruments
	  ◦ Prostheses
	• Complexity of devices, such as safety needles and robotics
	• Skill and experience of users
	• Safety features (user dependent or automatic)
	• Reuse of single-use devices

(continued)

Table 3-2. Selected Categories and Topics for an Infection Prevention and Control Risk Assessment (continued)

Risk Group	Risk Factors
Environmental issues	• Construction, renovation, and alterations • Notification of construction • ICRAs and construction permits • Utilities performance • Environmental cleaning and disinfection • Adequate environmental staff • Ventilation and utilities • Water systems and decorative water features • Isolation rooms
Emergency preparedness	• Staff education • Managing influx of infectious patients • Triaging patients • Isolation, barriers, and PPE • Utilities and supplies • Medications for prophylaxis and treatment • Security • Staff presence during emergencies
Resource limitations	• Nurse staffing • Other clinical and support staffing • Infection preventionist and hospital epidemiologist staffing • Laboratory support services • Environmental services and facilities

Organization's surveillance data and processes	• Trained and available staff
	• Clear and validated definitions
	• Monitoring device and procedure-related risks:
	  ○ Catheter-related bloodstream infections
	  ○ Ventilator-associated pneumonia
	  ○ Catheter-associated urinary tract infections
	  ○ Surgical site infections
	  ○ Gastrointestinal infections
	• Sepsis
	• MDROs
	• Lack of IT and data support

Education and communication	• Education of all staff on IPC strategies • Timely education for emerging diseases and MDROs • Communication of IPC information • Communication of emergency preparedness information • Intradepartmental communication

(continued)

Table 3-2. Selected Categories and Topics for an Infection Prevention and Control Risk Assessment (continued)

Risk Group	Risk Factors
Supplies and equipment	• Availability of supplies and equipment for patient care and IPC team • Education about appropriate use of supplies • Skill of staff using the equipment • Appropriate cleaning, disinfection, and sterilization • Safe storage of supplies and equipment

ICRA, infection control risk assessment; **ICU,** intensive care unit; **IPC,** infection prevention and control; **IT,** information technology; **IV,** intravenous; **MDRO,** multidrug-resistant organism; **NICU,** neonatal; **PPE,** personal protective equipment

Collecting and Using Data for the Risk Assessment

After the risk assessment team determines the general categories and selects the specific risks for evaluation, the team must collect and review data to perform the risk assessment. Many types and sources of data can be helpful, including the following:

- Infection surveillance and employee health data
- Information about the incidence of infections or infection-related deaths in patients or residents
- Findings from cluster or outbreak investigations
- IPC incident reports
- Equipment failures
- Sharps injuries
- Employee exposures or PPE use
- Data from departments such as finance, medical records, and admissions
- Data from local and state health departments

Resources for comparing surveillance data for infections include the NHSN,[45] the CMS, and the Outcome and Assessment Information Set (OASIS)[46] for nursing care centers. Many government agencies mandate the reporting of surveillance data, and these data are available in some states for organizational comparisons. Internationally, many countries have surveillance systems, such as the KISS system in Germany,[47] where ministries of health maintain databases created from all health care organizations in the country.[48]

Some professional organizations also collect surveillance data to help in performing clinical risk assessments for specific organisms, procedures, or infections. Currently, there is a lack of surveillance data for some settings, such

as home care, ambulatory surgery centers, and office-based practices, as well as in some countries. Valuable information may be found in the scientific literature.

Clinical Risk Assessment for Surgical Site Infections

Risk factors for surgical site infections (SSIs) are associated with the host and the perioperative factors in each of the phases of surgery—preoperative, intraoperative, and postoperative. Furthermore, some risk factors are modifiable, and others are not.[49-52] Early recognition of perioperative SSI risk factors and patient risk stratification are significant in developing predictive risk models that can assist surgeons in determining postsurgical risks for total hip procedures, for example, and the appropriateness of special prevention strategies for high-risk patients. This type of clinical risk assessment tool can also be used to educate patients on their individual risk of complications and to help them manage postoperative expectations and the potential for SSIs.

The American College of Surgeons, through the NSQIP,[53] has developed a risk assessment calculator tool to help surgeons, patients, and patients' families understand potential postsurgical outcomes based on data from thousands of patents and projected length of stay. The risk calculator is free and available online.

Analyzing Potential Risks

To help analyze potential risks, organizations should ask questions, including whether a known or potential risk is likely to occur. Another question is how severe the consequences of the risk would be. Yet another important issue is whether the organization is adequately prepared to handle the risk so that any negative effects are eliminated or minimized.

In addition to asking these questions, organizations may wish to consider other factors when analyzing potential risks, such as accreditation and regulatory issues from CMS survey guides[54,55] for ambulatory care as well as the OASIS program for long term care[46] and human, financial, organizational, or environmental effects.

Selecting Priority Infection Risks

Given the limited resources in many IPC programs, addressing every identified risk during a given time period is not always possible. Therefore, an organization should use resources wisely by first addressing issues with the most potential for serious harm. The organization must determine which risks should be prioritized for the IPC program during a given time period.

An organization may turn to its risk assessment team, advisory council, or IPC or patient safety/quality improvement and patient safety committee to balance data, experience, and information from knowledgeable staff in the organization and to select the risks that pose the greatest potential for morbidity or mortality. The team should set guidelines for determining priorities to provide consistency and avoid bias from emotional or personal agendas. The team should be able to articulate clearly why a particular risk has been prioritized or given a lower score.

Regardless of how the priorities are selected, the organization's leaders should determine approval and, if endorsed, provide the needed resources to implement the priorities. The approved priorities should then guide the development of measurable goals and objectives for the IPC plan. Tool 3-2 is helpful for prioritizing specific infection risks to the organization or to the community the organization serves, such as categories of multidrug-resistant organisms. Other assessment tools for particular settings such as hospitals, long term care facilities, outpatient settings, and hemodialysis facilities are included in the Resources section at the end of this chapter.

TRY THIS TOOL

Tool 3-2. Infection Prevention and Control Risk Assessment for Multidrug-Resistant Organisms (MDROs)

Reevaluating the Risk Assessment Process

As discussed earlier, risk identification and assessment are continuous processes that, at minimum, should be evaluated annually. However, it may be prudent and necessary for an organization to examine risks more frequently. Events such as an infectious outbreak in a long term care facility, a new cardiac surgery service in acute care, or an outbreak of hepatitis C in an outpatient endoscopy clinic would all prompt such a reevaluation. In addition, it may also be sensible to review how effectively the actual risk assessment process is being carried out.

After the risk assessment process is complete, writing goals and measurable objectives for the IPC program is essential to formulating the IPC plan and determining the activities of the infection surveillance, prevention, and control program. As with the risk assessment, engaging a team of knowledgeable people is best to create goals to address the risk priorities and use them as drivers for key activities.

Prioritizing Risks and Establishing Goals

Organizations should set and prioritize goals to minimize the possibility of transmitting infections. The IPC team can use the risk assessment results to develop the goals for the IPC program. The goals should be directly linked to the highest priorities to show a continuous process from analysis to action. For example, if the incidence of *Clostridioides difficile* is identified as a significant risk for the organization, there should be a goal to reduce the incidence. If one of the high priorities is to improve environmental cleaning, there should also be a goal for this effort.

The IPC plan will probably include other goals for maintaining the program that are not ranked as high priorities in the analysis but that are necessary for programmatic success and maintenance of established practices. Each goal should be accompanied by a measurable objective, an action plan, and an evaluation process to determine whether the objective has been met. A discussion of writing goals and objectives is found in Sidebar 3-6 on page 78. In addition, Tool 3-3 can be downloaded to help develop SMART (specific, measurable, action-oriented, realistic/relevant, and timely) goals and objectives that drive the IPC plan.

Sidebar 3-6. Writing Clear Goals and Measurable Objectives

Infection prevention and control (IPC) goals are general statements that establish intent, direction, and broad parameters for the desired achievements of an IPC program. For example, a goal might state the following:

The IPC program will reduce pneumonia in ventilated patients in the intensive care unit (ICU).

This goal clearly communicates intent, but because no specific numeric target or date exists, it is impossible to determine by what amount the pneumonias in the ICU will be reduced or the timeline for achieving this outcome. An organization must develop a measurable objective for each goal.

Objectives of the IPC program are statements of specific intent or desired achievements for the program. Objectives should state what will be achieved (in numeric values, when possible), provide a specific time frame when the action will be completed, and identify the population, location, or process being targeted.

A written objective should be measurable. Therefore, an objective for the previous goal could be stated as follows:

- The medical ICU will have zero ventilator-associated pneumonias for a period of at least three consecutive months by December 2021.
- Reduce ventilator-associated pneumonia by equal to or less than 50%, from 1.4/1,000 ventilator-days to 0.7/1,000 ventilator-days in the medical ICU (MICU) by June 2021.

Goals and measurable objectives establish targets for performance improvement activities and allow the care staff and the IPC program to evaluate progress and success or failure in these efforts (see Table 3-3 on page 79.) After goals and objectives have been established, they should be used to develop the IPC plan.

TRY THIS TOOL

Tool 3-3. Creating SMART Goals for IPC

Exposures to Pathogens

The actions that an organization takes to protect patients, residents, staff, visitors, and others from contact with potentially infectious organisms are critical. The use of aseptic technique, safe injection practices, hand hygiene, and PPE (such as gowns, gloves, masks, and respirators) falls into this category. Isolation procedures, engineering controls for airborne pathogens, barriers during construction, and safety hoods in the laboratory would be appropriate topics or issues to consider under this goal as well. (Many of these strategies are discussed in detail in Chapters 6 and 7.)

Infections Associated with Procedures

Patients are exposed to many procedures that are designed to diagnose, improve, or maintain health. As previously mentioned, some of these procedures carry significant risk for infection because they are invasive or complex in nature (for example, surgical procedures). The health status of the patient, the duration of the procedure, and the state of the wound (for example, clean or dirty) all influence whether a person may experience a postoperative SSI. For example, healthy patients having clean hernia repairs have a relatively low risk for SSI, whereas those having bowel surgery after trauma have a higher risk.

Because of the risks for infection associated with surgery, each area of care in the surgical services, including preoperative, perioperative, and postoperative settings, should have goals and related policies and procedures to ensure minimal infection risk to patients. This applies to inpatient and ambulatory surgery areas. Settings where invasive procedures are performed require constant vigilance from the IPC team to ensure that effective IPC policies and practices are in place. These settings can include, but are not limited to, the following:

- Interventional radiology
- Endoscopy and bronchoscopy settings
- Pain clinics
- Anesthesia
- Dermatology clinics
- Ear, nose, and throat clinics
- Dental offices

Table 3-3. Sample Goals and Objectives for the Infection Prevention and Control Plan

Goal	Examples of Measurable Objectives
Reduce ventilator-associated pneumonias (VAPs) in the intensive care unit (ICU)	• Reduce VAP by equal to or greater than 50%, from 1.4/1,000 ventilator-days to 0.7/1,000 ventilator-days in the medical ICU (MICU) by June 2020. • Achieve zero VAPs for a minimum of 3 months by January 2021 in the MICU. • Assess daily whether the need for a ventilator is documented for 98% of ICU ventilated patients by January 2021.
Decrease sharps injuries in employees.	• Reduce needlestick injuries among direct care and support staff by at least 60% from the 2019 rate within the first 6 months of 2020. • Reduce scalpel injuries in surgical staff by 80% from current rate with implementation of "pass zone" by July 2020.
Increase immunizations in the organization.	• Identify and immunize at least 90% of eligible staff. • Immunize 100% of eligible staff in the organization with influenza vaccine within 6 months of initiating a mandatory flu vaccine program.
Increase hand hygiene compliance.	• Achieve at least 95% compliance with hand hygiene policy on at least 80% of nursing units by October 2021.
Prevent transmission of infectious diseases in the organization.	• Achieve at least 98% compliance with contact isolation policy for patients with methicillin-resistant *Staphylococcus aureus* and *Clostridioides difficile* on all patient care units during 2021.
Maintain consistent cleaning of reusable patient equipment in the ICUs.	• Achieve at least 98% compliance with appropriate cleaning procedures for reusable direct care patient equipment during patient stay and at discharge in the MICU, surgical ICU, and neonatal ICU during 2021.
Infection prevention and control staff notify staff about construction, renovation, or alteration in facility before beginning work.	• Achieve equal to or greater than 95% notification to infection prevention and control staff before any construction, renovation, or alteration occurs in that facility for all appropriate (per policy) construction projects by January 2021.
Prepare for the response to an influx or risk of influx of infectious patients.	• Achieve equal to or greater than 90% of Hospital Emergency Incident Command System plan requirements related to infectious patients during at least three drills in 2021.

Infections Associated with Medical Devices and Supplies

The IPC program is responsible for overseeing the processes that ensure safe use of medical devices—such as syringes, intravenous needles and tubing, indwelling urinary catheters, bronchoscopes, and ventilators—and the appropriate management of equipment and sterile supplies. As such, the goals and associated policies and procedures related to cleaning, disinfection, sterilization, storage, and transport of equipment, sterile supplies, and single-use devices should be reviewed and approved by the IPC oversight body. Compliance with IPC practices should be monitored as delegated by the organization. This is an important topic to include in the risk assessment and in the IPC plan, as it is a commonly cited area of noncompliance on Joint Commission surveys.

Improving Hand Hygiene

Hand hygiene is addressed in National Patient Safety Goal® (NPSG) NPSG.07.01.01 and International Patient Safety Goal (IPSG) IPSG.5. Compliance with these goals is required for all accredited organizations. Goals and objectives related to hand hygiene may include a specified target for hand hygiene compliance, improved hand hygiene technique, and improved accessibility of hand hygiene products.[56-58] Joint Commission Center for Transforming Healthcare provides tools and resources for improving compliance with hand hygiene.

Finalizing the IPC Plan

When the risk assessment is completed, priorities are selected, and goals and objectives are established, the IPC team can finalize its IPC plan. The IPC plan is a written dynamic document designed to respond quickly to changes and demands in the health care environment. These changes may be related to issues such as emerging infectious diseases, new requirements for mandatory reporting of HAI information, an organization's acquisition of new services, or major construction projects. Creating measurable goals and objectives is critical for an effective IPC plan. Table 3-3 provides some examples of clear and measurable SMART goals and objectives for the IPC plan.

The IPC plan should be a clear, well-defined, and useful document that identifies priorities and needs, sets goals and objectives, lists strategies to meet the goals, and includes an evaluation process determined by the organization. The plan may include or append narratives, policies, procedures, protocols, practice guidelines, clinical paths, care maps, or other helpful documents. The plan should integrate evidence-based science or expert consensus, a written description of the activities, including surveillance, and a process for investigating a cluster or outbreak of infections. It may also include the communication strategies for getting IPC information to staff and independent practitioners, visitors, and the community and also reporting infections to the health department, the CDC, the ministry of health, or other agencies, as required.

> **TIP** The IPC plan should be a useful document that identifies priorities and needs, sets goals and objectives, lists strategies to meet the goals, and includes the evaluation process. The plan should be flexible, based on shifting priorities.

Using Evidence-Based Guidelines to Drive IPC Activities

Health care organizations should continuously update their IPC program and plan and ensure that its infection prevention and control activities are based on the best scientific evidence or expert consensus to guide decisions about patient care, maintenance of the environment, staff safety, and other elements of the program. As previously mentioned, many guidelines and guidance documents are available to help organizations in this effort. The IPC team should refer to these and other resources when developing and evaluating the IPC plan. Additional resources and examples for developing an IPC plan are provided at the end of this chapter.

The IPC plan is most helpful to staff if the activities are clearly stated in writing. The Joint Commission and JCI require all accredited programs to have some type of IPC plan. This requirement applies to single and multifacility organizations, to those organizations offering basic care, and those providing complex care services. It also applies to most JCI programs surveyed and those surveyed by The Joint Commission. An example of a multifacility organization would be one that provides acute inpatient care for adults and children, provides acute long-term care, has a behavioral health unit, and has many outpatient facilities—such as outpatient surgeries, pain clinics, and dialysis and rehabilitation centers. Each of these services requires a risk assessment that applies to the specific services offered and the geographic area.

IPs should check the standards for their setting to determine what is mandated and what is recommended. Having documentation of IPC program activities, priorities, goals, and objectives will help eliminate ambiguity as to how the program's resources will be allocated and used. The plan also helps to maintain focus. The plan or activities should be written in a simple style and be easily understandable and accessible to the IPC team and other staff who participate in the activities.

Key components of the IPC plan are the scope and methods for surveillance, which differ depending on the setting and populations served. Each organization should design a surveillance program based on its characteristics, populations, services, risks, and requirements and should prepare a written surveillance plan, as discussed in Chapter 4.

The surveillance plan may be a separate document or may be integrated into the IPC plan. See Sidebar 3-7, at right, for tips on writing the IPC plan. Although there is no nationally standardized method for identifying, collecting, managing, analyzing, and reporting data on infections, the CDC's NHSN surveillance methodology and criteria are used by many organizations in the United States and a variety of health care organizations worldwide. In addition to the NHSN HAI Surveillance Criteria,[45] definitions have been established for hemodialysis,[59] long term care,[60] and home health and hospice settings.[61] For international settings, surveillance is discussed in the JCI Standards manual and "International Patient Safety Goals" chapter.[62] As mentioned previously, some countries in the global community also use definitions from the WHO or use definitions of their own design.[63] Detailed information on designing and implementing a surveillance program can be found in Chapter 4.

Developing an Infection Prevention and Control Plan

The written IPC plan is the statement of the identified risks and risk priorities, goals, objectives, action plans, and evaluation method for the IPC activities and progress for a given time period, such as a year. The plan is driven

---

Sidebar 3-7. Tips for Writing an Infection Prevention and Control Plan

- Develop an outline and create a table of contents for the written IPC plan.
- Identify the local, state, and federal regulations and other requirements (that is, accreditation standards and IPC standards and guidelines) that are applicable to the specific heath care setting.
- Review the literature and hospital reports.
- Perform a risk assessment and identify and document the highest-risk priorities.
- Establish goals and develop measurable objectives.
- Develop strategies and set internal and external benchmarks to meet the IPC program's goals and objectives.
- Establish mechanisms for evaluating the effectiveness of the IPC program.
- Set up a system to be notified of any new services or procedures.
- Develop a timeline and assign responsibility for periodically reviewing the plan.
- Ask for review and comments from key staff, such as the infection prevention and control committee (IPCC), quality improvement and patient safety (QPS), nursing.
- Network with infection preventionists who practice in similar health care settings to obtain and share information needed to develop and maintain the IPC program.

---

in large part by the high priorities identified through the risk assessment process and other events, such as sentinel events and new science or regulations. The IPC plan is likely to be updated after each risk assessment is completed. Tool 3-4 provides a sample IPC plan template that can be customized for your organization. Tools 3-5 through 3-8 provide real-world examples of IPC plans and detailed risk assessments.

To develop an IPC plan, consider convening a group that will work collaboratively to contribute various perspectives and expertise to the process. In addition to the topics noted above, issues that should be addressed in the development process include the following:

- Effective and ongoing management of the IPC program
- Infection risks and prevention and control strategies in the clinical and support areas
- Surveillance activities and the written infection surveillance plan
- Outbreak investigation
- Written descriptions of the IPC activities
- Program evaluation process, as determined by the facility
- Occupational safety and health issues
- Emergency planning for IPC
- Communication of IPC information
- Applicable requirements of government, accrediting, and other organizations
- Leadership support and resources allocated

An organization may wish to include with the IPC plan relevant support documents. For example, the surveillance plan and the process for outbreak investigation may be integrated into an overall infection surveillance, prevention, and control plan or may stand as separate written documents and be referenced or placed in an appendix to the IPC plan. Other relevant policies or documents can be managed in the same way. The organization's emergency management plan may reside with another department

such as a facility emergency operations or management plan, and the infection prevention and control response to an influx of infectious patients can be incorporated into that plan and noted or cross-referenced in the IPC plan.

The organization may wish to have a separate IPC plan for each care setting (for example, inpatient, ambulatory surgery, outpatient physician offices or clinic, rehabilitation, hemodialysis, long term acute care). This is the clearest way to ensure that the specific challenges of each division are addressed. Alternatively, the organization may wish to combine the plans for all the sites into one document, being very clear about which goals and activities apply to the different settings. If the plan is being written for a multifacility system with several hospitals, many clinics, and other settings, it may be useful to coordinate selected overall objectives, projects, and studies, such as hand hygiene, while still allowing for the individual objectives for each setting.

Regardless of how an organization chooses to design its infection surveillance, prevention, and control plans, useful documents should be selected to guide activities and measure performance. Table 3-4 on page 83 provides content suggestions for a written IPC plan.

Evaluating the IPC Plan

Each organization should develop its own method for evaluating the IPC plan on a regular basis to ensure that it aligns with organizational performance methods and goals and that it is effective.

Once the plan is completed and approved, it is important to share it with the appropriate staff and departments, as it is these persons who will carry out the recommendations and the activities. Important committees include the IPC committee, the quality improvement and patient safety committee, nursing, medical staff groups, managers, and directors of affected services and administration/leadership.

Summary

This chapter describes and illustrates some key components of the infection surveillance, prevention, and control program related to best practices and Joint Commission Infection Prevention and Control standards and JCI standards. Topics included the following:

- The rationale, methods, and participation for the IPC risk assessment, which can take many forms and is the basis for the IPC plan

Table 3-4. Sample: Annual Hospital Infection Prevention and Control Plan

High-Risk Priority	IPC Goal	Measurable Objective	Method(s)	Evaluation	Participating Staff
CLABSI rate higher than 25% NHSN data	Reduce CLABSI in SICU and MICU	Achieve 30% reduction in SICU and MICU CLABSI from 4.6 to ≤ 1.0/1,000 device-days by December 2021	• Use evidence-based bundle for CLABSI PI team	• Monitor monthly • Report quarterly to staff and ICC	• ICU nursing staff IV team • ICU med staff infection prevention and control
High rate of sharps injuries in surgical staff	Reduce sharps injuries from scalpels	Reduce from 8/quarter to ≤1/quarter scalpel injuries in surgery by March 2021	PI team convened	• Monitor monthly • Report quarterly to OR staff	• OR staff employee health surgeons • Infection prevention and control
Readiness for influx of patients with communicable disease	Develop and test plan for influx of infectious patients with respiratory disease	Triage and care for up to 100 patients per day with respiratory illness in excess of normal admissions for three times during the months of August through October 2021	Develop triage and surge capacity plan with multidisciplinary team	• Test three times by December 2020 • 90% effective care for influx patients according to policy • Report to disaster planning committee	ER Staff: • Physicians • Administration • Admitting • Infection prevention and control • Other

CLABSI, central line–associated bloodstream infection; **ER,** emergency room; **ICC,** Infection Control Committee; **ICU,** intensive care unit; **IV,** intravenous; **MICU,** medical intensive care unit; **NHSN,** National Healthcare Safety Network; **OR,** operating room; **PI,** performance improvement; **SICU,** surgical intensive care unit

- The rationale for each health care setting to design and implement its own risk assessment and IPC plan based on its specific geographic location, population(s) served, services offered, resources, and risk priorities to ensure patient and staff safety
- The purpose for the infection prevention and control plan
- The process of developing measurable and SMART goals and objectives for an IPC plan based on the identified risks, evidence for best practices, mandates, and organizational and programmatic considerations
- Strategies for the risk-driven and evidence-based infection, prevention, and control plan for the many different health care settings
- The evaluation of the infection prevention and control plan
- Relevant Joint Commission standards, Joint Commission International standards, National Patient Safety Goals, and International Patient Safety Goals with practical examples for implementing the standards and goals
- Case studies from the literature to illustrate creative ideas and solutions for selected topics

Resources

Tools to Try

Tool 3-1. Consideration for Designing a Risk Assessment

Tool 3-2. Infection Prevention and Control Risk Assessment for Multidrug-Resistant Organisms (MDROs)

Tool 3-3. Creating SMART Goals for IPC

Tool 3-4. Sample Hospital Infection Prevention and Control Plan Template

Tool 3-5. UC Health: University of Colorado Infection Prevention and Control Plan

Tool 3-6. Missouri Baptist Medical Center Infection Prevention Risk Assessment and Priorities (BJC Healthcare)

Tool 3-7. Barnes-Jewish West County Hospital Risk Assessment and Infection Prevention Priorities (BJC Healthcare)

Tool 3-8. Banner Health Infection Prevention Risk Assessment

Risk Assessment and IPC Plan

- APIC. Yearlong Risk Assessment. Accessed Dec 16, 2020. https://apic.org/Resource_/TinyMceFileManager/Academy/ASC_101_resources/Risk_Assessment/Risk_Assessment_Example_2.docx

- APIC. Annual Risk Assessment and Plan for ASC. Accessed Dec 16, 2020. https://apic.org/Resource_/TinyMceFileManager/Education/ASC_Intensive/Resources_Page/ASC_Risk_Assessment_Template.docx

- CDC. Infection Control Plan for Outpatient Oncology Settings. Accessed Mar 31, 2020. https://www.cdc.gov/hai/pdfs/guidelines/basic-infection-control-prevention-plan-2011.pdf

- CDC. Infection Prevention and Control Assessment Tool for Acute Care Hospitals. Accessed Aug 20, 2020. https://www.cdc.gov/infectioncontrol/pdf/icar/hospital.pdf

- CDC. Infection Prevention and Control Assessment Tool for Long-term Care Facilities. Accessed Aug 20, 2020. https://www.cdc.gov/infectioncontrol/pdf/icar/ltcf.pdf

- CDC. Infection Prevention and Control Assessment Tool for Hemodialysis Facilities. Accessed Mar 31, 2020. https://www.cdc.gov/infectioncontrol/pdf/icar/dialysis.pdf

- Premier Safety Institute. Infection Control Risk Assessment. Accessed Aug 20, 2020. https://www.premiersafetyinstitute.org/safety-topics-az/building-design/infection-control-risk-assessment-icra/

- Wolters Kluwer. How to Perform an Infection Prevention and Control Risk Assessment. Accessed Aug 20, 2020. https://www.wolterskluwer.com/en/expert-insights/how-to-perform-an-infection-prevention-and-control-risk-assessment

- AHCA, NCAL. HVA Assessment Tool Template. Accessed Aug 20, 2020. https://www.ahcancal.org/Survey-Regulatory-Legal/Emergency-Preparedness/Documents/HVA%20template.pdf#search=HVA

- APIC. Content of an Infection Control Plan. Accessed Dec 16, 2020. https://apic.org/Resource_/TinyMceFileManager/Education/ASC_Intensive/Resources_Page/Content_of_an_Infection_Prevention_and_Control_Plan.pdf

- APIC. GHC Infection Control and Employee Health Plan, D-07-003. Accessed Dec 2020. https://apic.org/Resource_/TinyMceFileManager/Academy/ASC_101_resources/Policies-Protocols-Procedures/ISPC_EH_Plan_for_ASC-_sample_policy.doc

- CDC. Basic Infection Control and Prevention Plan for Outpatient Oncology Settings. Accessed Dec 2020. https://www.cdc.gov/hai/settings/outpatient/basic-infection-control-prevention-plan-2011/

- WHO. Guidelines on Core Components of Infection Prevention and Control Programmes at the National and Acute Health Care Facility Level. Accessed Aug 20, 2020. https://www.who.int/publications/i/item/9789241549929

- UNC Medical Center. Infection Control Guidelines for Adult and Pediatric Inpatient Care. Accessed Aug 8, 2020. http://spice.unc.edu/wp-content/uploads/2019/04/Infection-Control-Guidelines-Adult-and-Peds-IC0030.pdf

- CDC. Infection Control Assessment Tool for Acute Care Hospitals. https://www.cdc.gov/infectioncontrol/pdf/icar/hospital.pdf
- CDC. Infection Control Assessment Tool for Long-term Care Facilities. https://www.cdc.gov/infectioncontrol/pdf/icar/ltcf.pdf
- CDC. Infection Control Assessment Tool for Outpatient Settings. https://www.cdc.gov/infectioncontrol/pdf/icar/outpatient.pdf
- CDC. Infection Control Assessment Tool for Hemodialysis Facilities. https://www.cdc.gov/infectioncontrol/pdf/icar/dialysis.pdf

References

1. US Centers for Medicare & Medicaid Services (CMS). Accessed Dec 13, 2020. www.cms.gov

2. US Occupational Safety and Health Administration (OSHA). Accessed Dec 13, 2020. www.osha.com

3. US Centers for Disease Control and Prevention (CDC). Accessed Dec 13, 2020. www.cdc.gov

4. Association for Professionals in Infection Control and Epidemiology (APIC). Accessed Dec 13, 2020. www.apic.org

5. Society for Healthcare Epidemiology of America (SHEA). Accessed Dec 13, 2020. www.shea-online.org

6. Infectious Diseases Society of America (IDSA). Accessed Dec 13, 2020. www.idsociety.org

7. Arias KM. Implementing an effective surveillance program. In *The APIC/JCR Infection Prevention and Control Workbook*, 3rd ed. Oak Brook, IL: Joint Commission Resources, 2017.

8. Soule B, Nadzam D. Performance measures. In *The APIC Text of Infection Control and Epidemiology, Online*, 4th ed. Washington, DC: Association for Professionals in Infection Control and Epidemiology, 2014;17:1–12.

9. Schroder C, et al. Epidemiology of healthcare associated infections in Germany: Nearly 20 years of surveillance. *Int J Med Microbiol.* 2015;305(7):799–806.

10. Al-Mousa HH, et al., Impact of the International Nosocomial Infection Control Consortium (INICC) multidimensional approach on rates of ventilator-associated pneumonia in intensive care units of two hospitals in Kuwait. *J Infect Prev.* 2018;19(4):168–176. doi:10.1177/1757177418759745oi:10.1016/j.ijmm.2015.08.034.

11. Kelly T, Seller D, Ritter J. Mining real world data: Leveraging an infection surveillance system to quantify the impact of clinical interventions. *Am J Infect Control.* 2019 Jun;47(6):S48. DOI: https://doi.org/10.1016/j.ajic.20ai.04.120.

12. Kaya GK, et al. Framework to support risk assessment in hospitals. *Int J Qual Health Care.* 2019;31(5):393–401.

13. Kuntz JL, et al. Predicting the risk of *Clostridium difficile* infection upon admission: A score to identify patients for antimicrobial stewardship efforts. *Perm J.* 2016;20(1):20–25. doi:10.7812/TPP/15-049.

14. Stroever, S. Qualitative research methods. In *The APIC Text of Infection Control and Epidemiology*, 4th ed. Washington, DC: Association for Professionals in Infection Control and Epidemiology, 2014;19:1–17.

15. Zinatsa F, et al. Voices from the frontline: Barriers and strategies to improve tuberculosis infection control in primary health care facilities in South Africa. *BMC Health Serv Res.* 2018;18(1):269. doi:10.1186/s12913-018-3083-0. Accessed Dec 16, 2020. https://bmchealthservres.biomedcentral.com/articles/10.1186/s12913-018-3083-0

16. Cox L, et al. Some limitations of qualitative risk rating systems. *Risk Anal.* 2005 Jun;25(3):651–662. Accessed Dec 13, 2020. https://doi.org/10.1111/j.1539-6924.2005.00615m.x

17. The Joint Commission. The Joint Commission's Implementation Guide for NPSG .07.05.01 on Surgical Site Infection: The SSI Change Project. Accessed Dec 13, 2020. https://www.jointcommission.org/-/media/tjc/documents/resources/hai/implementation_guide_for_npsg_ssipdf.pdf

18. CDC. Public Health Professional Gateway: Do a SWOT Analysis: Evaluate a CoP. Accessed Dec 13, 2020. https://www.cdc.gov/phcommunities/resourcekit/evaluate/swot_analysis.html

19. Larson E, Aiello AE. Systematic risk assessment methods for the infection control professional. *Am J Infect Control*. 2006 Jun;34(5):323–326.

20. The Joint Commission. Sentinel Event Policy and Procedures. Accessed Dec 3, 2020. https://www.jointcommission.org/resources/patient-safety-topics/sentinel-event/sentinel-event-policy-and-procedures/

21. Chami K, et al. Guidelines for infection control in nursing homes: A Delphi consensus web-based survey. *J Hosp Infect*. 2011;79(1):75–89.

22. US Food and Drug Administration. Hazard Analysis Critical Control Point (HACCP) Principles and Application Guidelines. Accessed Dec 12, 2020. https://www.fda.gov/food/hazard-analysis-critical-control-point-haccp/haccp-principles-application-guidelines#app-c

23. US Food and Drug Administration. HAACP Principles and Application Guidelines. Accessed Dec 13, 2020. https://www.fda.gov/food/hazard-analysis-critical-control-point-haccp/haccp-principles-application-guidelines#

24. Quality-One. Healthcare FMEA (HFMEA). Accessed Dec 12, 2020. https://quality-one.com/hfmea/

25 The SAFER Matrix: A New Scoring Methodology. *Jt Comm Perspect*. 2016 May;36(5):1, 3.

26. TJC Launches New SAFER Scoring Matrix. *Hosp Peer Rev*. 2016 Jul;41(7):82–83.

27. The Joint Commission. Tracer Methodology. Accessed Dec 2, 2020. https://www.jointcommission.org/-/media/tjc/documents/fact-sheets/tracer-methodology-6-1-2020.pdf?db=web&hash=1AE38A490C184D0632EE6626605A221A

28. California Hospital Association. Hazard Vulnerability Assessment. Accessed Dec 12, 2020. https://www.calhospitalprepare.org/hazard-vulnerability-analysis

29. Apisarnthanarak A, et al. Hospital infection prevention and control issues relevant to extensive floods. *Infect Control Hosp Epidemiol*. 2013 Feb;34(2):200–206.

30. CDC. Healthcare Water System Repair and Recovery following a Boil Water Alert or Disruption of Water Supply. Accessed Nov 29, 2020. https://www.cdc.gov/disasters/watersystemrepair.html

31. Karkey A, et al. Outbreaks of *Serratia marcescens* and *Serratia rubidaea* bacteremia in a central Kathmandu hospital following the 2015 earthquakes. *Trans R Soc Trop Med Hyg*. 2018;112(10):467–472. doi:10.1093/trstmh/try077.

32. CDC. Preparedness and Safety Messaging for Hurricanes, Flooding, and Similar Disasters. Accessed Dec 10, 2020. https://www.cdc.gov/cpr/readiness/hurricane_messages.htm

33. APIC. Infection Prevention Tips for Flood and Hurricane Season. Accessed Dec 3, 2020. https://apic.org/wp-content/uploads/2019/02/Flood_and_hurricane_infection_prevention_tips.pdf

34. CDC. Remediation and Infection Control Considerations for Reopening Healthcare Facilities Closed Due to Extensive Water and Wind Damage. May 2007. Accessed Dec 12, 2020. https://stacks.cdc.gov/view/cdc/39588

35. David S, et al. Epidemic of carbapenem-resistant *Klebsiella pneumoniae* in Europe is driven by nosocomial spread. *Nat Microbiol*. 2019;4(11):1919–1929. doi:10.1038/s41564-019-0492-8.

36. Hopman J, et al. Risk assessment after a severe hospital-acquired infection associated with carbapenemase-producing *Pseudomonas aeruginosa*. *JAMA Netw Open*. 2019;2(2):e187665.

37. Herrera-Ibatá DM, et al. Quantitative approach for the risk assessment of African swine fever and classical swine fever introduction into the United States through legal imports of pigs and swine products. *PLOS ONE*. 2017 Aug;12(8):e0182850. https://doi.org/10.1371/journal.pone.0182850.

38. Stern AM, Cetron MS, Markel H. The 1918–1919 influenza pandemic in the United States: Lessons learned and challenges exposed. *Public Health Rep.* 2010;125(Suppl 3):6–8. doi:10.1177/00333549101250S303.

39. Morens DM, et al. Pandemic COVID-19 joins history's pandemic legion. *mBio.* 2020;11(3):e00812-20. doi:10.1128/mBio.00812-20.

40. Rebmann T, Vassallo A, Holdsworth JE. Availability of personal protective equipment and infection prevention supplies during the first month of the COVID-19 pandemic: A national study by the APIC COVID-19 task force. *Am J Infect Control.* 2021 Apr;49(4):434–437. doi:10.1016/j.ajic.2020.08.029.

41. Duffy J, et al. Mucormycosis outbreak associated with hospital linens. *Pediatr Infect Dis J.* 2014;33(5):472–476.

42. Lazary A, et al. Reduction of healthcare–associated infections in a long-term care brain injury ward by replacing regular linens with biocidal copper oxide impregnated linens. *Int J Infect Dis.* 2014;24:23–29. doi:10.1016/j.ijid.2014.01.022.

43. Howorth FH. Prevention of airborne infection during surgery. *Lancet.* 1985 Feb;1(8425):386–388. doi: 10.1016/s0140-6736(85)91399-6.

44. Chauveaux D. Preventing surgical-site infections: Measures other than antibiotics. *Orthop Traumatol Surg Res.* 2015 Feb;101(1 Suppl):S77–S83. doi: 10.1016/j.otsr.2014.07.028.

45. CDC, National Safety Healthcare Network (NHSN). CDC/NHSN Surveillance Definitions for Specific Types of Infections. Accessed Dec 1, 2020. https://www.cdc.gov/nhsn/pdfs/pscmanual/17pscnosinfdef_current.pdf

46. CMS. Outcome and Assessment Information Set (OASIS-D) Guidance Manual. Effective January 1, 2019. Accessed Dec 5, 2020. https://www.cms.gov/Medicare/Quality-Initiatives-Patient-Assessment-Instruments/HomeHealthQualityInits/Downloads/draft-OASIS-D-Guidance-Manual-7-2-2018.pdf

47. Bischoff P, et al. Surveillance of external ventricular drainage-associated meningitis and ventriculitis in German intensive care units. *Infect Control Hosp Epidemiol.* 2020 Apr;41(4):452–457.

48. Journal of Infectious Diseases & Therapy. Benchmarking of Healthcare-Associated Infections in Gulf Cooperation Council (GCC) States. Accessed Dec 13, 2020. https://www.omicsonline.org/proceedings/benchmarking-of-healthcareassociated-infections-in-gulf-cooperation-council-gcc-states-72495.html

49. WHO. WHO Global Guidelines for the Prevention of Surgical Site Infection. Accessed Dec 2, 2020. https://www.who.int/gpsc/SSI-outline.pdf

50. Ban KA, et al. Executive summary of the American College of Surgeons/Surgical Infection Society Surgical Site Infection Guidelines–2016 Update. *Surg Infect (Larchmt).* 2017 May/Jun;18(4):379–382. doi: 10.1089/sur.2016.214.

51. Soule BM. Evidence-based principles and practices to prevent surgical site infections. Oak Brook, IL: Joint Commission Resources, Jun 2018. Accessed Dec 2. 2020. http://jointcommissioninternational.org

52. Berríos-Torres SI, et al. Centers for Disease Control and Prevention guideline for the prevention of surgical site infection, 2017. *JAMA Surg.* 2017 Aug;152(8):784–791. doi: 10.1001/jamasurg.2017.0904. Erratum in *JAMA Surg.* 2017 Aug;152(8):803.

53. Florschutsz AV, et al. Surgical site infection risk factors and risk stratification. *J Am Acad Orthop Surg.* 2015 Apr;23(Suppl):S8–S11.

54. CMS. §482.42 Condition of Participation: Infection Prevention and Control and Antibiotic Stewardship Programs. In *State Operations Manual: Appendix A—Survey Protocol, Regulations and Interpretive Guidelines for Hospitals.* Accessed Mar 22, 2020. https://www.cms.gov/Regulations-and-Guidance/Guidance/Manuals/downloads/som107ap_a_hospitals.pdf

55. CMS. Conditions for Coverage (CfC): Infection Control. In *State Operations Manual Appendix L—Guidance for Surveyors: Ambulatory Surgical Centers* (Rev. 200, 2-12-20). Apr 1, 2015. Accessed Dec 12, 2020. https://www.cms. gov/Regulations-and-Guidance/ Guidance/Manuals/downloads/som107ap_l_ ambulatory.pdf

56. Gould DJ, et al. Interventions to improve hand hygiene compliance in patient care. *Cochrane Database Syst Rev.* 2017;9(9):CD005186. doi:10.1002/14651858.CD005186. Accessed Aug 20, 2020. https://doi.org/10.1002/14651858. CD005186.pub4

57. Ojanperä H, Kanste OI, Syrjala H. Hand-hygiene compliance by hospital staff and incidence of health-care–associated infections, Finland. *Bull World Health Organ.* 2020;98(7):475–483. doi:10.2471/BLT.19.247494.

58. The Joint Commission. Measuring Hand Hygiene Adherence: Overcoming the Challenges. 2009. Accessed Dec 13, 2020. https://www.jointcommission.org/assets/1/18/hh_ monograph.pdf

59. CDC. Tracking Infections in Outpatient Dialysis Facilities. Accessed Dec 2, 2020. https://www.cdc.gov/nhsn/dialysis/index.html

60. Stone ND, et al. Surveillance definitions of infections in long- term care facilities: Revisiting the McGeer Criteria. *Infect Control Hosp Epidemiol.* 2012 Oct; 33(10):965–977.

61. Embry FC, Chinnes LF. APIC-HICPAC Surveillance Definitions for Home Health Care and Home Hospice Infections. Feb 2008. Accessed Dec 13, 2020. http://www.apic.org/Resource_/ TinyMceFileManager/Practice_Guidance/HH-Surv-Def.pdf

62. Joint Commission International. "International Patient Safety Goals." In *Joint Commission International Accreditation Standards for Hospitals*, 7th ed. Oak Brook, IL: Joint Commission Resources, 2021.

63. Parmar. MM, et al. Airborne infection control in India: Baseline assessment of health facilities. *Indian J Tuberc.* 2015 Oct;62(4):211–217. doi: 10.1016/j. ijtb.2015.11.006.

Chapter 4

Planning and Implementing an Effective Surveillance Program

By Kathleen Meehan Arias, MS, MT(ASCP), SM(AAM), CIC, FAPIC

Disclaimer: Strategies, tools, and examples discussed in this book do not necessarily reflect Joint Commission or Joint Commission International requirements for all settings. Always refer to the most current standards applicable to your health care setting to ensure compliance.

Introduction

Infection prevention and control (IPC) surveillance refers to the ongoing and systematic collection, analysis, interpretation, and dissemination of health data to provide meaningful information that can be used to inform infection risks, epidemiologically important organisms, antimicrobial resistant organisms, emerging infectious diseases, and outbreaks so that measures and practices can be implemented to reduce IPC risks. Surveillance activities should be planned and implemented as an integral component of an overall IPC program.

Federal, local, state, and accrediting agencies require surveillance programs in a variety of health care settings, including hospitals, ambulatory surgery centers and other outpatient centers, long term care (LTC), dialysis, home care, rehabilitation, and behavioral health care and human services. One goal of an IPC program is to prevent health care–associated infections (HAIs). Surveillance data have effectively been used to reduce the occurrence of infections by identifying IPC risk factors, implementing and monitoring the use of risk-reduction measures, and assessing the effectiveness of IPC interventions.[1-4]

The purpose of this chapter is to identify Joint Commission and Joint Commission International (JCI) standards related to surveillance in the "Infection Prevention and Control" (IC) and "Prevention and Control of Infection" (PCI) chapters, respectively, and to provide strategies, examples, and best practices to meet those requirements. This chapter specifically discusses topics related to the following:

- Planning surveillance
- Implementing the surveillance plan
- Reporting and using surveillance data
- Outbreak identification, investigation, and control

The standards discussed in this chapter are listed in the boxes on the following pages. Some of the elements of performance (EPs) and measurable elements (MEs) are addressed in detail in other chapters, as noted, and are discussed here only as they relate to an organization's need to incorporate surveillance activities into an infection surveillance, prevention, and control program.

Relevant Joint Commission Standards Addressed in This Chapter

Note: These standards were in effect at the time of publication. They refer to Joint Commission standards effective January 1, 2021. Always consult the most recent version of Joint Commission standards for the most accurate requirements for your setting.

Planning for Surveillance

IC.01.03.01 The [organization] identifies risks for acquiring and transmitting infections.

EP 1 The [organization] identifies risk for acquiring and transmitting infections based on the following: Its geographic location, community, and population served; the care, treatment, and services it provides; and the analysis of surveillance activities and other infection control data.

IC.01.05.01 The [organization] has an infection prevention and control plan.

EP 2 The [organization's] infection prevention and control plan includes a written description of the activities, including surveillance, to minimize, reduce, or eliminate the risk of infection.

Implementing Surveillance

IC.02.01.01 The [organization] implements its infection prevention and control plan.

EP 1 The [organization] implements its infection prevention and control activities, including surveillance, to minimize, reduce or eliminate the risk of infection. (*See also* MM.09.01.01, EP 5)

EP 8 The [organization] reports infection surveillance, prevention, and control information to the appropriate staff within the [organization].

EP 9 The [organization] reports infection surveillance, prevention, and control information to local, state, and federal public health authorities in accordance with law and regulation.

EP 10 When the [organization] becomes aware that it transferred a patient who has an infection requiring monitoring, treatment, and/or isolation, it informs the receiving organization.

EP 11 When the [organization] becomes aware that it received a patient from another organization who has an infection requiring action, and the infection was not communicated by the referring organization, it informs the referring organization.

Note: *Infections requiring actions include those that require isolation and/or public health reporting or those that may aid in the referring organization's surveillance.*

IC.02.04.01 The [organization] offers vaccination against influenza to licensed independent practitioners and staff.

EP 9 The [organization] provides influenza vaccination rate data to key stakeholders which may include leaders, licensed independent practitioners, nursing staff, and other staff at least annually.

LD.03.02.01 The [organization] uses data and information to guide decisions and to understand variation in the performance of processes supporting safety and quality.

Outbreak Investigation

IC.01.05.01 The [organization] has an infection prevention and control plan.

EP 5 The [organization] describes, in writing, the process for investigating outbreaks of infectious disease. (*See also* IC.02.01.01, EP 5)

IC.02.01.01 The [organization] implements its infection prevention and control plan.

EP 5 The [organization] investigates outbreaks of infectious disease. (*See also* IC.01.05.01, EP 5)

Relevant Joint Commission International (JCI) Standards Addressed in This Chapter

Note: These standards were in effect at the time of publication. They refer to the *Joint Commission International Accreditation Standards for Hospitals, seventh edition,* ©2020. Always consult the most recent version of Joint Commission International standards for the most accurate requirements for your hospital or medical center setting.

Planning for Surveillance

PCI.5 The hospital uses a risk-based data-driven approach in establishing the focus of the health care–associated infection and prevention program.

ME 1 The hospital establishes the focus of the program through the collection and tracking of data related to respiratory tract, urinary tract, intravascular invasive devices, surgical sites, epidemiologically significant diseases and organisms, and emerging or reemerging infections with the community.

ME 2 The data collected in respiratory tract, urinary tract, intravascular invasive devices, surgical sites, epidemiologically significant diseases and organisms, and emerging or reemerging infections with the community are analyzed to identify priorities for reducing rates of infection.

PCI.5.1 The hospital identifies areas at high risk for infection by conducting a risk assessment, develops interventions to address these risks, and monitors the effectiveness.

ME 1 The hospital completes and documents a risk assessment, at least annually, to identify and prioritize areas at high risk for infections.

Implementing Surveillance

PCI.1. One or more individuals oversee all infection prevention and control activities. This individual(s) is qualified in infection prevention and control practices through education, training, experience, certification, and/or clinical authority.

ME 5 The hospital reports infection prevention and control program results to public health agencies as required.

ME 6 The hospital takes appropriate action on reports from relevant public health agencies.

PCI.12.1 The hospital develops and implements a process to manage a sudden influx of patients with airborne infections and when negative-pressure rooms are not available.

ME 2 The hospital develops and implements a process for managing an influx of patients with contagious diseases.

PCI.14 The infection prevention and control process is integrated with the hospital's overall program for quality improvement and patient safety, using measures that are epidemiologically important to the hospital.

ME 2 The hospital collects and analyzes data for the infection prevention and control activities, and the data include epidemiologically important infections.

ME 3 The hospital uses monitoring data to evaluate and support improvements to the infection prevention and control program at least annually.

ME 4 Monitoring data include benchmarking infection rates.

ME 5 The infection prevention and control program documents monitoring data and provides reports of data analysis to leadership on a quarterly basis.

PCI.15 The hospital provides education on infection prevention and control practices to staff, physicians, patients, families, and other caregivers when indicated by their involvement in care.

(continued)

ME 4 The hospital communicates findings and trends from quality improvement activities to all staff and included as part of staff education.

Outbreak Investigation

PCI.4. The hospital designs and implements a comprehensive infection prevention and control program that identifies the procedures and processes associated with the risk of infection and implements strategies to reduce infection risk.

ME 3 The hospital identifies those processes associated with infection risk.

Strategies for Planning a Surveillance Program

One of the first steps in planning or updating an organization's surveillance program is to identify the leaders, managers, and others who can influence health care practices or provide technical support for data collection, management, and analysis. The organization should then assemble a working group to plan and provide ongoing support for the surveillance program. This group should be composed of the person (or persons) responsible for the daily management of the IPC program and individuals from a variety of patient/resident care services and support services, depending on the organization's needs, size, and scope of care. These individuals are typically from patient/resident care services, medical staff, nursing, laboratory, pharmacy, quality assurance/performance improvement, and information/data management services. The group should be delegated the following responsibilities:

- Identifying the essential components of an effective surveillance plan that aligns with the organization's needs, external requirements, and accreditation standards
- Creating a written surveillance plan that includes these essential components
- Incorporating the written surveillance plan into the organization's written IPC plan (see Chapter 3)
- Supporting the implementation and assessment of surveillance and IPC activities

The standards do not specify the elements of an effective surveillance program in a health care organization. However, much has been published about surveillance for a variety of health care settings and the elements that should be included.[5-13] Those responsible for planning, developing, managing, and implementing the surveillance program should refer to those publications and the additional resources listed at the end of this chapter.

When developing a surveillance program, ensure that the essential components listed in Sidebar 4-1 on page 93 are considered.

Using Surveillance Activities and Data to Identify Infection Risks

One of the main purposes for conducting surveillance is to provide meaningful information for an organization to identify risks so that IPC activities to reduce those risks can be determined and implemented. An important step when planning the surveillance program is selecting appropriate health-related events (indicators) to monitor.[5]

Before an organization can plan or update its surveillance program, it should conduct a facility risk assessment. Detailed methods for conducting the risk assessment are described in Chapter 3. Those developing the program should identify what events and indicators to monitor, based on the following:

- Facility risk assessment
- Federal, local, state, accrediting, public health, and other relevant agency requirements, including mandatory reporting requirements
- Availability of the data needed
- Available staff and other resources (for example, information technology, informatics)
- Quality assurance/performance improvement initiatives
- Organizational needs and objectives

Sidebar 4-1. Components of an Effective Surveillance Program

1. Assess and define the population(s) to be monitored (for example, the types of patients most commonly served, the most common diagnoses, the most frequently performed surgical or invasive procedures, and whether the organization's strategic plan focuses on particular groups of patients, such as those at increased risk for infection).
2. Choose the events/indicators to be monitored (for example, processes or outcomes such as treatment costs, length of stay, mortality, and other events of importance to the organization or those most relevant to the population served). It is rarely feasible to conduct organizationwide surveillance for all events.
3. Identify published and validated surveillance criteria/case definitions. For example, if surveillance is conducted for primary bloodstream infections associated with central line use in the surgical intensive care unit in order to compare the organization's findings to data from the Centers for Disease Control and Prevention (CDC) National Healthcare Safety Network database, the CDC case definition for primary bloodstream infections should be used. The definition should be standardized, previously published, and validated for accuracy, consistency, and reproducibility.
4. Select the surveillance methodology (for example, active, passive, prospective, retrospective).
5. Determine the time period for observation.
6. Identify data elements to be collected (for example, patient charts/records, communication with care providers, admission diagnosis reports, surgical schedule/database).
7. Determine methods for data collection, management, analysis, and reporting.
8. Identify recipients of surveillance data and reports. Surveillance data should be shared with those health care providers who are most able to positively affect and improve patient care. Reporting should be systematic and timely.
9. Design interpretive surveillance reports.
10. Use surveillance findings in quality assurance/performance improvement activities.
11. Develop and implement a written surveillance plan, using all of the above components.
12. Design and implement a method for periodically evaluating the effectiveness of the surveillance program. The surveillance program should be evaluated regularly alongside the overall infection prevention and control plan.

The surveillance program should measure outcomes of health care, processes (practices) of health care, and events of importance to the organization.[5-10] Choose measures that provide information to be used in performance improvement initiatives related to IPC practices and outcomes. Some measures should focus on staff. Monitor both high-risk, high-volume events and low-volume high-risk events in specific populations, as identified by the facility risk assessment. Select infections and other events for which there are previously published and validated criteria that reflect generally accepted definitions of the disease or event being monitored. Criteria have been published for defining HAIs in a variety of health care settings, including hospitals, long term care, and home care.[10-13]

When possible, monitor infections for which there are nationally available benchmark data that can be used for meaningful comparison. For example, the US Centers for Disease Control and Prevention (CDC) National Healthcare Safety Network (NHSN)[11] focuses on data related to infections associated with medical devices (bloodstream infections, central line–insertion practices, ventilator-associated events), procedure-associated infections (surgical site infections), antimicrobial use and resistance, multidrug-resistant organisms, and Novel Coronavirus 2019/COVID-19. Ensure that all individuals who conduct surveillance activities and identify HAI cases apply recognized surveillance criteria precisely and consistently. A thorough discussion of the essential elements and activities of IPC surveillance programs is beyond the scope of this chapter. For additional information on developing and implementing surveillance programs in a variety of health care settings, refer to the articles and supplemental resources listed at the end of this chapter.[5-13]

Examples of the types of surveillance events and performance measures to monitor can be found in Table 4-1 on pages 95–96. In addition to these events, some organizations use active surveillance to monitor specific organisms (for example, methicillin-resistant *Staphylococcus aureus* or carbapenem-resistant *Enterobacteriaceae*) or diseases (for example, hepatitis B or COVID-19). Active surveillance involves taking prospective steps to identify patients who have or may develop HAIs by using standardized definitions, predetermined criteria, and protocols that result in risk-adjusted HAI incidence rates.

If rates are to be calculated, ensure that data for both the numerator (number of persons with a specified condition) and the denominator (total number of persons at risk for that condition) are available. Tips for choosing surveillance events and performance measures can be found in Sidebar 4-2.

Elements of a Written Surveillance Plan

In addition to incorporating the essential components noted in Sidebar 4-1, the written surveillance plan should also include the following:

- Surveillance program purpose, goals, and measurable objectives (*See* Chapter 3 for a discussion on how to create goals and measurable objectives.)
- Description of applicable reporting requirements of local, state, federal, and other relevant agencies
- Reason for selecting each event monitored (See examples in Table 4-1.)
- Process and frequency used to evaluate the surveillance program

The elements in a surveillance plan will depend on the type and needs of the organization. It is necessary to conduct a risk assessment and identify organizational needs, relevant regulations, and accreditation and other requirements prior to developing both the surveillance and IPC plans. Once the written surveillance plan is completed, it must be incorporated into, or attached to, the organization's IPC plan, as discussed in Chapter 3. An example of how the surveillance plan can be

incorporated into the overall IPC plan can be found in Tool 4-1. In addition, Tool 4-2 provides guidelines for developing an infection surveillance, prevention, and control (ISPC) program and a written ISPC plan.

Table 4-1. Examples of Types of Surveillance Events and Performance Measures to Monitor

Outcome Measures	Potential Reasons for Selecting Measure
Device-associated infections, such as central line–associated bloodstream infection, catheter-associated urinary tract infections, and ventilator-associated pneumonia	• Monitor and improve patient outcomes • National data available from NHSN to compare the organization's performance with that of others • Internal organization performance improvement requirement • Public/mandatory reporting requirement • Other external requirement*
Surgical site infections following a specific operative procedure, such as hip and knee replacements and cardiac thoracic surgeries	• Monitor and improve patient outcomes • Internal organization performance improvement requirement • Public/mandatory reporting requirement • External requirement*
Sharps injuries and blood/body fluid exposures in staff	• Monitor and improve • Internal organization performance improvement requirement • External requirement*
Infection or colonization with a specific organism (e.g., MRSA, VRE, MDRO gram-negative organisms, *Clostridium difficile*, respiratory syncytial virus, rotavirus)	• Monitor occurrence rates in patients and residents • Detect occurrence to trigger implementation of measures to prevent transmission • External requirement*
Process Measures	
Staff compliance with infection prevention protocols, such as the following: • Hand hygiene • Standard precautions • Transmission-based precautions • Central line insertion, maintenance, and removal • Urinary catheter indications, insertion, maintenance, and removal • Safe injection, infusion, and medication handling practices • Use of PPE • Instrument/medical device processing • Sterilization quality assurance testing • Environmental cleaning and disinfection • Communicable disease reporting • Antimicrobial prescribing and administration • Installing and maintaining barriers during construction and renovation projects • Disposal, storing, and handing of regulated medical/infectious waste	• Monitor and improve staff adherence to recommended practices • Internal organization performance improvement requirement • External requirement*

(continued)

Table 4-1. Examples of Types of Surveillance Events and Performance Measures to Monitor (continued)

Other Events	Potential Reasons for Selecting Measure
Influenza immunization rates in staff, residents, or patients	• Monitor and improve staff compliance with the organization's influenza immunization program • Monitor compliance with CMS or other external requirement*
Syndromes or organisms indicative of an emerging infectious disease or bioterrorist event	• Public health recommendation to detect emerging infectious diseases • External requirement*
Quality assurance testing (e.g., monitoring of negative airflow in airborne infection isolation rooms, biological monitoring of sterilizers, testing of high-level disinfectants)	• Monitor and ensure staff adherence to required practices • Internal organization performance improvement requirement • External requirement*
Patients or residents admitted with an antibiotic-resistant organism	• Detect occurrence to trigger implementation of measures to prevent transmission
Compliance with requirement that the organization notifies a receiving facility when it has transferred a patient/resident who has an infection requiring monitoring, treatment, and/or isolation	• Detect occurrence so appropriate actions can be taken by the receiving organization

* External reporting requirements include those of local, state, federal, public health, and accrediting agencies.

CMS, Centers for Medicare & Medicaid Services; **MRSA,** methicillin-resistant *Staphylococcus aureus*; **NHSN,** National Healthcare Safety Network; **OSHA,** US Occupational Safety and Health Administration; **PPE,** personal protective equipment; **VRE,** vancomycin-resistant enterococci

Evaluating the Components of the Surveillance Program

An organization must periodically evaluate its surveillance program to assess its ability to meet its needs and objectives. It should compare the program's structure and activities with the organization's needs and with current evidence-based practices and published recommendations for surveillance programs in similar settings. The evaluation should also consider changes in the organization's identified IPC risks, such as the occurrence of emerging infectious diseases, an increase in antibiotic-resistant organisms, and new services and procedures provided by the organization.

Those evaluating the surveillance program should ask the following questions:
• Does the program contain all essential elements? (See the list in Sidebar 4-1.)
• Are data collected, managed, analyzed, and reported by knowledgeable staff qualified by training and experience?
• Are the data needed easily available?
• Are surveillance activities able to identify infections associated with care, treatment, or services?
• Are surveillance activities conducted in accordance with published recommendations for surveillance programs in similar settings?
• Does the program meet the latest requirements of local, state, federal, accrediting, and other relevant agencies?

- Have surveillance findings been used effectively to improve adherence to IPC practices and reduce and control HAIs? (*See Chapter 11 for a discussion of this topic.*)
- Are resources (staff and other resources) adequate to meet the surveillance needs of the organization?

The evaluation of the surveillance program should be documented in writing, including an assessment of the allocation of adequate staff and other resources. Additional information on developing and implementing surveillance programs in a variety of health care settings is provided in the supplemental resources and articles listed at the end of this chapter.[5–10,14]

Table 4-2 on pages 98–99 is a checklist that health care organizations can use when developing and evaluating a surveillance program for a health care facility.

Implementing the Surveillance Program

Joint Commission Standard IC.02.01.01 and JCI standards PCI.1, PCI.5, PCI.14, and PCI.15 require that accredited organizations implement their IPC plan. Eleven EPs fall under this Joint Commission standard; however, this chapter discusses only the five EPs that relate to surveillance activities (EPs 1 and 8–11). Other EPs under this standard are discussed in subsequent chapters and are discussed here only briefly.

One of the main functions of a surveillance program is to provide information for an organization to identify IPC risks in patients, residents, and staff. There are many published reports that demonstrate how surveillance data can identify potential problems and risk factors for infection, implement IPC measures, and document the reduction of infection rates in a variety of health care settings.[1–4] Refer to Chapter 6 for information on implementing practices to reduce the risk of infection.

Surveillance is used to monitor IPC practices and outcomes in patients and residents. Written surveillance reports should be disseminated periodically to the following staff within the organization:
- Leaders, managers, and frontline health care staff who can affect IPC practices in the organization to improve outcomes
- Administrators, members of the board of directors, and medical directors who can support performance

improvement activities and the staff and other resources of the IPC program

A well-written report can provide critical information to stimulate performance improvement activities. Tool 4-4 provides guidance for developing an informative surveillance report. This tool can be downloaded and used as a guideline for all types of health care settings.

The following examples show how an organization can demonstrate compliance with these requirements:
- A long term care facility provides meeting minutes demonstrating that the person responsible for the IPC program attends quality assurance/performance improvement or quality improvement and patient safety committee meetings. This individual regularly provides a written report to the committee and discusses surveillance findings that may identify potential areas for improvement.
- IPC staff participate in leadership rounds with leaders and frontline staff to discuss unit-based data on HAIs and evidence-based IPC measures to prevent them.[15]

IPC staff should also prepare a comprehensive written annual report for the administrator and members of the committee with oversight of the infection surveillance, prevention, and control program. (Note that for JCI accredited organizations, a quarterly report to leadership is required.)

Tool 4-5 provides a sample table of contents for an annual report of the infection surveillance, prevention, and control program. The comprehensive report should summarize the IPC department's activities for a calendar year combined with the surveillance plan for the following year. Appendixes can describe the findings of the program's monitored events, such as HAIs, antimicrobial stewardship, staff immunization rates, and sharps injuries and exposures to staff. Tool 4-6 is a sample summary

Table 4-2. Checklist for Developing and Assessing a Surveillance Program

	Yes	No	If No, note plan for remediation
The surveillance program includes the following essential elements:			
1. Facility risk assessment (populations and services defined and risks identified)			
2. Outcome, process, and other events/indicators to be monitored			
3. Identification of surveillance requirements of state, federal, accrediting, and other relevant agencies			
4. Defined surveillance criteria/case definitions that include validated, published definitions for health care–associated infections (HAIs)			
5. Time period for observation determined			
6. Identification of data elements to be collected			
7. Methods for data collection and management			
8. Methods for data analysis			
9. Process for reporting infection surveillance, prevention, and control information within the organization and to external agencies/organizations			
10. Identification of recipients of surveillance data and reports			
11. Use of interpretive surveillance reports			
12. Use of surveillance findings in quality assurance/ performance improvement activities			
13. Written surveillance plan			
14. Method for periodically evaluating effectiveness of the program			

(continued)

Table 4-2. Checklist for Developing and Assessing a Surveillance Program (continued)

The written surveillance plan includes all the above elements plus the following:			
	Yes	**No**	**If No, note plan for remediation**
1. Surveillance program purpose, goals, and measurable objectives			
2. Description of applicable reporting requirements of state, federal, accrediting, and other relevant agencies			
3. Reason for selecting each event monitored (outcome, process/practice, and other)			
4. Process and frequency for reporting influenza vaccination rates to staff and other key stakeholders			
5. Process and frequency for evaluation of the surveillance program, including requirement for written documentation of evaluation			
Program evaluation questions			
	Yes	**No**	**If No, note plan for remediation**
Does the program contain all the elements listed above?			
Are data collected, managed, analyzed, and reported by knowledgeable staff qualified by training and experience?			
Are the data needed easily available?			
Do surveillance activities identify infections associated with care, treatment, or services in the facility?			
Are surveillance activities conducted in accordance with published recommendations for surveillance programs in similar settings?			
Does the program meet the latest requirements of state, federal, accrediting, and other relevant agencies?			
Have surveillance findings effectively been used to improve adherence to infection prevention practices and reduce the risk/occurrence of HAIs?			
Are staff and other resources adequate to meet the surveillance needs of the organization?			
Is there written documentation of the program evaluation?			

Source: Arias Infection Prevention and Control Consulting. Used with permission.

report on prioritized risks, objectives, IPC strategies, and evaluation of effectiveness. Tool 4-7 is a sample surveillance tool for long term care facilities that can be customized for other settings. See the Supplemental Resources section at the end of this chapter for setting-specific surveillance resources and guides.

TRY THESE TOOLS

Tool 4-5. Sample Table of Contents for ISPC Program Annual Report and Plan

Tool 4-6. Sample Infection Prevention and Control (IPC) Surveillance Plan Summary

Tool 4-7. Vancouver Island Health Authority: Daily Infection Prevention and Control Surveillance Tool for Long Term Care Facilities

---

Timely Reporting of Infection Information Data

Infection preventionists (IPs) and health care organizations play a vital role in providing information and data to local, state, and federal public health authorities. Communitywide outbreaks have been recognized after IPs and other health care workers have reported surveillance findings and diseases to local and state health departments.[16] Timely reporting of disease occurrence is critical to identify and control outbreaks and rapidly spreading epidemics, as demonstrated during the COVID-19 pandemic caused by the severe acute respiratory syndrome coronavirus 2 (SARS-CoV-2). During the COVID-19 pandemic, health care organizations helped to reduce the risk of communitywide spread by reporting cases to public health authorities, who used the data to monitor spread and target IPC measures.

In addition to public health authorities, health care organizations are required to report a variety of infection surveillance information to other external organizations. For example, health care organizations must meet mandatory reporting requirements for reporting HAIs and other data to external quality measurement agencies. Requirements for reporting data to external organizations are discussed in more detail in Chapter 10.

Some examples of how an organization can show compliance with the requirements to report information to external organizations include the following:

- The organization's surveillance plan describes its reporting program to the CDC NHSN, as required by its state health care quality agency.
- The organization can provide examples of the reports it receives from NHSN.
- The IP at a long term care facility periodically distributes to its medical and nursing staff a list of diseases and conditions that must be reported to the local health department. The IP maintains a database of reported cases.

Transmission of infections between health care facilities happens when an infectious patient or resident is transferred between facilities and the necessary IPC practices are not used. When a Joint Commission–accredited organization becomes aware that it has transferred to another facility a patient or resident who has an infection requiring monitoring, treatment, or isolation, it must inform the receiving organization. JCI-accredited organizations should follow local regulations. An example of appropriate reporting would be the following: When a nursing home transfers a resident known to be colonized with a carbapenem-resistant *Enterobacteriaceae* to an acute care hospital, it notifies the hospital in writing that the resident is colonized with this organism and must be treated with contact precautions.

A health care facility must have a protocol for informing a referring facility that it has received one of its patients or residents who has an infection requiring action when the infection was not communicated by the referring facility. This allows the referring facility to determine if any actions are needed to prevent the transmission of the infection among its staff, patients, or residents.

An example of appropriate follow-up would be the following: A hospital admits a patient from a behavioral health center and discovers at admission that the patient has a urinary tract infection caused by a multidrug-resistant *Acinetobacter baumannii*; however, the infection was not reported to the hospital. Because this patient should have been on contact precautions, and this was not the case at admission, the hospital follows its written protocol and notifies the behavioral health center about the infection. This will allow the behavioral health center to implement any IPC actions needed. This requirement is discussed in more detail in Chapter 9.

Additional Surveillance Concerns

Immunization is critical in preventing transmission of flu virus in health care facilities. The Joint Commission standards related to influenza immunization are discussed in more detail in Chapter 10. It is important to note in this chapter the significant role of IPC staff in providing influenza vaccination rates to key leaders and managers by including this information in their annual ISPC report.

Because JCI-accredited organizations are required to send an IPC data report to leadership on a quarterly basis, influenza vaccination rate data should be in this report if such data are identified as a priority based on the risk assessment and communicated to all staff as part of the staff education.

HAIs are a significant cause of morbidity and mortality.[17] A well-executed surveillance program is integral to an organization's quality assurance, performance improvement, and quality improvement and patient safety programs because it involves monitoring both the occurrence of HAIs and the adherence to the IPC practices to prevent them. IPC staff should regularly provide interpretive surveillance reports to leaders and managers and serve as either leaders or participants in performance improvement initiatives.

The following is an example of how surveillance data can identify a problem and stimulate performance improvement activity: The IP at a large health care system identifies three new cases of hepatitis C infection in patients undergoing dialysis at an off-site dialysis center. The IP immediately reports these findings to the administrator and physician in charge of the center. Subsequently, the administrator convenes a multidisciplinary staff team to review IPC practices related to hemodialysis at the center and to identify potential risks, including any noncompliance with recommended IPC measures that may place patients at risk of developing hepatitis C.

Using Information Technology and Informatics for the Surveillance Program

Information technology (IT) and informatics are key to infection prevention and control.[18] IT can be used to retrieve, exchange, store, analyze, and disseminate surveillance data and reports. Informatics can assist with surveillance, prevention, and public health activities.[19] Studies show that electronic surveillance systems and automated data collection programs can provide increased data sensitivity and specificity compared to traditional surveillance methods.[20-21]. IPC staff should use IT and computer-assisted surveillance systems when available to increase efficiency and reduce time spent on data collection and analysis. IPC staff should work with staff in their organization, including administrative leadership, who can assist them in identifying, purchasing, and incorporating these systems into the surveillance program.

Investigating Outbreaks of Infectious Disease

Only a small proportion of HAIs are related to outbreaks.[22] Most outbreaks in health care settings are suspected when routine surveillance activities detect a cluster of cases, an unusual organism, or an apparent increase in the occurrence of an organism; when a clinician diagnoses an unusual disease; or when a health care provider or laboratory worker notices a cluster of cases. IPC staff are important in recognizing and investigating potential outbreaks.

Joint Commission Standard IC.02.01.01, EP 5 requires an organization to investigate outbreaks of infectious disease within the organization and to have written documentation about how it will investigate outbreaks. JCI Standard PCI.4, ME 3 requires an organization to identify processes or procedures associated with any infection risks (for example, infectious disease outbreaks).

Some recommended steps in an outbreak investigation are outlined in Sidebar 4-3[23] on page 102. Although these steps are in numerical order, in practice, several steps are generally performed simultaneously. However, to avoid unnecessary work, the first three steps should be completed first. IPC activities to prevent additional transmission should be identified and implemented as soon as possible. These actions should be based on the known or suspected organism or disease responsible for the outbreak. Information on identifying, investigating, managing, and preventing outbreaks is included in the references at the end of this chapter and on many health department websites.

Organizations should document and describe, in writing, the process for investigating outbreaks of infectious disease. The IP's role in outbreak identification, investigation, and management involves forming partnerships with internal and external stakeholders, such as patient care units, laboratories, and public health agencies. Should an outbreak occur or be suspected, having a preapproved written plan will guide IPC activities and alleviate confusion. During plan development, the organization should convene a multidisciplinary team to delineate the outbreak investigation steps, define responsibilities, and identify team members who will participate in the response. The team should include staff from various disciplines (such as administrators, managers, direct care providers, the laboratory, and support services staff) in the planning process. A multidisciplinary team identifies needs and potential problem areas and can educate all involved about their role in outbreak identification and management.

Sidebar 4-3.
Recommended Steps in an Outbreak Investigation

1. Verify the diagnoses of cases.
2. Establish the existence of an outbreak.
3. Construct a working case definition.
4. Find cases (retrospectively and prospectively) and record information.
5. Describe cases: person, place, time.
6. Develop hypotheses to explain the occurrence of cases.
7. Conduct special studies as needed (for example, microbiological/other laboratory studies).
8. Test the hypotheses (perform an analytical study).
9. Refine and reevaluate the hypotheses.
10. Implement control and prevention measures.
11. Maintain surveillance for additional cases.
12. Communicate findings.
13. Prepare a final outbreak investigation report.

Source: Adapted from US Centers for Disease Control and Prevention (CDC). Lesson 6. Investigating an outbreak. In *Principles of Epidemiology in Public Health Practice: An Introduction to Applied Epidemiology and Biostatistics,* 3rd ed. Atlanta: CDC, 2012.

Issues in the outbreak management plan include the following:

- Actions when an outbreak is suspected or confirmed, including immediate notification of management
- How to conduct a risk assessment to identify affected persons
- Communication strategies
- Formation of an outbreak response team
- Coordination with the organization's emergency response team, as needed, to respond to a widespread outbreak or pandemic
- Identification and implementation of immediate control measures appropriate to the mode of transmission of the suspected or causative organism
- Responsibilities for implementing control measures
- How to obtain administrative approval for measures and additional resources
- Assessment of the need to obtain specimens to identify cases
- Development of a protocol for specimen collection, handling, testing, and reporting, when needed
- How to document all aspects of an outbreak and its management
- Notification of the appropriate public health authorities
- Management of confidentiality issues
- Actions to conclude the outbreak, including preparation of a final outbreak report
- Actions to prevent a similar outbreak in the future

After an outbreak has ended, the outbreak response team should review how the outbreak was identified and controlled and prepare a written report. The report should describe the event, how it was recognized and managed, and the actions taken to resolve the problem. It should also identify who prepared the report and to whom it was provided. The outbreak management plan should be modified based on the lessons learned from the investigation. In addition, any insights into the need for practice changes should be incorporated into the IPC program policies and procedures.

When applicable to demonstrate compliance, an organization could provide an example of a report that documents how the organization identified and investigated a cluster of an organism, such as methicillin-resistant *Staphylococcus aureus*, or a cluster of a disease, such as gastroenteritis.

The IP should be involved in the activities of the emergency response team. In the case of a widespread infectious disease outbreak or a pandemic, such as the

COVID-19 pandemic, it may be necessary to activate the organization's emergency response team, as discussed in Chapter 5.

> **TIP** A heath care organization should have a written plan for outbreak management. Although it may not seem necessary, having a preapproved plan will guide IPC activities and alleviate confusion during an outbreak.

Summary

Surveillance is a critical component of an IPC program. As demonstrated during the COVID-19 pandemic, timely recognition and reporting of disease are essential to control outbreaks and rapidly spreading epidemics. This chapter provides strategies for health care organizations to develop, implement, and assess an effective surveillance program that can reduce the risk of infections in patients, residents, staff, visitors, and the community.

Resources

Tools to Try

Tool 4-1. Outline for an Infection Surveillance, Prevention, and Control (ISPC) Plan

Tool 4-2. Guidelines for Developing an Infection Surveillance, Prevention, and Control (ISPC) Program and a Written ISPC Plan

Tool 4-3. Checklist for Developing and Evaluating a Surveillance Program for a Health Care Facility

Tool 4-4. Outline for Presenting Surveillance Findings and Developing an Interpretive Surveillance Report

Tool 4-5. Sample Table of Contents for ISPC Program Annual Report and Plan

Tool 4-6. Sample Infection Prevention and Control (IPC) Surveillance Plan Summary

Tool 4-7. Vancouver Island Health Authority: Daily Infection Prevention and Control Surveillance Tool for Long Term Care Facilities

Websites

- US Centers for Disease Control and Prevention (CDC). National Healthcare Safety Network (NHSN). Accessed Dec 21, 2020. https://www.cdc.gov/nhsn/

- CDC. Outbreak Investigations in Healthcare Settings. Accessed Dec 21, 2020. http://www.cdc.gov/hai/outbreaks/index.html

- The Joint Commission. Infection Prevention and Control Resources. Accessed Dec 21. 2020. https://www.jointcommission.org/resources/patient-safety-topics/infection-prevention-and-control

- The Association for Professionals in Infection Control and Epidemiology. Accessed Dec 21, 2020. https://apic.org

Supplemental Resources

See *APIC Text of Infection Control and Epidemiology.* (Washington, DC: Association for Professionals in Infection Control and Epidemiology) for information on the following topics:

- Overview of infection prevention programs
  - McCarty J, Steinfeld, S. Chapter 1: Infection Prevention and Control Programs
  - Bienvenu S, Moody J. Chapter 6: Healthcare Informatics and Information Technology

- Epidemiology, surveillance, performance, and patient safety measures
  - Arias KM. Chapter 11: Surveillance
  - Campbell EA, Eichhorn CL. Chapter 12: Outbreak Investigations
  - Bronson-Lowe D, Bronson-Lowe C. Chapter 13: Descriptive Statistics
  - Soule BM, Nadzam DM. Chapter 17: Performance Measures

Reingold AL. Outbreak investigations—A perspective. *Emerg Infect Dis.* 1998 Jan–Mar;4(1):21–27. Accessed Dec 21, 2020. http://wwwnc.cdc.gov/eid/article/4/1/98-0104

US Centers for Disease Control and Prevention (CDC). Summary of Infection Prevention Practices in Dental Settings: Basic Expectations for Safe Care. Accessed Dec 21, 2020. https://www.cdc.gov/oralhealth/infectioncontrol/pdf/DentalEditable_TAG508.pdf

Ontario Agency for Health Protection and Promotion (Public Health Ontario), Provincial Infectious Diseases Advisory Committee. *Best Practices for Surveillance of Health Care- associated Infections in Patient and Resident Populations*, 3rd ed. Toronto, ON: Queen's Printer for Ontario, 2014. Accessed Dec 21, 2020. https://www.publichealthontario.ca/-/media/documents/B/2014/bp-hai-surveillance.pdf?la=en

See pages 79–81 of the above document for a self-assessment tool that can assist an organization in identifying best practices to include in its surveillance program.

- CDC. Outline for Healthcare–Associated Infection (HAI) Outbreak Investigation Toolkit. Accessed Dec 21, 2020. https://www.cdc.gov/hai/outbreaks/outbreaktoolkit.html

Data Collection Forms and Instructions
- CDC. Outline for Healthcare-Associated Infections Surveillance, Apr 2006. Accessed Dec 21, 2020. https://www.cdc.gov/nhsn/PDFS/OutlineForHAISurveillance.pdf

- CDC. Guide to Infection Prevention for Outpatient Settings: Minimum Expectations for Safe Care. Sep 2016. Accessed Dec 21, 2020. https://www.cdc.gov/infectioncontrol/pdf/outpatient/guidechecklist.pdf

- CDC. Infection Prevention and Control Assessment Tool for Long-term Care Facilities. Version 1.3.1, September 2016. Accessed Dec 21, 2020. https://www.cdc.gov/infectioncontrol/pdf/ICAR/LTCF.pdf

- CDC. Lesson 6. Investigating an outbreak. Self-Study Course SS1978. In *Principles of Epidemiology in Public Health Practice: An Introduction to Applied Epidemiology and Biostatistics*, 3rd ed. Atlanta: CDC, 2012. Accessed Dec 21, 2020. https://www.cdc.gov/csels/dsepd/ss1978/index.html

- CDC. *Morbidity and Mortality Weekly Report (MMWR)*, *MMWR Recommendations and Reports, MMWR Surveillance Summaries*, and *MMWR Supplements* (published electronically). Accessed Dec 21, 2020. These are good sources of information on outbreaks, emerging infectious diseases, and infection control measures. To subscribe, go to https://www.cdc.gov/mmwr/mmwrsubscribe.html

- US Centers for Medicare & Medicaid Services. (CMS) Hospital Infection Control Worksheet. Accessed Dec 21, 2020. https://www.cms.gov/Medicare/Provider-Enrollment-and-Certification/SurveyCertificationGenInfo/Downloads/Survey-and-Cert-Letter-15-12-Attachment-1.pdf

- CMS. Ambulatory Surgical Center (ASC) Infection Control Surveyor Worksheet: Exhibit 351. July 17, 2015. Accessed Dec 21, 2020. https://www.cms.gov/Regulations-and-Guidance/Guidance/Manuals/downloads/som107_exhibit_351.pdf

- CMS. CMS Long Term Care (LTC) Infection Control Worksheet LTC Facility Self-Assessment Tool. Accessed Dec 21, 2020. https://qsep.cms.gov/data/252/A._NursingHome_InfectionControl_Worksheet11-8-19508.pdf

- World Health Organization. Global Outbreak Alert and Response Network (GOARN). Accessed Dec 21, 2020. https://www.who.int/ihr/alert_and_response/outbreak-network/en Provides worldwide information on outbreaks and emerging infectious diseases.

- Multi-year series of case studies in the *American Journal of Infection Control* on using the CDC National Safety Healthcare Network definitions for HAI surveillance. For an example, see Cali S, et al. Health care–associated infection studies project: An *American Journal of Infection Control* and National Healthcare Safety Network data quality collaboration. *Am J Infect Control*. 2020;48:443–445.

References

1. Yokoe DS, et al. A compendium of strategies to prevent healthcare–associated infections in acute care hospitals: 2014 updates. *Infect Control Hosp Epidemiol.* 2014;35(5):S1–31. Accessed Dec 21, 2020. https://pubmed.ncbi.nlm.nih.gov/25376067

2. Blot K, et al. Prevention of central line–associated bloodstream infections through quality improvement interventions: A systematic review and meta-analysis. *Clin Infect Dis.* 2014;59(1):96–105.

3. Koll BS, et al. Prevention of hospital-onset *Clostridium difficile* infection in the New York metropolitan region using a collaborative intervention model. *J Healthc Qual.* 2014 May–Jun;36(3):35–45.

4. Hendersohn DM, et al. A collaborative, systems-level approach to eliminating health care–associated MRSA, central-line-associated bloodstream infections, ventilator-associated pneumonia, and respiratory virus infections. *J Healthc Qual.* 2012 Sep–Oct;34(5):39–47.

5. Lee TB, et al. Recommended practices for surveillance: Association for Professionals in Infection Control and Epidemiology (APIC), Inc. *Am J Infect Control.* 2007 Sep;35(7):427–440. Accessed Dec 21, 2020. http://www.apic.org/Resource_/TinyMceFileManager/Practice_Guidance/AJIC-Surveillance-2007.pdf

6. US Centers for Disease Control and Prevention. Outline for Healthcare-Associated Infections Surveillance. Apr 2006. Accessed Dec 21, 2020. http://www.cdc.gov/nhsn/PDFS/OutlineForHAISurveillance.pdf

7. Arias KM. Chapter 2: Surveillance. In *APIC Text of Infection Control and Epidemiology.* Washington, DC: Association for Professionals in Infection Control and Epidemiology, 2016.

8. Scheckler WE, et al. Requirements for infrastructure and essential activities of infection control and epidemiology in hospitals: A consensus panel report. *Am J Infect Control.* 1998 Feb;26(1):47–60.

9. Friedman C, et al. Requirements for infrastructure and essential activities of infection control and epidemiology in out-of-hospital settings: A consensus panel report. *Am J Infect Control.* 1999 Oct;27(5):418–430.

10. Smith PW, et al. SHEA/APIC guideline: Infection prevention and control in the long-term care facility. *Infect Control Hosp Epidemiol.* 2008 Sep;29(9):785–814. Accessed Dec 21, 2020. https://www.ncbi.nlm.nih.gov/pmc/articles/PMC3319407/

11. Centers for Disease Control and Prevention. National Healthcare Safety Network (NHSN) Patient Safety Component Manual, 2021. Accessed Dec 21, 2020. https://www.cdc.gov/nhsn/pdfs/pscmanual/pcsmanual_current.pdf

12. Stone ND, et al. Surveillance definitions of infections in long-term care facilities: Revisiting the McGeer criteria. *Infect Control Hosp Epidemiol.* 2012 Oct;33(10):965–977. Accessed Dec 21, 2020. http://www.jstor.org/stable/10.1086/667743

13. Association for Professionals in Infection Control and Epidemiology. APIC-HICPAC Surveillance Definitions for Home Health Care and Home Hospice Infections. Feb 2008. Accessed Dec 21, 2020. http://www.apic.org/Resource_/TinyMceFileManager/Practice_Guidance/HH-Surv-Def.pdf

14. Ontario Agency for Health Protection and Promotion (Public Health Ontario), Provincial Infectious Diseases Advisory Committee. *Best Practices for Surveillance of Health Care-associated Infections in Patient and Resident Populations*, 3rd ed. Toronto: Queen's Printer for Ontario, 2014. Accessed Dec 21, 2020. http://www.publichealthontario.ca/en/eRepository/Surveillance_3-3_ENGLISH_2011-10-28%20FINAL.pdf

15. Knobloch MJ, et al. Leadership rounds to reduce health care–associated infections. *Am J Infect Control.* 2018;46(3)303–310.

16. Beaudoin A, et al. Invasive Group A Streptococcus infections associated with liposuction surgery at outpatient facilities not subject to state or federal regulation. *JAMA Intern Med.* 2014;174(7):1136–1142.

17. Agency for Healthcare Research and Quality. Estimating the Additional Hospital Inpatient Cost and Mortality Associated with Selected Hospital-Acquired Conditions. Nov 2017. Accessed Dec 14, 2020. https://www.ahrq.gov/hai/pfp/haccost2017-results.html

18. Billings C, et al. Advancing the profession: An updated future-oriented competency model for professional development in infection prevention and control. *Am J Infect Control.* Jun;47(6):602–614. Accessed Dec 21, 2020. https://apic.org/wp-content/uploads/2019/05/June-2019-AJIC-Article-APIC-Competency-Model.pdf

19. Bienvenu S, Moody J. Chapter 6: Healthcare Informatics and Information Technology. In *APIC Text of Infection Control and Epidemiology.* Washington, DC: Association for Professionals in Infection Control and Epidemiology.

20. Russo PL, et al. Impact of electronic healthcare–associated infection surveillance software on infection prevention resources: A systematic review of the literature. *J Hosp Infect.* 2018;99(1):1–7.

21. Stachel A, et al. Implementation and evaluation of an automated surveillance system to detect hospital outbreak. *Am J Infect Control.* 2017;45:1372–1377.

22. Beck-Sague C, Jarvis WR, Martone WJ. Outbreak investigations. *Infect Control Hosp Epidemiol.* 1997 Feb;18(2):138–145.

23. US Centers for Disease Control and Prevention (CDC). Lesson 6. Investigating an outbreak. Self-Study Course SS1978. In *Principles of Epidemiology in Public Health Practice: An Introduction to Applied Epidemiology and Biostatistics,* 3rd ed. Atlanta: CDC, 2012. Accessed Dec 21, 2020. https://www.cdc.gov/csels/dsepd/ss1978/index.html

Chapter 5

Planning for and Managing Infectious Disease Emergencies

By Ruth Carrico, PhD, DNP, FNP-C, CIC, FSHEA, FNAP, and Terri Rebmann, PhD, RN, CIC, FAPIC

Disclaimer: Strategies, tools, and examples discussed in this book do not necessarily reflect Joint Commission or Joint Commission International requirements for all settings. Always refer to the most current standards applicable to your health care setting to ensure compliance.

Introduction

Prior to 2020, pandemic influenza (avian, swine, or other novel influenza strain) and Ebola virus disease were the primary infectious disease examples used to demonstrate a potential influx of infectious patients into health care facilities. Scenarios involving these examples made it clear that an influx of infectious patients can originate from only a single case and have a profound impact on health care operations. In early 2020, the importance of planning for infectious disease emergencies and the need for organizational, community, and cross-facility planning came into sharp focus. The first cases of SARS-CoV-2 infection and resultant COVID-19 showed the entire world the ferocity of a novel infection and demanded attention and collaboration across all health care settings worldwide. The novel coronavirus pandemic identified gaps in existing preparedness and reinforced the critical need to plan in partnership with public health and the full spectrum of health care facilities and settings.

Although, at the time of this writing, we remain in the midst of the COVID-19 pandemic, it can be reasonably anticipated that surges of infectious diseases will continue, resulting in continued stressors on all aspects of health care. It is, therefore, vital to pay close attention to the strategies, examples, and best practices in this chapter to ensure that infection prevention and control (IPC) programs are firmly aligned with emergency preparedness counterparts. The relationship among infection prevention and control, emergency preparedness, and emergency management is embedded in the Joint Commission and

Joint Commission International (JCI) requirements addressed in this chapter. This relationship underscores the need for a strong multidisciplinary approach to IPC that is both internal and external. Both infection prevention and control and emergency management standards focus on the impact infectious patients can have on the health care setting, the health care workforce, and respective communities and illustrate how adequate planning is steeped in cross-facility collaboration and multisector engagement.

The COVID-19 pandemic exposed challenges in procurement, selection, and use of personal protective equipment (PPE), which is important in preventing infection and transmission of infection among health care workers and from patient to patient. Other areas of importance involve environmental infection prevention and control and hygiene, care of equipment, specimen collection and testing, hand hygiene, and underappreciated aspects of transmission prevention such as social distancing and use of universal source control interventions by health care workers and the general public.

Joint Commission Infection Prevention and Control (IC) Standard IC.01.06.01 and JCI Prevention and Control of Infection (PCI) Standard PCI.12.2 underscore the need to plan, communicate, and interact with internal and external partners. Where applicable, the organization—through its individual leadership structure—should know its existing capabilities for responding to an influx of infectious patients and be able to evaluate those capabilities in relation to anticipated needs and identified weaknesses.

The activities and plans used by the infection prevention and control function in all settings, including public health, long term care, outpatient care, and dialysis settings, must continue to be dynamic, visible, and comprehensive. The requirements addressed in this chapter promote the type and intensity of planning that will ensure thoughtful response and care during times that challenge the entire organization and the local community.

Planning for an Influx of Infectious Patients

The health care organization is an important resource for the continued functioning of a community. An organization's ability to deliver care, treatment, and services is threatened when it is ill-prepared for a real or potential epidemic or infection that is likely to require expanded or extended care capabilities either during a short patient encounter or over a prolonged period. Therefore, it is important for an organization to plan how to do the following:

- Prevent the introduction of the infection into the organization.
- Quickly recognize a potentially infectious patient.
- Recognize if existing patients have become infected or have the potential for infection.
- Contain the risk or spread of the infection.
- Protect the health care workers from recognized and unrecognized exposure.

- Communicate critical information rapidly, effectively, and inclusively.
- Use existing capabilities to serve the needs of the community.

An organization's planned response to an infectious disease emergency should be grounded in competent IPC practices of the health care worker and should build upon evidence-based principles and prevention activities and processes in everyday best practices. However, novel pathogens provide challenges to existing practice, and competence also includes the ability to recognize how microorganisms are transmitted and select and use appropriate interventions even if they extend beyond what is recognized as everyday best practices. During infectious disease emergencies, the demand on resources may overcome the supply. During these times, an IP must think critically about priorities of safe care while being flexible with carefully selected best practices. The COVID-19 pandemic brought uncertainty and lack of confidence in basic IPC practice, further underscoring the importance of developing a solid infection control foundation in the practice of every health care worker.

The planned response to an influx of infectious patients may comprise a broad range of options, including, the following:

- Temporarily halting of services and/or admissions
- Delaying transfer or discharge

Relevant Joint Commission International (JCI) Standards Addressed in This Chapter

Note: These standards were in effect at the time of publication. They refer to the *Joint Commission International Accreditation Standards for Hospitals, seventh edition,* ©2020. Always consult the most recent version of Joint Commission International standards for the most accurate requirements for your hospital or medical center setting.

Prevention and Control of Infection (PCI)

PCI.12.2 The hospital develops, implements, and evaluates an emergency preparedness program to respond to the presentation of global communicable diseases.

ME 1 Hospital leaders, along with the individual(s) responsible for the infection prevention and control program, develop and implement an emergency preparedness program to respond to global communicable diseases that provides processes for: (a) communication with organizations participating in worldwide surveillance activities; b) development and implementation of segregation and isolation strategies; c) training, including demonstration, on the use of personal protective equipment appropriate to infectious disease; (d) development

and implementation of communication strategies; e) identification and assignment of staff roles and responsibilities; and f) response to emerging or reemerging infections within the community.

ME 2 The hospital identifies the first points of patient entry into the hospital system and targets education on early recognition and prompt action.

ME 3 The hospital evaluates the entire program at least annually and, when applicable, involves local, regional, and/or national authorities.

ME 4 At the conclusion of every drill or tabletop exercise, debriefing of the evaluation is conducted.

ME 5 Follow-up actions identified from the evaluation process and debriefing are developed and implemented.

- Cohorting patients (that is, grouping together patients exposed to or infected with the same laboratory-confirmed pathogen)
- Rapidly triaging and placing patients
- Limiting and/or screening nonessential people within the facility, including staff and visitors
- Conserving PPE, including rationing, disinfection, and limited reuse (Note that international health care settings should follow local/national regulations.)
- Rapidly deploying new testing and/or treatment options
- Fully activating the organization's operations/emergency management plans.

The actual response depends on issues such as the extent to which the community is affected by the infection, the types of services the organization offers, and the organization's capabilities. However, an influx of infectious patients may occur without regard to an organization's capabilities. Therefore, the importance of

TIP An organization's ability to deliver care, treatment, and services is threatened when the organization is ill prepared for a real or potential epidemic or infection that is likely to require expanded or extended care capabilities over a prolonged period. Therefore, an organization must plan how to prevent the introduction of the infection into the organization, how to quickly recognize if existing patients have become infected, and/or how to contain the spread of the infection. Health care workers must be protected, and their short- and long-term physical and mental health resulting from such an event must be recognized and prioritized.

cross-facility planning with public health involvement is paramount to protecting the health care infrastructure.

The rationale for these standards recognizes the following important factors:

- Health care organizations are important to the essential infrastructure of their community. Maintaining a health care process is an important social strength. Loss of adequate health care has a severely destabilizing effect on a community.
- A health care organization must plan to be able to carry out its mission during challenging situations.
- The planning process includes identifying and developing strategies to prevent the introduction of infection, recognizing such situations, and promoting activities and systems that can contain infectious events. Containment also involves preventing transmission to others (health care workers, patients, visitors) within the facility.
- The response of an individual health care organization depends on a variety of factors, including the impact of the event on the community, the types of services it offers, and its capabilities.
- An organization's ability to respond is directly related to its health care workforce's ability to competently apply IPC practices. Their skills need to be hardwired.

> **TIP** A health care organization is an important part of the essential infrastructure of its community. Maintaining a health care process is an important social strength. Loss of adequate health care has a severely destabilizing effect on a community.

Not every facility in every setting will use these standards in the same manner. An organization has to be realistic about its capabilities and challenges as it prepares for infectious disease emergencies; it needs to coordinate with other health care organizations in its community. By exercising and evaluating these plans, an organization works to protect patients, families, and its community.

Exploring the Standards

Joint Commission and JCI standards for managing infectious disease emergencies are designed to form connections with other standards and to recognize that there are both complex and complicated linkages and relationships among and between standards. This weaving together of the standards mirrors the comprehensive relationships that must be present and functional as part of the processes of care.

The requirements related to responding to an influx of potentially infectious patients are those that deal with the organization's ability to respond to an emergency. Specifically, Standard EM.01.01.01 states that *the [organization] engages in planning activities prior to developing its written Emergency Operations Plan*. In addition, Standard FMS.11 in the JCI manual requires that *the hospital develops, maintains, and tests an emergency management program to respond to internal and external emergencies and disasters that have the potential of occurring within the hospital and community*. The elements of performance (EPs) and measurable elements (MEs) for these standards underscore the direct relationship between infection prevention and control through assessment of risk, communication with external partners, and maintenance of an inventory of supplies and equipment, including personal protective equipment.

The process of the hazard vulnerability analysis should be familiar to the infection preventionist (IP), as it is similar to the risk assessment used to develop and evaluate an IPC program. A health care organization must perform a risk assessment for vulnerabilities related to emergency management to customize both the IPC plan and the emergency management plan based on unique characteristics, such as geographic setting, community resources, populations served, and ability to receive supplies during a crisis. (See Chapter 3 for a more detailed discussion of risk assessment.)

Recognizing a Potential Influx of Infectious Patients

Some organizations may ensure that they obtain current clinical and epidemiological information on new infections that could cause a potential influx of patients by communicating trends identified in their own organization and community with other health care organizations. Other sources of information include reviewing antibiograms; assessing reportable disease summaries or reports from the federal, state, and local health department; sharing health alert messages from public health officials with facility staff; conducting syndromic surveillance; and identifying emerging infections or changes in susceptibilities of organisms by reviewing antimicrobial utilization or communicating with clinical pharmacists. An organization would be wise to incorporate the aforementioned data/information into its risk assessment.

An influx of infectious patients in any care setting poses a risk to the health care facilities, staff, patients, and others; therefore, facilities should be prepared to recognize symptoms of illness, follow public health guidance, and screen patients for infectious symptoms and illnesses of public health concern.

There also should be a protocol for an infectious disease risk assessment of patients brought to a facility from other countries for treatment. The risk assessment should be based on the endemic illnesses in the individual's country of origin or newly recognized illnesses that can affect both local and global health.

Emerging infections in other parts of the world should be included in planning and communication, given the continued acceleration of international travel, movement of vectors for infection (for example, mosquitoes), and variations in public health program capabilities (for example, immunization, testing methods to identify novel pathogens). Transmissible infections anywhere in the world should be recognized as a concern and considered in emergency response planning.

Communicating to Staff About a Potential Infectious Patient Influx

Information about emerging infections that may cause an influx of potentially infectious patients should be communicated to staff and licensed independent practitioners. This can be done using newsletters, e-mail, and other types of communication. Such communication should include changes in patient presentation or clinical course when an infectious agent or process is identified. Methods of communication should enable the sharing of relevant information before, during, and after an influx of patients (see also Chapter 9).

Capturing the Response to an Influx of Infectious Patients

Written policies and procedures, program plans, training courses, checklists, and signage—as well as evidence of communication regarding these policies, procedures, and plans—should be available for review and reference. If decisions are made regarding acceptance of patients, this should be communicated clearly—internally and externally. Plans should include the processes and

procedures to follow when confronted with the influx and how staff and the community will handle situations if the facility declines to accept patients. It is important to recognize in planning activities that patients with an infectious disease may still enter the facility, despite efforts to redirect them or prevent admission.

If the organization decides to accept an influx of potentially infectious patients, then the organization needs to describe in writing its methods for managing these patients over an extended period of time. Written policies, procedures, and plans should be in place that demonstrate the multidisciplinary scope and involvement necessary to manage infectious patients over time and to protect frontline health care workers. There should be evidence of communication and work with the organization's emergency management function. There also should be evidence of staff training and education regarding these activities. The ability of staff to perform in a competent and safe manner should be included as an evaluative component of the training and education provided.

Addressing Emergency Management

The cornerstones of emergency management include preparedness, recognition, response, recovery, and mitigation; communication is an essential component. Although distinct, these cornerstones are part of a continuous and interconnected process that should be viewed as cyclic and not linear. Figure 5-1 on page 112 shows this cyclic process. The sections that follow examine these components more closely.

Emergency planning—particularly planning for emergencies that involve infectious diseases—is never finished; it is an ongoing process that evolves as threats change and gaps in planning are identified. In this way, emergency planning is aligned with continuous process evaluation and improvement and is part of a state of readiness. An effective emergency management program incorporates continuous process evaluation and improvement into all aspects of the plan and provides a mechanism for evaluation and improvement. IPs should be aware of their roles in this process.

Readiness and Preparedness

An emergency is not the time to determine whether health care workers are competent to prevent transmission of infection to others and themselves. Safe care techniques

Figure 5-1. Elements of a Continuous Emergency Management Program

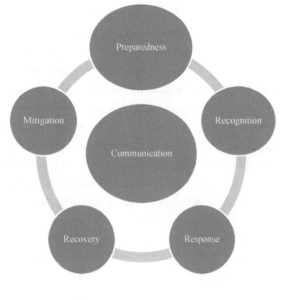

Sidebar 5-1. Infection Prevention and Control Competency Statements for Hospital-Based Health Care Workers

1. Describe the role of microorganisms in disease.
2. Describe how microorganisms are transmitted in health care settings.
3. Demonstrate standard and transmission-based precautions for all patient contact in health care settings.
4. Describe occupational health practices that protect the health care worker from acquiring infection.
5. Describe infection prevention practices that prevent the health care worker from transmitting infection to a patient.
6. Demonstrate the ability to solve problems and apply knowledge to recognize, contain, and prevent infection transmission.
7. Describe the importance of health care preparedness for natural or human-caused infectious disease disasters.

Source: Carrico R, et al. Infection prevention and control competencies for hospital-based healthcare personnel. *Am J of Infect Control.* 2008 Dec; 36(10):691–701.

and standard precautions must be part of the daily practice of every health care worker in every health care discipline. Competencies can be defined as a combination of knowledge, attitude, and skills demonstrated by the health care worker. For example, a set of IPC competencies for hospital-based health care workers has been proposed by Carrico, Rebmann, and colleagues and is shown in Sidebar 5-1, at right. These competencies address the constructs recognition, response, containment, and communication as integral parts of routine as well as emergency response practice and may be adapted for other settings, as needed. Standardization across disciplines and settings in a given community can assist the IP in implementing competency-based education. (*See* Sidebar 5-2 on page 113 for education topics for staff, patients, and visitors related to emergency management.) Examples of such standardized practices include the ability of the health care worker to select, don (put on), use, doff (take off), and dispose of PPE in a safe manner.

PPE is a recognized asset in preventing contact with blood or other body fluids, when used correctly. To ensure safety, health care workers must be proficient in PPE use every time they use it. That means proper technique must be incorporated into daily practice so there is consistency

and reliability in their work. (*See* Chapter 6 for additional discussion of PPE.)

In 2017, the CDC's Healthcare Infection Control Practices Advisory Committee published *Core Infection Prevention and Control Practices for Safe Healthcare Delivery in All Settings* (CDC, 2017). This document contains widely agreed-upon best practices that constitute standards of care applicable in all settings where health care is delivered. Such practices apply during routine as well as emergency situations. (*See* Sidebar 5-3 on page 114 for a list of these core practices.)

Another important consideration is the evaluation and capabilities of the physical plant—or the care environment—and the need to involve the facility's

Sidebar 5-2. Infection Prevention and Control Education Topics Related to Emergency Management—for Staff, Patients, and Visitors

- Screening/triage procedures (including self-screening for staff during a biological event)
- Patient decontamination procedures
- Patient management (placement/isolation, patient cohorting, transport and discharge protocols, and so on)
- Disease-specific information on bioterrorism agents, emerging infections, and pandemic influenza
- Transmission-based precautions and isolation procedures
- Respiratory hygiene and cough etiquette
- Personal protective equipment (PPE) use and reuse
- Decontamination of respirators, when applicable (for staff only)
- Hand hygiene
- Quarantine
- Procedures for obtaining, handling, and processing patient specimens for laboratory testing, including how to coordinate testing through the Laboratory Response Network
- Cleaning and disinfection of toys that are shared between children in the facility
- Procedures to follow during times when visitation is restricted
- Occupational health/safety procedures
- Surge capacity issues that affect infection transmission (for example, negative pressure surge capacity, lack of PPE)
- Organizational emergency management plan protocols and procedures that affect infection transmission
- Postmortem care
- Food and water safety, including times when utilities may be not available
- Sanitation control, such as cleaning and disinfection of laundry, linens, medical equipment, and environmental surfaces
- Waste management, including times when routine pickup is not available
- Pet management
- Infection prevention and control protocols for alternative care sites owned/operated by the hospital/ health care organization
- Social distancing measures
- Knowledge and use of different types of face masks

Source: Adapted from Rebmann T. 2008 APIC Emergency Preparedness Committee. APIC state-of-the-art report: The role of the infection preventionist in emergency management. *Am J Infect Control.* 2009 May;37(4):271–281.

emergency management system early in the planning process. All health care organizations will not need (or be able) to address this requirement in the same manner. Instead, each organization should evaluate its capabilities and role in the community with respect to health care delivery and services provided.

A thorough evaluation of the limitations and capabilities of the building(s), utilities, ventilation systems,

equipment, and supplies allows emergency planners to determine pockets of need, prioritize activities, and budget accordingly for improvements or enhancements. Existing abilities to promote adherence with respiratory hygiene or "cough etiquette" through provision of masks, tissue, and environmental cleaning and disinfection should be evaluated, along with indicators that target implementation or change in the existing process.

In some settings, understanding the ventilation system in the physical plant may be an important responsibility for the IP. Figure 5-2 on page 115 shows a typical air distribution system for a single-patient room. The figure shows the typical location of supply and return air ducts and the relationship between airflow and patient bed location. Figure 5-3 on page 116 shows that a single patient care area is often supplied with air from more than one air handling unit. When investigating appropriate patient placement, it may be important to know under what conditions air space is shared between patients. Tool 5-1 offers guidance for improvising isolation to accommodate a surge capacity for an influx of infectious patients who do not have an airborne-spread disease. Chapter 7 discusses the environment of care in more detail.

TRY THIS TOOL

Tool 5-1. Guidelines for Improvising Isolation During Influx of Patients with Non-Airborne Infectious Disease

Recognition of an Infectious Disease Emergency

Recognition of an infectious disease and an infectious patient allows the organization to identify and contain an infectious patient before the disease is transmitted to other patients, staff, and the community. The goal should be to have regular care practices that minimize transmission, recognize key indicators or symptoms, and initiate the response portion of the plan as early as possible. (See Tools 5-2 and 5-3 for guidance related to emergency recognition and response.) Recognition may involve identifying patients presenting with specific types of signs, symptoms, or complaints. A list of symptoms and syndromes often associated with infectious diseases is outlined in Sidebar 5-4 on page 117. Health care workers should be trained on these symptoms and syndromes so that they can quickly identify potentially contagious individuals and implement appropriate control measures. After staff recognize these patients, response activities can begin, such as appropriate use of PPE, isolation, cohorting, and so on. Care processes and systems that incorporate safety measures are great assets in early recognition.

Figure 5-2. Air Distribution in a Single-Patient Room

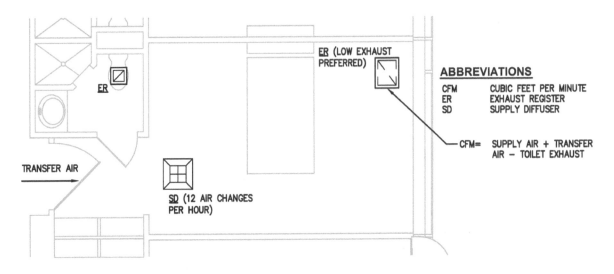

TYPICAL SINGLE OCCUPANCY AIR DISTRIBUTION
(100% OUTSIDE AIR SYSTEM)

This illustration depicts the transfer and exchange of air in a single occupancy hospital room.

Source: Graphic provided by Jim Hemmer PE, Luckett & Farley, Louisville Kentucky. Used with permission.

TRY THESE TOOLS

Tool 5-2. Occupational Health Considerations for Emergency Preparedness

Tool 5-3. Notification Procedures for Health Care Professionals to Report Known or Potential Bioterrorism Incidents

As discussed in the example below, practices implemented in one hospital demonstrate how care processes and systems change were key to early recognition of infectious patients. However, each health care facility needs to evaluate its unique risks and implement programs to address them. The program described in this example may not be suitable for all facilities, but it demonstrates the conceptual basis for the approach.

Example

University Hospital is a 404-bed Level 1 trauma center with large oncology and women's health services in the United States. Its active infectious diseases service operates the largest comprehensive HIV/AIDS clinic in the region. In the early 1990s, the hospital employee health department noted a subtle increase in tuberculosis (TB) skin test conversions among staff. Investigation revealed that there were several cases of active TB with delayed diagnosis. The most common reason for the delayed diagnosis was that the patients presented with symptoms consistent with community-acquired pneumonia (CAP), and although TB infection was on the differential diagnosis, it was not a primary consideration, and airborne preventive strategies were not immediately initiated. Diagnostic testing was performed on day two or three of hospitalization. This delay in diagnostic testing without prevention strategies led to workplace exposures for health care workers. A systems change was initiated. The investigation helped leaders recognize the shifting population and the increased risks for health care workers. A protocol was developed so that all patients admitted with CAP were immediately placed in airborne infection isolation until TB was ruled out. This system change resulted in a process that supported rapid

Figure 5-3. Schematic of Multiple Air Handlers Servicing a Single Patient Care Area

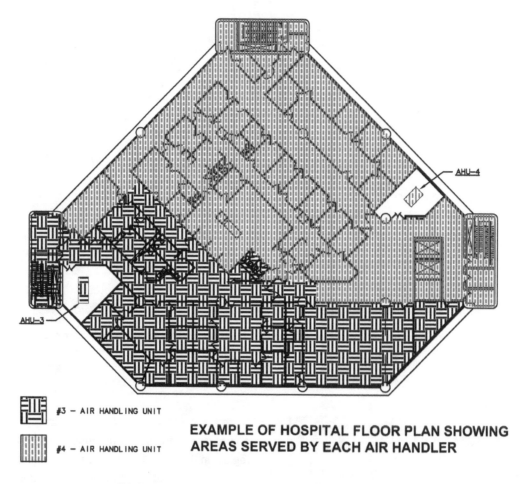

#3 – AIR HANDLING UNIT

#4 – AIR HANDLING UNIT

EXAMPLE OF HOSPITAL FLOOR PLAN SHOWING AREAS SERVED BY EACH AIR HANDLER

This figure depicts the placement of air-handling units in a hospital.

Source: Graphic provided by Jim Hemmer PE, Luckett & Farley, Louisville Kentucky. Used with permission.

evaluation so that isolation could be quickly discontinued once a transmissible cause was ruled out.

Over the next decade, patients with unsuspected TB were isolated through this early risk identification process. The approach supported this prevention activity and the safety of the care environment in a positive way. It resulted in the isolation of patients with influenza-related pneumonia, further improving the safety of the care environment for patients, staff, and visitors. Health care workers were well trained to obtain optimal respiratory specimens for laboratory testing in a safe manner. This process

underscores the risks of undetected respiratory infection transmission to staff and the potential relationships between patient illness and staff illness. Consequently, staff are aware that a patient with a cough represents a potential risk, and using personal protective equipment is part of routine patient care. The lessons learned from this TB experience have resulted in a culture of safety, which was valuable during the COVID-19 pandemic response, and highlighted the need for best practice approaches embedded into routine practice for ongoing preparation for an unsuspected infectious disease exposure.

Sidebar 5-4. Symptoms and Syndromes That Indicate an Infectious Patient

- Flu-like illness, consisting of fever, body aches, headache, and so forth
- Cough, with or without sputum (Bloody sputum is particularly worrisome.)
- Upper respiratory symptoms, such as nasal drainage, watery eyes, sinus pain/pressure, and so forth
- Rash, regardless of whether it is itchy (Rash with fever is particularly worrisome.)
- Loose or unformed stools (Bloody stools are particularly worrisome.)
- Watery or explosive diarrhea stools (Bloody stools are particularly worrisome.)
- Stiff or very sore neck (Stiff or sore neck with fever is particularly worrisome.)
- Red eye or drainage from eye(s)
- Open wound or lesion, regardless of whether it is draining (Actively draining wounds/lesions are particularly worrisome.)
- Severe bleeding disorder with no discernable source

Response to an Infectious Disease Emergency

Emergency management efforts require early recognition to facilitate prompt response. The University Hospital example demonstrates the need for early recognition and early risk identification processes that enable prompt response. After a risk is identified, the facility may activate its infectious disease emergency response plan. During response to a situation involving a known or suspected infectious patient(s), containment is a primary initiative. Containment can be accomplished by isolating or quarantining the patient, initiating PPE use by the health care worker, masking the patient if his or her condition allows and warrants source control by this method, cohorting with other patients having a shared

diagnosis, or using combinations of these actions. Although accomplishing a common goal of limiting spread of an infectious disease, *isolation* and *quarantine* have different meanings:

- **Isolation:** Separation and confinement of individuals known or suspected (based upon signs, symptoms, or laboratory findings) to be infected with a contagious disease to prevent them from transmitting the disease to others
- **Quarantine:** Compulsory physical separation, including restriction of movement, of populations or groups of *healthy* individuals who have potentially been exposed to a contagious disease

Tools 5-4 through 5-7 provide response resources. Additional information about isolation and quarantine is available on the CDC Emergency Preparedness and Response website at http://emergency.cdc.gov/preparedness/quarantine.

Response may also include implementing an incident management system, as needed. Implementing an incident management system requires that the organization identify and train individuals who can perform functions 24 hours a day, 7 days a week, 365 days per year.

TRY THESE TOOLS

Tool 5-4. Infectious Substance Exposure Response Form

Tool 5-5. Managing Exposure to *Bordetella pertussis*

Tool 5-6. Managing Exposure to Measles Virus

Tool 5-7. Phone Script and Decision Algorithm for Possible COVID-19

Each situation needs to be evaluated, and response activities should be specific to the cause or suspected cause, modes of transmission, and individuals involved. Figure 5-4 shows an algorithm used to manage and place patients who require airborne precautions. Infectious diseases that require airborne precautions include, but are not limited to measles, Severe Acute Respiratory Syndrome (SARS), varicella (chickenpox), and *Mycobacterium tuberculosis*. Responding to and

Figure 5-4. Patient Management and Placement for Airborne Precautions

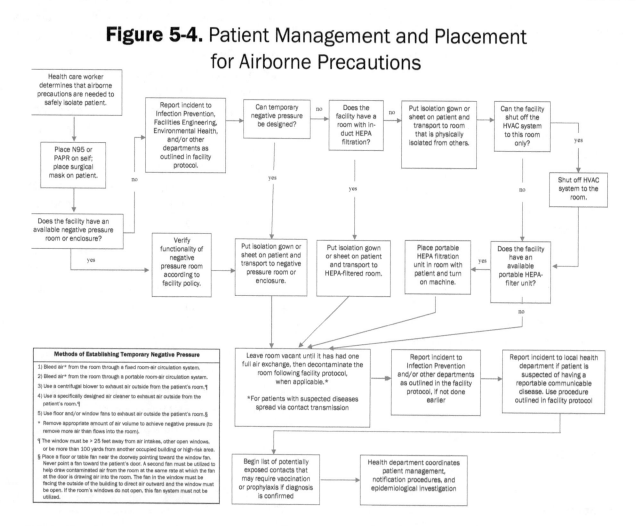

This algorithm shows one approach to managing and placing patients who require airborne precautions. **HEPA**, high-efficiency particulate air; **HVAC**, heating, ventilating, and air conditioning; **PAPR**, powered air purifying respirator

Source: Adapted from Rebmann T. Management of patients infected with airborne-spread diseases: An algorithm for infection control professionals. *Am J Infect Control.* 2005 Dec;33:571–579.

preventing airborne transmission of infectious disease requires personal respiratory protection for the health care worker and special ventilation and air handling.

Response to an infectious disease emergency might require increasing surge capacities beyond a facility's existing capabilities. This may include allocating additional or new physical space for patients or altering the care environment, such as increasing negative pressure surge capacity environments to allow for airborne infection isolation. The complexities in implementing these strategies underscore the need for

planning. Sidebar 5-5 on page 119 may be helpful in planning containment activities. Tool 5-8 offers guidance on preventing transmission of particular infections.

TRY THIS TOOL

Tool 5-8. Guide for Preventing Transmission of Selected Infections

---

Sidebar 5-5. Preparing for an Influx of Infectious Patients Requiring Airborne Infection Isolation

An influx of patients requiring an airborne infection isolation (negative airflow) environment might exceed an organization's physical plant capabilities. The following may aid in evaluating current processes and identifying opportunities and strengths to include in the emergency management plan. While not a comprehensive list, it should initiate a dialogue between an infection preventionist, the facility emergency manager, facilities engineering staff, the safety officer, and executive staff:

- Identify existing airborne infection isolation (negative airflow) environments and determine capacity.
- Consult current American Society of Heating, Refrigerating and Air-Conditioning Engineers documents to assist in evaluating airflow, filtration, and existing capabilities of the existing heating, ventilating, and air conditioning (HVAC) system
- Ensure status of negative airflow by using current industry standard testing procedures.
- Evaluate the existing seal of each room. Check seals around windows and electrical outlets.
- Select an appropriate area for surge capacity (wing or separate building), considering the following:
  - The existing HVAC system operation and capabilities
  - Location of adjacent populations in all directions, particularly high-risk areas such as oncology and nurseries
  - Controlled access for traffic patterns
  - Accessibility from areas of first patient encounter (for example, emergency department, admissions)
  - The existing utility and service capabilities:
    - Electrical outlets on emergency backup power
    - Oxygen delivery
    - Medical gas
    - Suction
    - Sinks
    - Commodes
- Develop a floor plan that indicates blocks of rooms/areas served by each air handler.
- Develop a plan that indicates blocks of rooms/areas served by each ventilation exhaust fan.
- Develop a schematic for each air-handling unit system, indicating flow to each room, return airflow, associated exhaust system, and any recirculation pattern. This information may prompt you to reconsider your initial selection of an appropriate area.
- Identify where air is exhausted and ensure that it is at least 25 feet away from any air intake and 100 yards from other entrances into the facility.
- Evaluate existing equipment, including ventilators, portable suction, and additional oxygen tanks.
- Evaluate existing supplies, including personal protective equipment and suction supplies.

Refer to the Patient Management and Placement for Airborne Precautions algorithm (Figure 5-4) for additional information when identifying additional airborne isolation surge capacity.

Source: Ruth M. Carrico, PhD, DNP, APRN, FNP-C, CIC FSHEA, FNAP, Center of Excellence for Research in Infectious Diseases (CERID), University of Louisville School of Medicine, 2020. Used with permission.

Communication

Adequate and inclusive communication is an essential component of an organization's emergency response process. Communication should occur among individuals in the organization as well as with external agencies and partners. In situations involving an infectious patient(s), direct communication with the local health department should be included in the initial response. Organizations should not bypass their local health department in an effort to speed communications. One of the many responsibilities of the local public health system is to ensure that knowledge is shared with those individuals and organizations that can be of assistance. Failing to adhere to this chain of communication can add confusion and interrupt important organizational and agency links. The 24-hour contact number for the local health department should be in an organization's emergency response plans. Including other external partners in the communication process is also paramount to an effective plan. Identification of assistance with environmental hygiene or environmental laboratory support may be valuable additions to the risk assessment as well as to the communication plan.

Organizations must also consider methods or equipment used in the communication process. As an organization evaluates existing communication capabilities and develops future plans, representatives from departments that control information systems should be involved. Organizations should recognize that in times of crisis, usual methods of communication may fail, so backup or redundant measures should be considered, tested, and evaluated.

Protection and Care for Health Care Workers

An infectious disease that affects the general public will certainly affect health care workers. Health care workers deal with the risk of transmission while performing their job responsibilities and outside of work during family and community interactions. The COVID-19 pandemic demonstrated the risk of serious illness and even death among health care workers. There should be programs and processes to recognize and minimize risk, such as respirator fit testing and training for proper donning and doffing of PPE, and also to monitor the health of the workforce. Occupational health plans should include testing, furloughs return-to-work protocols, workers'

compensation (if the exposure is attributable to job responsibilities), and active communication and reporting in accordance with public health law. Also, it should be recognized that health care workers may have more than one job and more than one employer. This brings additional complexity and requires active and ongoing communication between health care workers and all their places of employment, as appropriate. Coordinating situations in which health care workers must be furloughed or in isolation due to illness requires a new level of transparency and communication. Health care organizations also should have a collaborative plan for large-scale immunization of their workforce. More information regarding occupational health programs is provided in Chapter 10. In addition, Tools 5-9 through 5-11 offer guidance on PPE and keeping health care workers safe.

TRY THESE TOOLS

Tool 5-9. Guidelines for Extending the Use and Reuse of Respiratory Protection (N95 Respirators and Surgical/Procedure Masks) During an Infectious Disease Disaster

Tool 5-10. Inventory Form for IPC Equipment and Supplies Stockpile

Tool 5-11. Guidelines for Calculating Personal Protective Equipment Stockpile

---

TIP An organization should not bypass its local health department to speed communications. One of the many responsibilities of local and state public health systems is to ensure that information is shared with individuals and organizations essential to emergency response. Failing to adhere to this chain of communication can delay the public health response, potentially causing confusion and interrupting important organizational and agency collaboration that is critical for patient and public health.

Recovery and Mitigation

Recovery from a disaster or public health emergency and mitigation for future events are important parts of emergency management because both include opportunities for the health care organization to identify needs for returning to normal and reducing the risk of future emergencies. During the COVID-19 pandemic, recovery and mitigation happened concurrently with response operations in an effort to restore a new sense of normalcy. The ability to establish a new normal, as seen during the COVID-19 pandemic, may require a fine balance between adherence to nonpharmaceutical interventions (physical distancing, mask compliance, and hand hygiene) among community members and measured reopening guided by community leaders.

Unfortunately, when a health emergency is prolonged, fatigue can set in among members of the community, including health care workers, making recovery difficult and increasing the risk of infection. Therefore, the infectious disease emergency response plan should include strategies for supporting the mental well-being of providers and patients. During the COVID-19 pandemic, professional organizations developed and launched a variety of interventions focused on the mental health and well-being of health care workers. See the Supplemental Resources section at the end of this chapter for a link to such resources compiled by the Technical Resources Assistance Center of the US Department of Health and Human Services.

Resource allocation can be a critical limiting factor for health care organizations during an emergency, leading to conservation measures during the response phase that deviate from routine best practices. During recovery, it is important to plan for eliminating conservation measures, communicating about how to return to normal best practices, and performing audits for adherence. To mitigate any issues with returning to normal too quickly, IPs should collaborate with supply chain partners to assess impact.

Recovery—marking the conclusion of an infectious disease emergency—may not be as clear-cut as discharging the last patient with the disease from the facility, or finding that all persons at risk do not develop the disease at the conclusion of the incubation period. The disease may became a new fact of life. Therefore, emergency management is a continuum. Health care organizations must continuously prepare to respond to provide safe care to their communities.

Case Study

Considerations for Responding to a Potential Infectious Disease Emergency

The following scenario provides a model for implementation in a given facility and how that facility can demonstrate compliance with accreditation requirements when planning for infectious disease emergencies. The US Centers for Disease Control and Prevention has developed a Comprehensive Hospital Preparedness Checklist for Novel Coronavirus 2019 (COVID-19) to help acute care facilities assess and improve preparedness and response to a communitywide outbreak of COVID-19. A link to this resource is provided in the Supplemental Resources section at the end of this chapter.

The emergency department (ED) charge nurse notifies the nursing supervisor of his concern about the number of patients he believes have been seen in the ED during the past several days. By his assessment, volumes are growing, which he noticed has increased throughput times. Admissions from the ED to patient care areas are slower than usual, and the waiting area seems overburdened with patients exhibiting respiratory symptoms.

(continued)

Considerations for Responding to a Potential Infectious Disease Emergency (continued)

The nursing supervisor notes the evening's census and reviews information from the previous several days. She notes an increase in the number of patients seen in the ED with respiratory symptoms and also significantly more patients requiring admission for those symptoms tonight than the night before. Consulting with the ED physician and hospitalist on call, she contacts the infection preventionist (IP) to discuss the situation. The IP includes a representative from microbiology in the discussion to determine if a particular organism has been identified that may affect patient placement decisions. The IP also reaches out to the local public health department and proactively includes someone from engineering who can answer questions regarding ventilation systems and verification of negative pressure patient environments.

The group formulates a list of questions to guide their immediate response and for longer-term planning:

- Is there a need to house some or all of these patients in an airborne infection isolation room that includes negative airflow?
- If staff are caring for patients who are coughing, are they selecting and using appropriate personal protective equipment?
- Given the just-in-time approach for stocking supplies, is there enough respiratory protective equipment? Are weekend deliveries possible if additional items are needed?
- Is the impact on the environment being appropriately assessed so that environmental services staff are involved in the cleaning and disinfection decisions?
- Has the hospital discharged patients with these symptoms?
- Has the hospital transferred patients with these symptoms to other health care facilities, including local long term care facilities? What communication needs to occur with these facilities?
- What public health guidance needs to be incorporated into the hospital's internal response plans and external communications?

This case demonstrates some of the complexities of an effective infection prevention and control (IPC) program:

- Education of the organizational decision maker's (nursing supervisor's) ability to capture information that can be transformed into data that guides decisions (census, syndromic surveillance)
- Early involvement of the IP
- Active evaluation of the appropriateness of the care environment (with environmental services and physical plant input)
- Active evaluation of supply levels and availabilities
- Evaluation of the capabilities of the physical facility

This case also demonstrates the need to ensure that health care workers are knowledgeable about and competent in applying IPC practices as a routine part of their job performance. This involves the ability to think critically and make effective use of limited resources—skills likely to be needed during an actual emergency.

Summary

To comply with Joint Commission Standard IC.01.06.01 and JCI Standard PCI.12.2, organizations should plan for small-scale (individual facility) as well as larger-scale (community) responses to infectious disease emergencies. They must engage in comprehensive planning that addresses the different phases of emergency management—preparedness, recognition, response, recovery, and mitigation—with communication being critical in each phase. An effective program includes staff competent in applying standard IPC precautions in their daily work. Recognizing that many health care staff members work in more than one facility, promoting standardization increases the ability of staff to adhere to IPC best practices. Working with the facility emergency manager, local emergency management agencies, local hospital associations, and other area health care organizations helps an organization promote harmony and can be the basis for long-term collaboration.

Resources

Tools to Try

Tool 5-1. Guidelines for Improvising Isolation During Influx of Patients with Non-Airborne Infectious Disease

Tool 5-2. Occupational Health Considerations for Emergency Preparedness

Tool 5-3. Notification Procedures for Healthcare Professionals to Report Known or Potential Bioterrorism Incidents

Tool 5-4. Infectious Substance Exposure Response Form

Tool 5-5. Managing Exposure to _Bordetella pertussis_

Tool 5-6. Managing Exposure to Measles Virus

Tool 5-7. Phone Script and Decision Algorithm for Possible COVID-19

Tool 5-8. Guide for Preventing Transmission of Selected Infections

Tool 5-9. Guidelines for Extending the Use and Reuse of Respiratory Protection (N95 Respirators and Surgical/Procedure Masks) During an Infectious Disease Disaster

Tool 5-10. Inventory Form for IPC Equipment and Supplies Stockpile

Tool 5-11. Guidelines for Calculating Personal Protective Equipment Stockpile

Supplemental Resources

- The Joint Commission. _Emergency Management in Health Care: An All-Hazards Approach._ 4th ed. Oak Brook, IL: Joint Commission Resources, 2019.

- CDC. Emergency Preparedness and Response. Resources for Emergency Health Professionals. Clinician Outreach and Communication Activity (COCA). Accessed Sep 12, 2020. https://emergency.cdc.gov/coca/calls/index.asp

- New York State Department of Health. Biological Emergencies. Accessed Sep 12, 2020. https://www.health.ny.gov/environmental/emergency/health_care_providers/biological_emergencies.htm

- American Psychiatric Association. Disaster and Trauma Resources. Accessed Sep 12, 2020. https://www.psychiatry.org/psychiatrists/practice/professional-interests/disaster-and-trauma

- Association for Professionals in Infection Control and Epidemiology. The APIC Text Online. Accessed Sep 12, 2020. https://text.apic.org/the-apic-text-online

- ASHRAE. ASHRAE Epidemic Task Force, 2020. Accessed Apr 2021. https://www.ashrae.org/file%20library/technical%20resources/covid-19/ashrae-healthcare-c19-guidance.pdf

- Heymann D. _Control of Communicable Diseases Manual_, 20th ed. Washington DC: American Public Health Association, 2014.

- Saint Louis University. Institute for Biosecurity. Accessed Apr 2021. https://www.slu.edu/public-health-social-justice/centers_institutes/institute_bsdp.php

- US Department of Health and Human Services. Pandemic Influenza Plan, 2017. Accessed Apr 2021. https://www.cdc.gov/flu/pandemic-resources/pdf/pan-flu-report-2017v2.pdf

- Rebmann T, et al. Infection Prevention and Control for Shelters During Disasters. 2008. Accessed on Sep 12, 2020. http://www.apic.org/Professional-Practice/Emergency-Preparedness

- Infection Prevention for Alternate Care Sites. 2009. Accessed Sep 12, 2020. http://apic.org/Professional-Practice/Emergency-Preparedness/

- Rebmann T, et al. Infection Prevention for Ambulatory Care Centers During Disasters. 2013. Accessed Sep 12, 2020. http://www.apic.org/Professional-Practice/Emergency-Preparedness

- CDC. Comprehensive Hospital Preparedness Checklist for Coronavirus Disease 2019 (COVID-19). Accessed Jan 9, 2021. https://www.cdc.gov/coronavirus/2019-ncov/hcp/hcp-hospital-checklist.html

- CDC. Healthcare Infection Control Practices Advisory Committee. Core Infection Prevention and Control Practices for Safe Healthcare Delivery in All Settings—Recommendations of the Healthcare Infection Control Practices Advisory Committee (HICPAC). 2017. Accessed Apr 2021. https://www.cdc.gov/hicpac/pdf/core-practices.pdf

- CDC. Personal Protective Equipment (PPE) Burn Rate Calculator. Accessed Sep 12, 2020. https://www.cdc.gov/coronavirus/2019-ncov/hcp/ppe-strategy/burn-calculator.html

- CDC. Implementing Filtering Facepiece Respirator (FFR) Reuse, Including Reuse After Decontamination, When There Are Known Shortages of N95 Respirators. Oct 19, 2020. Accessed Sep 12, 2020. https://www.cdc.gov/coronavirus/2019-ncov/hcp/ppe-strategy/decontamination-reuse-respirators.html

- CDC. Optimizing Personal Protective Equipment (PPE) Supplies. 2020. Accessed Sep 12, 2020. https://www.cdc.gov/coronavirus/2019-ncov/hcp/ppe-strategy/

- CDC/NIOSH. Personal Protective Equipment. Accessed Sep 12, 2020. https://www.cdc.gov/niosh/ppe/

- CDC. Considerations for Alternate Care Sites. 2020. Accessed Sep 12, 2020. https://www.cdc.gov/coronavirus/2019-ncov/hcp/alternative-care-sites.html

- National Personal Protective Technology Laboratory (NPPTL). Healthcare Respiratory Protection Resources. 2020. Accessed Sep 12, 2020. https://www.cdc.gov/niosh/npptl/hospresptoolkit/fittesting.html

- US Department of Health and Human Services. Topic Collection: COVID-19 Behavioral Health Resources. Accessed Jan 9, 2021. https://asprtracie.hhs.gov/technical-resources/115/covid-19-behavioral-health-resources/

Chapter 6

Implementing Clinical Strategies to Reduce Infection Risk

By Loretta L. Fauerbach, MS, FSHEA, FAPIC, CIC, and
Elizabeth E. Tremblay, MPH, CPH, CIC

Disclaimer: Strategies, tools, and examples discussed in this book do not necessarily reflect Joint Commission or Joint Commission International requirements for all settings. Always refer to the most current standards applicable to your health care setting to ensure compliance.

Introduction

Infection prevention and control (IPC) activities must be collaborative and include all parties that are part of the practice being addressed. Through this collaboration, successful implementation of IPC practices can occur. Communication to staff and patients is imperative so that each person knows his or her role in the prevention and control activity. Policies and procedures should be readily available to all. With this mindset, a successful IPC program can exist. This chapter addresses the requirements for clinical strategies to reduce infection risk in various settings and discusses successful strategies and applications. Relevant IPC implementation requirements are addressed in Joint Commission Standards IC.02.01.01 through IC.02.03.01 and Joint Commission International (JCI) Standards PCI.4, PCI.5, and PCI.12 through PCI.14.

Relevant Joint Commission Standards Addressed in This Chapter

Note: These standards were in effect at the time of publication. They refer to Joint Commission standards effective January 1, 2021. Always consult the most recent version of Joint Commission standards for the most accurate requirements for your setting.

IC.02.01.01 The [organization] implements its infection prevention and control plan.

EP 1 The [organization] implements its infection prevention and control activities, including surveillance, to minimize reduce or eliminate the risk of infection. (*See also* MM.09.01.01, EP 5)

EP 2 The [organization] uses standard precautions, including the use of personal protective equipment, to reduce the risk of infection. (*See also*

EC.02.02.01, EP 4) **Note:** *Standard precautions are infection prevention and control measures to protect against possible exposure to infectious agents. These precautions are general and applicable to all patients.*

EP 3 The [organization] implements transmission-based precautions in response to the pathogens that are suspected or identified within the [organization's] service setting and community.

(continued)

(continued)

EP 5 The [organization] investigates outbreaks of infectious disease. (*See also* IC.01.05.01, EP 5)

IC.01.02.01 [Organization] leaders allocate needed resources for the infection prevention and control program.

EP 3 The [organization] provides equipment and supplies to support the infection prevention and control program.

MM.09.01.01 The [organization] has an antimicrobial stewardship program based on current scientific literature.

EP 1 Leaders establish antimicrobial stewardship as an organizational priority. (*See also* LD.01.03.01, EP 5)

EP 4 The [organization] has an antimicrobial stewardship multidisciplinary team that includes the following members, when available in the setting:
- Infectious disease physician
- Infection preventionist(s)
- Pharmacist(s)
- Practitioner

Relevant Joint Commission International (JCI) Standards Addressed in This Chapter

Note: These standards were in effect at the time of publication. They refer to the *Joint Commission International Accreditation Standards for Hospitals, seventh edition*, ©2020. Always consult the most recent version of Joint Commission International standards for the most accurate requirements for your hospital or medical center setting.

PCI.3, ME 3 Hospital leadership approves and allocates resources required for the infection prevention and control program.

PCI.4, ME 3 The hospital identifies those processes associated with infection risk.

PCI.5, ME 2 The data collected in respiratory tract, urinary tract, intravascular invasive devices, surgical sites, epidemiologically significant diseases and organisms, and emerging or reemerging infections with the community are analyzed to identify priorities for reducing rates of infection.

PCI.12, ME 1 The hospital utilizes a process to isolate patients with infectious diseases, and staff use transmission-based precautions, in accordance with recommended guidelines.

PCI.13, ME 1 The hospital identifies situations in which personal protective equipment is required and ensures that it is available at any site of care at which it could be needed.

PCI.14, ME 2 The hospital collects and analyzes data for the infection prevention and control activities, and the data include epidemiologically important infections.

MMU.1.1, ME 1 The hospital develops and implements a program for antibiotic stewardship that involves infection prevention and control professionals, physicians, nurses, pharmacists, trainees, patients, families, and others.

ME 4 There is a mechanism to oversee the program for antibiotic stewardship. (*see also* GLD.9, ME 1)

The standards addressed in this chapter require an organization to implement its IPC plan using evidence-based strategies to reduce IPC risks. An IPC plan must be enacted for change to occur and for the organization's IPC program to effectively minimize, reduce, or eliminate the risk of infection.[1-3] As discussed in previous chapters, the IPC team should perform a risk assessment in order to develop an effective IPC plan that meets the needs of the organization. These standards represent the umbrella under which basic components of the IPC program fall.

The Role of Surveillance

Surveillance is a basic component of an IPC program because it provides data to identify infections in the facility and can be used to direct prevention strategies to reduce the risk of those infections. Surveillance in hospitals and long-term care organizations may be implemented using the National Healthcare Safety Network (NHSN) definitions and strategies[4] or criteria determined by local regulators (for example, ministries or departments of health).

Implementation of proven strategies is critical for the success of a program. Simply identifying strategies or writing policies and procedures will not ensure compliance with recommended practices. The field of implementation science has evolved and become an asset to IPC programs. According to Moir, implementation science is the study of the components necessary to promote authentic adoption of evidence-based interventions, thereby increasing their effectiveness.[5] Using good implementation methods helps to ensure sustainability of the evidence-based practice. By implementing the right interventions, an organization can improve patient outcomes and reduce infection risks for its patients, residents, and staff.

Multiple resources from literature, professional associations, health care improvement initiatives, accrediting organizations, and government agencies describe successful infection prevention interventions and implementation strategies. In addition, the Society for Healthcare Epidemiology of America (SHEA) has been involved in developing implementation education and tools for Novel Coronavirus 2019 (SARS-CoV-2/COVID-19) and other emerging pathogens. An Outbreak Response Tool Kit can be accessed at https://ortp.guidelinecentral. com/covid-19/.

Standard Precautions

Standard precautions are IPC measures and activities that protect against possible exposure to infectious agents. These precautions are general and are applicable to all (for example, patients, clients, and residents). Standard precautions include appropriate handling of hazardous materials and wastes and thus the linkage between infection prevention and control standards and those found in the "Environment of Care" chapter of *The Joint Commission Comprehensive Accreditation Manual* and in the "Facility Management and Safety" chapter of the JCI *Standards for Hospitals*.

Joint Commission–accredited organizations are required to use standard precautions universally across the continuum of health care, including outpatient and ambulatory care settings, hospitals, laboratories, home care, hospice, behavioral health and human services, long term care facilities (nursing home/care centers), and dialysis facilities.[6] For further information regarding standard precautions, refer to the website of the Centers for Disease Control and Prevention (CDC) at https://www.cdc.gov/hai/.

Standard precautions—including use of personal protective equipment (PPE) to prevent exposure to blood and body fluids, safe injection practices and medication handling, and respiratory and cough etiquette—reduce the risk of infection and prevent the transmission of pathogens.[6] The following sections take a closer look at these components.

Standard Precautions Strategies

Each health care setting may have unique needs for precautions based on the care, treatment, and services provided in its particular care setting. For example, behavioral health care and human services settings may need to develop practices for distributing alcohol-based hand rubs (ABHRs) to individuals served individually rather than having the product available from wall-mounted dispensers, for example. This action may be taken to prevent the container from being used as a projectile or to prevent the client from attempting to ingest the product. The IPC plan and risk assessment should include any unique situations related to the care environment and how those situations should be addressed (see Chapter 3).

Safe Injection Practices

Unsafe injection practices affect about 150,000 patients each year.[7] Between 2001 and 2011, there were multiple outbreaks of bacterial and viral infections associated with unsafe injection practices, as reported by the US Centers for Disease Control and Prevention (CDC). Each year, such outbreaks occur in outpatient settings such as ambulatory surgery centers and physician offices.

As part of overall efforts to reduce harm from unsafe injection practices, the CDC offers guidelines related to safe injection practices to reduce the risk of infectious and noninfectious adverse events in both patients and health care providers. Safe injection practices are part of standard precautions and protect patients and providers.[6] These practices are required by the US Centers for Medicare & Medicaid Services (CMS) and The Joint Commission as well as JCI.

The CDC initiated the One & Only Campaign as a public health effort to eliminate unsafe injection practices. Through targeted education and awareness, the One & Only Campaign empowers patients and health care providers to insist on safe injection practices—every time and for every patient. Information on this campaign is included in the Resources section at the end of this chapter. In 2016, the Association for Professionals in Infection Control and Epidemiology (APIC) updated its position paper "Safe Injection, Infusion, and Medication Vial Practices in Health Care."[7] Infection preventionists (IPs) may need to assess whether safe injection practices are in place in their organization. Additional tools and information about this topic are listed in the Resources section at the end of this chapter.

The CDC website for injection safety provides a toolkit for health care providers that addresses best practices for notifying patients exposed or potentially exposed to bloodborne or other pathogens. Regardless of whether the exposure occurs as a result of unsafe injection practices or lapses in basic infection control, facilities should be prepared to communicate the potential risks to all parties involved.

Safe Use of Needles, Syringes, and Intravenous Delivery Systems

Safe injection practices apply to proper use of needles, cannulas that replace needles, and intravenous delivery systems and include the following recommended strategies:

- Use aseptic techniques to avoid contaminating sterile injection equipment. Follow proper infection control practices while preparing and administering medications.
- Do not administer medications from the same syringe to multiple patients, even if the needle or cannula on the syringe is changed.
  - Needles, cannulas, and syringes are sterile, single-use items; do not reuse them for other patients or to access a medication or solution that might be used for a subsequent patient.
  - Use a fluid infusion and administration set (for example, intravenous bags, tubing, connectors) for one patient only and dispose of it appropriately after use.
- After a device has been used to enter or connect to a patient's intravenous infusion bag or administration set, consider the syringe or needle/cannula to be contaminated.
- Use of single-dose/single-use vials is strongly encouraged by the CDC for patient safety. Assign medication packaged as a multidose vial to a single patient whenever possible. Figure 6-1 shows a poster from the One & Only Campaign that can be used in facilities to encourage and implement safe injection practices.

Medication Management

In addition to managing needles and syringes, safe practices for handling medication (unopened and opened) vials are also delineated in the One & Only Campaign and in the APIC position paper for safe injection practices.[7] Ideally, medication vials should be used in one care area and not transported to another because of the difficulty in maintaining chain of custody and sterility.

Respiratory Hygiene and Cough Etiquette

Policies related to respiratory hygiene and cough etiquette aim to contain respiratory secretions of individuals who demonstrate signs and symptoms of respiratory infection. They prevent the transmission of respiratory illnesses from people who enter health care settings with cough, congestion, and/or rhinorrhea. To comply with respiratory hygiene and cough etiquette policies, an individual should do the following:

- Cover his or her nose/mouth when coughing or sneezing.
- Use tissues to contain respiratory secretions and dispose of tissues in the nearest waste receptacle after use.

Figure 6-1. CDC Poster for the One & Only Campaign

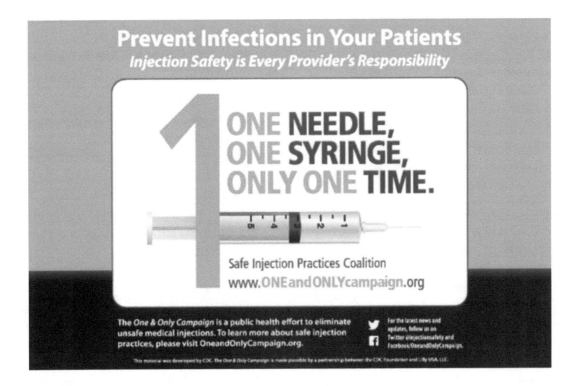

Source: CDC. The One & Only Campaign. Accessed Mar 13, 2020. https://www.cdc.gov/injectionsafety/one-and-only.html

- Clean hands after having contact with respiratory secretions and contaminated objects/materials. This can be accomplished by hand washing with non-antimicrobial or antiseptic soap and water or by using ABHRs.

See the CDC website for posters and more information at https://www.cdc.gov/flu/professionals/infectioncontrol/resphygiene.htm for posters and more information.

To encourage proper respiratory hygiene and cough etiquette, health care facilities and IPs should ensure the availability of tissues and hand hygiene supplies. An IP, in collaboration with other health care staff, should identify where and how to provide access to these critical supplies. There should also be a system to ensure availability of critical supplies at all times.

TIP Creative signage on respiratory hygiene and cough etiquette helps alert visitors and patients to adhere to the organization's IPC policies. Signs may be placed in waiting areas and at entrances to the facility to remind everyone about the need to contain respiratory illnesses—such as the flu—and the importance of hand hygiene.

Personal Protective Equipment (PPE)

PPE provides barriers to protect health care workers and to reduce the risk of transmission of pathogens, prevent exposure to potentially infectious material, and reduce cross-contamination during patient care activities. The CDC provides posters and guidance on PPE in health care settings (see https://www.cdc.gov/sharpssafety/).[8] This site links to additional resources such as the *Workbook for Designing, Implementing, and Evaluating a Sharps Injury Program*, videos, slides, and posters that demonstrate safe and proper use of PPE. Such materials provide helpful teaching aids for training, such as on how to don (put on) and doff (remove) PPE.[9,10] Additional resources are provided at the end of this chapter.

To reduce infection risk, health care organizations should identify the minimum required PPE for protection (based on identified risks associated with specific tasks and infections) and should provide those supplies. Monitoring compliance with PPE use helps ensure staff and patient safety. Additional information on managing supply and optimizing use of PPE during a pandemic, such as COVID-19 or a sudden influx of infectious patients, is discussed later in this chapter. Preventing breaches in PPE protocols, such as those associated with wearing PPE incorrectly or removing PPE in a way that leads to self-contamination, is critical for health care worker safety and for preventing contamination, which could lead to secondary transmission, as was reported during initial care of Ebola patients in the United States. As a result of lessons learned following Ebola disease outbreaks, additional recommendations—called *enhanced precautions*, to ensure that all skin is covered—were created to reduce risk of exposure to staff.

The CDC also provides recommendations for IPC practices in particular settings, such as outpatient settings and long term care facilities, for example. A guide to IPC in outpatient settings is available at https://www.cdc.gov/infectioncontrol/pdf/outpatient/guide.pdf.[11]

Long term care facilities have increased in number and scope of services provided in areas that include both medical and personal care to individuals who are unable to live independently. The facilities may be referred to as long term care facilities, nursing homes, skilled nursing facilities, and assisted living facilities. It is estimated that 1 to 3 million serious infections occur annually in these settings. The CDC has guidelines and recommendations for IPC in these facilities and in various nursing care

procedures at https://www.cdc.gov/longtermcare/index.html.

Face Shields

A face shield is designed to protect the eyes of caregivers from contamination. The CDC recommends that in addition to a face shield, the user also wear a mask due to limited data to determine if a face shield alone protects from the spray of respiratory droplets.

The CDC recommends the following prevention strategies related to face shields:

- Hands should be washed before and after removing the face shield, and users should avoid touching their eyes, nose, and mouth when removing it.
- Disposable face shields should only be worn for a single use and disposed of according to manufacturer instructions.
- Reusable face shields should be cleaned and disinfected after each use according to manufacturer instructions or by following the CDC's face shield cleaning instructions, available at https://www.cdc.gov/coronavirus/2019-ncov/hcp/ppe-strategy/eye-protection.html.
- Plastic face shields are not recommended for newborns and infants (see https://www.cdc.gov/coronavirus/2019-ncov/prevent-getting-sick/cloth-face-cover-guidance.html).

Transmission-Based Precautions

Although standard precautions provide the most basic intervention for preventing and controlling transmission of infectious agents during patient care, standard precautions can be enhanced through transmission-based precautions. This includes contact precautions, droplet precautions, and airborne isolation, as recommended in the CDC/HICPAC isolation guidelines for specific infectious agents.[6] The CDC has specific microorganism recommendations for managing patients with these unique pathogens. See the Resources list at the end of this chapter for specific sites.

The current CDC transmission-based isolation guideline is applicable across the continuum of care.[6] Organism-specific IPC recommendations are also available for organisms such as vancomycin-resistant *Enterococci* (VRE), methicillin-resistant *Staphylococcus aureus* (MRSA),[12] and *Burkholderia cepacia*.[13] Many states, such as North Carolina and Michigan, also have specific documents regarding the management of multidrug-resistant organisms (MDROs). (See "Key Infection Prevention Documents" in the Resources section at the end of this chapter.)

The CDC's *Facility Guidance for Control of Carbapenem-Resistant Enterobacteriaceae (CRE), November 2015 Update—CRE Toolkit* reviews strategies and validation for acute and long term care settings, including surveillance and specific IPC components.[14] The components are hand hygiene, contact precautions based on level of acuity, including postacute care, use of devices, lab notification, interfacility communication, antimicrobial stewardship programs, patient and staff cohorting, screening of contacts of CRE patients, active surveillance testing, and chlorhexidine gluconate (CHG) bathing.[14]

The CDC guidelines provide recommendations for the continuum of health care, and each facility must evaluate its practice setting and determine how best to implement and sustain transmission-based precautions and manage MDROs.[14] The IP can be a key ally to assist the leaders responsible for practice in a specific area within the continuum of care in this evaluation and implementation process.

Although the Agency for Healthcare Research and Quality (AHRQ) *Carbapenem-Resistant Enterobacteriaceae (CRE) Control and Prevention Toolkit* is related to a specific MDRO, it is an implementation primer that can be useful to the IP when implementing prevention and control initiatives.[15] The AHRQ CRE Toolkit addresses six areas that can be used alone or in conjunction with the other sections, based on the health care organization's specific needs. The sections include the following:
- Assessing Your Readiness for Change
- Starting Your Project
- Putting Your Intervention into Practice
- Implementing Best Practices
- Measuring the Impact of Your Intervention
- Implementing and Sustaining Your Intervention

Within the AHRQ toolkit are worksheets and tools to aid IPs and clinical leaders in facilitating implementation.

Each health care setting has its own unique microbial flora patterns, which reflect its community's and referring institutions' microbiology. Unique concerns often arise in specialized settings such as pediatrics, intensive care units, long term care facilities, rehabilitation units, and home health agencies.[14,16] The emergence of community-acquired MRSA adds another dimension to the complexity

of IPC in all health care settings.[17] An organization should be able to demonstrate how it applies transmission-based practices to prevent and control transmission of pathogens in its service settings.[18] (More information on this topic can be found in Chapter 12. In addition, download Tool 6-1.)

TRY THIS TOOL

Tool 6-1. Compliance Check Sheet for Isolation Precautions

Additional resources to assist organizations in refining their management of MDROs and other infectious organisms are provided at the end of this chapter.[19] Furthermore, Septimus et al. discuss a horizontal approach to IPC, which uses basic measures to prevent and control a wide range of MDROs, including universal gloving, gowning, high-touch cleaning, and CHG bathing.[20]

Demonstrating Isolation Strategy Implementation

The successful implementation of isolation strategies can be demonstrated through audits or surveillance that show trends in epidemiologically significant organisms. For example, increases in MDROs may indicate noncompliance or system failures with isolation and other IPC practices.[21] In 2020, the COVID-19 pandemic highlighted areas of noncompliance with recommended prevention strategies, including isolation. The ongoing assessment of adherence to appropriate isolation practices, which includes feedback to those who can affect practices and implementation of action plans to improve performance, can be used to demonstrate compliance with isolation requirements.

Compliance with transmission-based precautions and enhanced precautions is critical for the safety of patients, visitors, and staff. Minor infractions can have deadly consequences, as noted during the COVID-19 pandemic. Monitoring of practice must be built into daily routine activities. It must become part of the culture of the organization and must be considered an important commitment to everyone's safety and well-being.

PPE Use During Transmission-Based Precautions

PPE use has been of paramount importance during the COVID-19 pandemic to prevent and control transmission and spread of the deadly SARS-CoV-2/Novel Coronavirus 2019. The CDC offers recommendations for managing hospitalized patients with known or suspected cases of this virus. During training and orientation in health care organizations, proper PPE use should be taught and competency determined by demonstration. Sidebar 6-1 lists a number of IPC resources for managing COVID-19.

In addition, the CDC has amended its guidance for long term care facilities to address COVID-19 in those settings. Currently, changes in recommendations include the following:

Sidebar 6-1. IPC Resources for Managing COVID-19

The Centers for Disease Control and Prevention (CDC) provides a number of resources related to COVID-19, including the following:
- Interim Clinical Guidance for Management of Patients with Confirmed Coronavirus Disease (COVID-19). Accessed Dec 10, 2020. https://www.cdc.gov/coronavirus/2019-ncov/hcp/clinical-guidance-management-patients.html
- Interim Infection Prevention and Control Recommendations for Healthcare Personnel During the Coronavirus Disease 2019 (COVID-19) Pandemic. Accessed Dec 10, 2020. https://www.cdc.gov/coronavirus/2019-ncov/hcp/infection-control-recommendations.html
- How COVID-19 Spreads. Accessed Dec 10, 2020. https://www.cdc.gov/coronavirus/2019-ncov/prevent-getting-sick/how-covid-spreads.html

Posters are available to guide your PPE donning and doffing process. For example, see Figure 6-22[2] on pages 133–134. These posters are available for distribution within your facility as part of your COVID-19 response plan. See https://www.cdc.gov/coronavirus/2019-ncov/downloads/A_FS_HCP_COVID19_PPE.pdf.

- Tiered recommendations to address nursing homes in different phases of COVID-19 response
- Added recommendations to assign an individual to manage the facility's IPC program
- Added guidance about new requirements for nursing homes to report to the NHSN
- Added recommendations to create a plan for testing residents and health care personnel for SARS-CoV-2

During the COVID-19 outbreaks in 2020, CMS issued several memorandums related to nursing home practices in response to the severe effects that the virus had on the health and well-being of nursing care center staff and residents. Outbreaks in nursing care centers are associated with high rates of infection, morbidity, and mortality in this vulnerable population. Table 6-1 on page 135 lists some targeted directives from CMS for responding to COVID-19 in nursing care centers.

In addition, a CMS *Toolkit on State Actions to Mitigate COVID-19 Prevalence in Nursing Homes*[23] offers guidance and can be found at https://www.cms.gov/files/document/covid-toolkit-states-mitigate-covid-19-nursing-homes.pdf. CMS also has a helpful checklist for long term care facilities/nursing homes (*see* CMS Publication 12SOW-QI-Q11-061720a).

As stated earlier, health care workers should be able to articulate and demonstrate their competency regarding when and how to use PPE. It is important to understand staff attitudes and knowledge to help design education programs and interventions to ensure compliance.[24] No matter the health care setting, all health care workers must protect themselves by using PPE appropriately. The CDC offers posters and videos that demonstrate the appropriate sequences for donning and doffing PPE.[25]

Masks for Source Control

Face masks became a critical tool for preventing disease in communities through transmission by droplets and aerosols during the COVID-19 pandemic. Choices for face protection include surgical masks, respirators, face shields, and eye protection, and, in nonmedical situations, cloth masks for protection against COVID-19.[26,27] The US Occupational Safety and Health Administration provides guidance for protection of health care workers. Figure 6-3 on page 136 offers tips for wearing procedure masks in nonsurgical health care settings.[10]

Figure 6-2. CDC Poster: Use Personal Protective Equipment When Caring for Patients with Confirmed or Suspected COVID-19

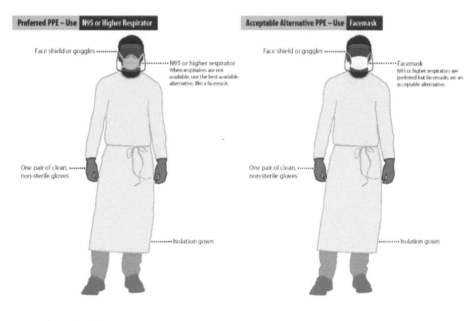

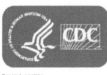

Source: Centers for Disease Control and Prevention (CDC). Accessed Dec 10, 2020.
https://www.cdc.gov/coronavirus/2019-ncov/downloads/A_FS_HCP_COVID19_PPE.pdf

(continued)

Figure 6-2. CDC Poster: Use Personal Protective Equipment When Caring for Patients with Confirmed or Suspected COVID-19 (continued)

Donning (putting on the gear):

More than one donning method may be acceptable. Training and practice using your healthcare facility's procedure is critical. Below is one example of donning.

1. **Identify and gather the proper PPE to don.** Ensure choice of gown size is correct (based on training).
2. **Perform hand hygiene using hand sanitizer.**
3. **Put on isolation gown.** Tie all of the ties on the gown. Assistance may be needed by another HCP.
4. **Put on NIOSH-approved N95 filtering facepiece respirator or higher (use a facemask if a respirator is not available).** If the respirator has a nosepiece, it should be fitted to the nose with both hands, not bent or tented. Do not pinch the nosepiece with one hand. Respirator/facemask should be extended under chin. Both your mouth and nose should be protected. Do not wear respirator/facemask under your chin or store in scrubs pocket between patients.*

   » **Respirator:** Respirator straps should be placed on crown of head (top strap) and base of neck (bottom strap). Perform a user seal check each time you put on the respirator.
   » **Facemask:** Mask ties should be secured on crown of head (top tie) and base of neck (bottom tie). If mask has loops, hook them appropriately around your ears.

5. **Put on face shield or goggles.** When wearing an N95 respirator or half facepiece elastomeric respirator, select the proper eye protection to ensure that the respirator does not interfere with the correct positioning of the eye protection, and the eye protection does not affect the fit or seal of the respirator. Face shields provide full face coverage. Goggles also provide excellent protection for eyes, but fogging is common.
6. **Put on gloves.** Gloves should cover the cuff (wrist) of gown.
7. **HCP may now enter patient room.**

Doffing (taking off the gear):

More than one doffing method may be acceptable. Training and practice using your healthcare facility's procedure is critical. Below is one example of doffing.

1. **Remove gloves.** Ensure glove removal does not cause additional contamination of hands. Gloves can be removed using more than one technique (e.g., glove-in-glove or bird beak).
2. **Remove gown.** Untie all ties (or unsnap all buttons). Some gown ties can be broken rather than untied. Do so in gentle manner, avoiding a forceful movement. Reach up to the shoulders and carefully pull gown down and away from the body. Rolling the gown down is an acceptable approach. Dispose in trash receptacle.*
3. **HCP may now exit patient room.**
4. **Perform hand hygiene.**
5. **Remove face shield or goggles.** Carefully remove face shield or goggles by grabbing the strap and pulling upwards and away from head. Do not touch the front of face shield or goggles.
6. **Remove and discard respirator (or facemask if used instead of respirator).*** Do not touch the front of the respirator or facemask.

   » **Respirator:** Remove the bottom strap by touching only the strap and bring it carefully over the head. Grasp the top strap and bring it carefully over the head, and then pull the respirator away from the face without touching the front of the respirator.
   » **Facemask:** Carefully untie (or unhook from the ears) and pull away from face without touching the front.

7. **Perform hand hygiene after removing the respirator/facemask** and before putting it on again if your workplace is practicing reuse.

Facilities implementing reuse or extended use of PPE will need to adjust their donning and doffing procedures to accommodate those practices.

www.cdc.gov/coronavirus

Source: Centers for Disease Control and Prevention (CDC). Accessed Dec 10, 2020.
https://www.cdc.gov/coronavirus/2019-ncov/downloads/A_FS_HCP_COVID19_PPE.pdf

Table 6-1. CMS Nursing Home Directives in Response to COVID-19

Date	Description
March 2020	QSO-20-14-NH: Guidance for restricting facility visitation for all visitors and nonessential health care personnel except for certain compassionate care situations, such as end-of-life.
May 2020	Nursing Home Reopening Recommendations
June 2020	Frequently asked questions that expand on previously issued documents such as outdoor visits, compassionate care situations, and communal activities
September 2020	CMS testing rules
	Visitation guidance to allow nursing homes to safely facilitate in-person visitation to address the psychological needs of residents
	CMS-approved Civil Money Penalty (CMP) and funds to purchase outdoor visitation equipment and indoor visitation safety measures
	Visitation access based on the county's positivity rate
	Universal Eye Protection

Two examples—one from the *Journal of the American Medical Association*, within a Boston hospital system and the other from CDC's *Morbidity and Mortality Weekly Report* (MMWR),[28-30]—showed that adherence to universal masking policies reduced transmission of SARS-CoV-2, the virus that causes COVID-19. Similarly, the World Health Organization (WHO) has also published guidance on when and how to use masks to halt the COVID-19 transmission.[31]

It is important to note, however, that cloth face coverings are not PPE. They are not surgical masks or N95 respirators, both of which should be reserved for use by health care workers and other medical first responders (see Figure 6-4 on page 137).[33] Use of cloth face coverings is an additional step, recommended by the CDC to the general public, to help slow the spread of COVID-19. Both the CDC and the WHO recommend wearing masks combined with social distancing and other COVID-19 preventive measures when in public.

WHO and CDC guidance for the general public includes the following[27,32]:

- People should wear masks in public settings and when around people who don't live in the same household, especially when other measures, such as social distancing, are difficult to maintain.
- Masks are a critical step to help prevent people from getting and spreading COVID-19.
- Masks are most likely to reduce the spread of COVID-19 when they are widely used by people in public settings. (Note that in February 2021, the CDC issued a requirement for face masks on planes, buses, trains, and other forms of public transportation into, within, or out of the US and in US transportation hubs, such as airports, to reduce and control the spread of COVID-19.)
- Masks should not be worn by children under the age of 2 or anyone who has trouble breathing or is unconscious, incapacitated, or otherwise unable to remove the mask without assistance.
- Masks with exhalation valves or vents should not be worn to help prevent the person wearing the mask from spreading COVID-19 to others (source control).

It is also important to recognize that a mask is contaminated after use and that it should be carefully removed to decrease spread and further risk of contamination. Masks should be stored appropriately and, if they are reusable, they should also be cleaned and disinfected appropriately.

Figure 6-3. Do's and Don'ts for Wearing Procedure Masks in Non-Surgical Healthcare Settings

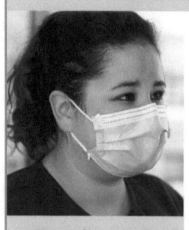

Do's & Don'ts

For wearing procedure masks in non-surgical healthcare settings

Procedure mask
(also called an isolation mask)

Disposable mask that protects the wearer from droplets that might be infectious. A version of this mask with a built-in face shield to protect against splashes is also available.

The Occupational Safety & Health Administration (OSHA) may update guidance related to masks as emerging pathogens arise and new recommendations are developed. Be on the lookout for updates by visiting the OSHA website or consult your facility's infection prevention or occupational health department.

Learn more: **www.osha.gov/SLTC/ respiratoryprotection/guidance.html**

Do

✓ Make sure to wear your mask to protect yourself from infectious droplets that may occur when patients cough, sneeze, laugh, or talk.

✓ Check to make sure the mask has no defects, such as a tear or torn strap or ear loop.

✓ Bring both top ties to the crown of head and secure with a bow; tie bottom ties securely at the nape of neck in a bow.

✓ Remove the mask when no longer in clinical space and the patient intervention is complete.

✓ For ear loop mask, remove the mask from the side with your head tilted forward. For tied masks, remove by handling only the ties, and untie the bottom tie followed by the top tie.

✓ Properly dispose of the mask by touching only the ear loops or the ties. Perform hand hygiene before and after removing a surgical mask or any type of personal protective equipment such as your gloves and gown.

Don't

✗ DON'T use for protection against very small particles that float in the air (e.g., TB, measles, or chickenpox).

✗ DON'T wear if wet or soiled; get a new mask.

✗ DON'T crisscross ties.

✗ DON'T leave a mask hanging off one ear or hanging around neck.

✗ DON'T reuse; toss it after wearing once.

✗ DON'T touch the front of the mask, as it is contaminated after use.

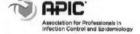 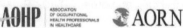

APIC — Association for Professionals in Infection Control and Epidemiology | ANA — AMERICAN NURSES ASSOCIATION | AOHP — ASSOCIATION OF OCCUPATIONAL HEALTH PROFESSIONALS IN HEALTHCARE | AORN

Source: APIC. Do's and Don'ts for Wearing Procedure Masks in Non-Surgical Healthcare Settings. Accessed May 25, 2021. http://www.apic.org/Resource_/TinyMceFileManager/consumers_professionals/APIC_DosDontsofMasks_hiq.pdf

Figure 6-4. Understanding the Difference Between a Surgical Mask and an N95 Respirator

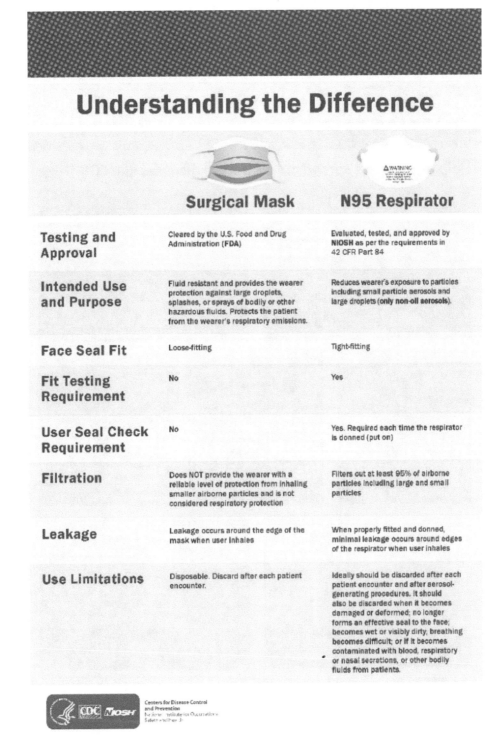

Source: CDC/NIOSH. Understanding the Difference. Accessed May 25, 2021.
https://www.cdc.gov/niosh/npptl/pdfs/UnderstandDifferenceInfographic-508.pdf

A successful IPC program can be achieved when all elements are implemented consistently. Using posters, signs, and media can help remind everyone of the key elements of infection prevention. Figure 6-5 is an example of a poster to help prevent and control the spread of respiratory diseases such as COVID-19.[34]

Figure 6-5. CDC Poster: Stop the Spread of Germs

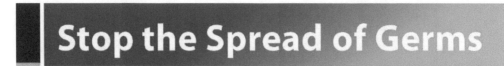

Stop the Spread of Germs

Help prevent the spread of respiratory diseases like COVID-19.

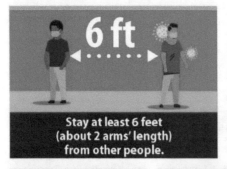

Stay at least 6 feet (about 2 arms' length) from other people.

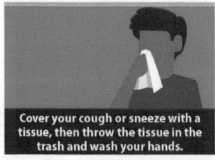

Cover your cough or sneeze with a tissue, then throw the tissue in the trash and wash your hands.

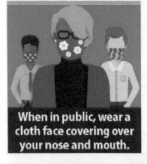

When in public, wear a cloth face covering over your nose and mouth.

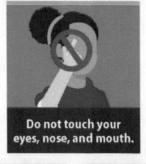

Do not touch your eyes, nose, and mouth.

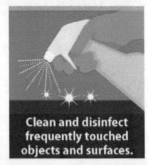

Clean and disinfect frequently touched objects and surfaces.

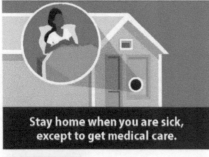

Stay home when you are sick, except to get medical care.

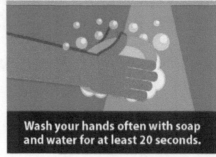

Wash your hands often with soap and water for at least 20 seconds.

cdc.gov/coronavirus

Source: CDC. Stop the Spread of Germs. 2020. Accessed Sep 20, 2020. https://www.cdc.gov/coronavirus/2019-ncov/downloads/stop-the-spread-of-germs.pdf

PPE Availability and Compliance with Use Recommendations

The availability of PPE supplies at the point of use is critical. Facilities should assess their process measures for overall compliance with recommended practices, including availability of supplies as well as the appropriate use of PPE.[6] Each unit or department should be able to demonstrate that it has a mechanism to ensure replacement of supplies when needed. Noncompliance is often fueled by PPE inaccessibility.

During the COVID-19 pandemic, severe PPE shortages created the potential for exposures to health care workers, putting workers and patients at risk. The CDC provides strategies to optimize PPE and PPE supplies in health care settings. These strategies offer a continuum of options using the framework of surge capacity when PPE supplies are stressed, running low, or absent. When using these strategies, health care facilities should:

- Consider these options and implement them sequentially
- Understand their current PPE inventory, supply chain, and utilization rate
- Train health care staff on PPE use and have them demonstrate competency with all PPE used to perform their job responsibilities
- As PPE availability returns to normal, promptly resume standard practices

As stated earlier, nursing homes were especially challenged during the COVID-19 pandemic, particularly with having the appropriate type and volume of PPE needed when the number of COVID-19 cases in the US was rapidly increasing.[35] Strategies for planning for a surge of infectious patients must be applied across the continuum of care. Figure 6-6 illustrates a framework for optimizing PPE.[36]

Investigating Infectious Disease Outbreaks

One important component of an IPC program is planning for managing an outbreak. Outbreaks can be related to the following:

- Health care–associated infections (HAIs) being transmitted in the health care setting
- Foodborne outbreaks caused by contaminated food and sometimes associated with the source of fruits, vegetables or meat, and dairy products
- Community-acquired infections that lead to an outbreak not related to health care, such as measles, MRSA, or norovirus transmitted in daycare centers or on cruise ships.

An organization's IPC plan should include how to investigate an outbreak, communicate information about the outbreak, and notify and collaborate with public health officials. The IP is often an important partner with public health officials and can report suspected community-acquired infections or foodborne outbreaks. Refer to Chapters 4 and 5 for more details on this topic.

The CDC provides many resources that are helpful in planning for and implementing clinical procedures to manage an outbreak. The site https://cdc.gov/outbreaks/index.html provides a current list of outbreaks, including US-based outbreaks, international outbreaks, and travel

Figure 6-6. Framework for Optimizing PPE

Conventional Capacity
strategies that should already be in place as part of general infection prevention and control plans in healthcare settings

Contingency Capacity
strategies that can be used during periods of anticipated PPE shortages

Crisis Capacity*
strategies that can be used when supplies cannot meet the facility's current or anticipated PPE utilization rate
*Not commensurate with U.S. standards of care

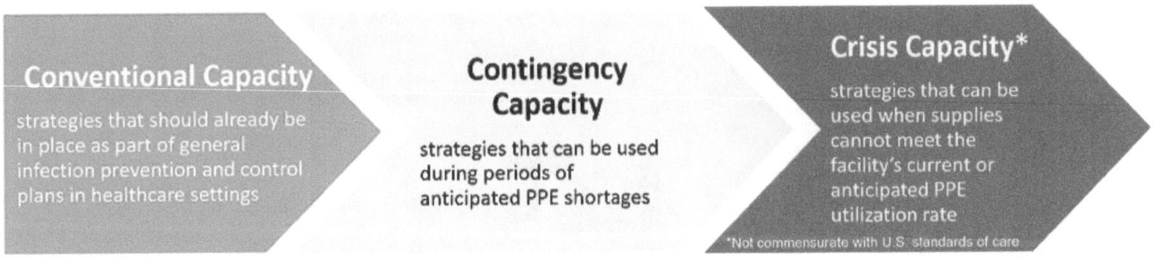

Source: CDC. Summary for Healthcare Facilities: Strategies for Optimizing the Supply of PPE During Shortages. Accessed May 25, 2021. https://www.cdc.gov/coronavirus/2019-ncov/hcp/ppe-strategy/strategies-optimize-ppe-shortages.html

Figure 6-7. Steps in a Foodborne Outbreak Investigation

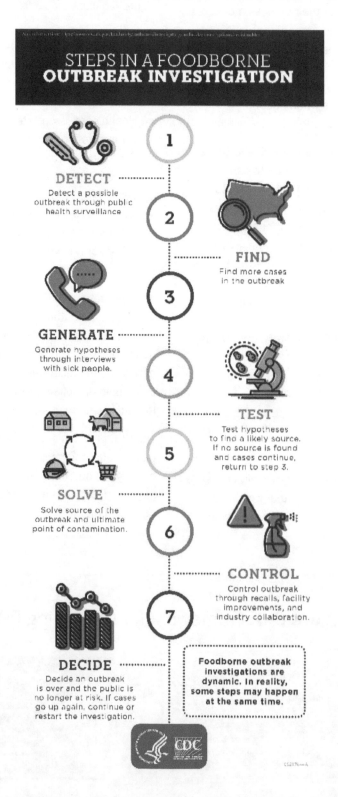

notices affecting international travel. The site also provides links to additional information related to understanding outbreaks, investigating outbreaks, and the CDC's role in global health security, including the following:

- Investigating Outbreaks: Using Data to Link Foodborne Disease Outbreaks to a Contaminated Source. May 25, 2016. Accessed May 25, 2021. https://www.cdc.gov/foodsafety/outbreaks/investigating-outbreaks/index.html
- Steps in a Foodborne Outbreak Investigation. Accessed May 25, 2021. https://www.cdc.gov/foodsafety/outbreaks/investigating-outbreaks/investigations/index.html

Figure 6-7 shows the steps in investigating a foodborne illness outbreak. The CDC has issued 10 steps used by epidemiologists to investigate outbreaks. The guidelines aim to ensure rapid and accurate evaluation of an outbreak to contain the disease as quickly as possible and prevent harm to the public. Guidelines may be found at https://www.verywellhealth.com/what-is-an-outbreak-epidemiology-101-1958752.

In addition, SHEA has published guidance for acute-care organizations in responding to an outbreak and incident management. The article "Outbreak Response and Incident Management: Shea Guidance and Resources for Healthcare Epidemiologists in United States Acute-Care Hospitals" is available in the December 2017 edition of the *Journal of Infection Control and Hospital Epidemiology*.[37]

Table 6-2 and Table 6-3 provide resources related to COVID-19 in a variety of health care and clinical settings.

Table 6-2. Resources for COVID-19 Response

Source	Resources

Centers for Disease Control and Prevention (CDC) guidance	• Coronavirus Disease 2019 (COVID-19) Guidance Documents. Accessed Dec 10, 2020. https://www.cdc.gov/coronavirus/2019-ncov/communication/guidance-list.html?Sort=Date%3A%3Adesc
	
	• Interim Infection Prevention and Control Recommendations for Patients with Suspected or Confirmed Coronavirus Disease 2019 (COVID-19) in Healthcare Settings
	Key concepts in this guidance:
	   ◦ Limit how germs can enter the facility.
	   ◦ Isolate symptomatic patients as soon as possible.
	   ◦ Protect health care personnel.
	
	Accessed Dec 10, 2020. https://www.cdc.gov/coronavirus/2019-ncov/infection-control/control-recommendations.html
	
	• Overview of Testing for SARS-CoV-2 (COVID-19). Accessed Dec 10, 2020. https://www.cdc.gov/coronavirus/2019-ncov/hcp/testing-overview.html
	
	(continued)

Table 6-2. Resources for COVID-19 Response (continued)

Source	Resources
CDC printable materials	• Print Resources. This website contains a wide variety of printable flyers, posters, fact sheets, and infographics for communication of information regarding COVID-19. Accessed Dec 10, 2020. https://www.cdc.gov/coronavirus/2019-ncov/communication/factsheets.html • Stop the Spread of Germs: Help Prevent the Spread of Respiratory Diseases like COVID-19. Accessed Dec 10, 2020. https://www.cdc.gov/coronavirus/2019-ncov/downloads/stop-the-spread-of-germs.pdf • Please Read Before Entering (COVID-19 symptom flyer/poster for outside clinic). Accessed Dec 10, 2020. https://www.cdc.gov/coronavirus/2019-ncov/downloads/Please-Read.pdf • 10 Things You Can Do to Manage Your COVID-19 Symptoms at Home. Accessed Dec 10, 2020. https://www.cdc.gov/coronavirus/2019-ncov/downloads/10Things.pdf • Symptoms of Coronavirus (COVID-19). Accessed Dec 10, 2020. https://www.cdc.gov/coronavirus/2019-ncov/downloads/COVID19-symptoms.pdf • How to Protect Yourself and Others. Accessed Dec 10, 2020. https://www.cdc.gov/coronavirus/2019-ncov/prevent-getting-sick/prevention-H.pdf • Get Your Clinic Ready for Coronavirus Disease 2019 (COVID-19). Accessed Dec 10, 2020. https://www.cdc.gov/coronavirus/2019-ncov/downloads/Clinic.pdf • Use Personal Protective Equipment (PPE) When Caring for Patients with Confirmed or Suspected COVID-19. Accessed Dec 10, 2020. https://www.cdc.gov/coronavirus/2019-ncov/downloads/A_FS_HCP_COVID19_PPE_11x17.pdf • Use Personal Protective Equipment (PPE) When Caring for Patients with Confirmed or Suspected COVID-19. Accessed Dec 10, 2020. https://www.cdc.gov/coronavirus/2019-ncov/downloads/A_FS_HCP_COVID19_PPE.pdf
CDC preparedness checklists	• Comprehensive Hospital Preparedness Checklist. Accessed Dec 10, 2020. https://www.cdc.gov/coronavirus/2019-ncov/downloads/HCW_Checklist_508.pdf • Healthcare Professional Preparedness Checklist for Transport and Arrival of Patients with Confirmed or Possible COVID-19. Accessed Dec 10, 2020. https://www.cdc.gov/coronavirus/2019-ncov/downloads/hcp-preparedness-checklist.pdf

(continued)

Table 6-2. Resources for COVID-19 Response (continued)

Source	Resources
Joint Commission COVID-19 resources	• Coronavirus (COVID-19). Accessed Sep 14, 2020. https://www.jointcommission.org/COVID-19/ • Interpreting Joint Commission Standards: FAQs. Accessed Apr 26, 2021. https://www.jointcommission.org/standards/standard-faqs/?utm_source=TJC%20Website&utm_medium=optimize&utm_campaign=tjc-home-connect&ref=tjchc56
Minnesota Centers for Enhanced Response (CER)	• Minnesota CER Assessment Tool. This tool provides an assessment to aide in evaluating the capacity to respond to high-consequence infectious diseases. Accessed Aug 24, 2020. https://www.health.state.mn.us/diseases/hcid/certool.pdf
Occupational Safety and Health Administration (OSHA)	• Control and Prevention. Recommendations for control and prevention of COVID-19. Accessed Aug 24, 2020. https://www.osha.gov/SLTC/covid-19/controlprevention.html#healthcare
Society for Healthcare Epidemiology of America (SHEA)	• Novel Coronavirus 2019 (COVID-19) Resources for healthcare epidemiologists, infection preventionists, and other medical professionals responding to COVID-19. Accessed Aug 24, 2020. https://www.shea-online.org/index.php/practice-resources/priority-topics/emerging-pathogens/novel-coronavirus-2019-2019-ncov-resources
US Environmental Protection Agency (EPA)	Preparation for Coronavirus Disease: How Should US Hospitals Prepare for Coronavirus Disease 2019 (COVID-19)? This list includes products that meet the EPA's criteria for use against SARS-CoV-2, the novel coronavirus that causes the disease COVID-19.[39] An infection preventionist, materials management, or the environmental service leader should check if a product's EPA registration number is included on this list when deciding which product to purchase and use for disinfection against COVID-19. It is important to match the EPA registration number with the product label to be sure that it can be used against SARS-CoV-2. Products may be marketed and sold under different brand names, but if they have the same EPA registration number, they are the same product. • About List N: Disinfectants for Use Against SARS-CoV-2. Accessed Aug 24, 2020. https://www.epa.gov/pesticide-registration/list-n-disinfectants-use-against-sars-cov-2 • Frequently Asked Questions About List N: Disinfectants for Use Against SARS-CoV-2. Accessed Apr 1, 2020. https://www.epa.gov/coronavirus/frequent-questions-about-coronavirus-disease-covid-19#disinfectants
Association for Professionals in Infection Control and Epidemiology (APIC)	• APIC Coronavirus FactSheet. Accessed Aug 24, 2020. https://apic.org/wp-content/uploads/2020/02/02420_Coronavirus_HiresNoBleed.pdf

Note: COVID-19 resources are evolving daily. All resources listed here are current as of their specified access date but are subject to modification/removal by their respective organizations as new/updated information becomes available.

Table 6-3. COVID-19 Infection Prevention for Varied Practice Settings

Source	Resources
Centers for Disease Control and Prevention (CDC) dental care settings	• Interim Infection Prevention and Control Guidance for Dental Settings During the Coronavirus Disease 2019 (COVID-19) Pandemic. Accessed Dec 10, 2020. https://www.cdc.gov/coronavirus/2019-ncov/hcp/dental-settings.html
CDC dialysis facilities	• Additional Guidance for Infection Prevention and Control Recommendations for Patients with Suspected or Confirmed COVID-19 in Outpatient Hemodialysis Facilities. Accessed Aug 17, 2020. https://www.cdc.gov/coronavirus/2019-ncov/hcp/dialysis.html • Coronavirus Disease 2019 (COVID-19) Outpatient Dialysis Facility Preparedness Assessment Tool. Accessed Aug 17, 2020. https://www.cdc.gov/coronavirus/2019-ncov/downloads/COVID-19-outpatient-dialysis.pdf • Preparing Your Dialysis Facility for Coronavirus Disease 2019 (COVID-19). Accessed Aug 17, 2020. https://www.cdc.gov/coronavirus/2019-ncov/downloads/hcp/fs-COVID19-Dialysis-Facility.pdf
CDC long term care	• Checklist for Nursing Homes and Other Long-Term Care Facilities. Accessed Apr 1, 2020. https://www.cdc.gov/coronavirus/2019-ncov/downloads/novel-coronavirus-2019-Nursing-Homes-Preparedness-Checklist_3_13.pdf
CDC long term care facilities and nursing homes	• Interim Infection Prevention and Control Recommendations to Prevent SARS-CoV-2 Spread in Nursing Homes. Accessed Aug 17, 2020. https://www.cdc.gov/coronavirus/2019-ncov/hcp/long-term-care.html • Applying COVID-19 Infection Prevention and Control Strategies in Nursing Homes. Recorded Webinar. Accessed Aug 17, 2020. https://emergency.cdc.gov/coca/calls/2020/callinfo_061620.asp
Podiatry	• American Podiatric Medical Association (APMA). COVID-19 Resources. Accessed Aug 17, 2020. https://www.apma.org/PracticingDPMs/covid19.cfm • CDC. Guide to Infection Prevention for Outpatient Podiatry Settings. Accessed Aug 17, 2020. https://www.cdc.gov/infectioncontrol/pdf/Podiatry-Guide_508.pdf • CDC. A Quick Guide to CDC's Guide to Infection Prevention for Outpatient Podiatry Settings. Accessed Aug 17, 2020. https://www.cdc.gov/infectioncontrol/pdf/Pocket-Podiatry-Guide_508.pdf

Medical Equipment, Supplies, and Resources

A publication developed by the Healthcare Infection Control Practices Advisory Committee (HICPAC) provides guidance on evaluating medical devices for infection prevention and safety standards.[39] This guidance provides algorithms for IPs to evaluate all aspects of products.

Materials management should partner with infection prevention and patient care areas in ensuring the safety, procurement, storage, and distribution of supplies. The IP should actively participate in reviewing and selecting supplies as they contribute to infection prevention strategies. The IP should ensure that practices are in place for proper cleaning, disinfection, and/or sterilization, as appropriate, of medical devices. Devices should not put the patient at risk due to malfunction and/or design. Another aspect of product evaluation is determining if the device and its packaging are designed in a way to facilitate clean and/or sterile use.

Supplies such as ABHRs, PPE, disinfectants registered with the Environmental Protection Agency (EPA) or local and state agencies, and sharps containers are typically the first items identified as key for infection prevention. But devices that are known to be linked to HAIs, such as urinary catheter supplies, central venous lines, ventriculostomy catheters, surgical skin preparations, and sterile drapes, are also critical to infection prevention. The IP's role in product evaluation and introduction of new products is paramount. In some cases, the IP's input and approval are built into the initial review of any new product. Chapter 8 provides a more detailed discussion of medical equipment and supplies related to IPC efforts.

Antimicrobial Stewardship

As applicable for the health care setting, an organization should have an antimicrobial stewardship program that is based on current scientific literature. Leadership plays a key role when ensuring the structure, budget, and resources are available to support an effective and efficient antimicrobial stewardship program (ASP). Leaders provide the authority for the program to take action and improve the use of antimicrobials.

Knowledgeable, proficient experts should participate in the ASP across the continuum of care. Quite often leaders may need to establish contracts with outside experts to serve on their ASP team if experts are not employed within their facility. Critical access hospitals, home care, and long term care facilities often need to contract experts to assist their ASP. The role of the ASP team member should include providing expertise related to ongoing patient treatment questions.

Implementing Antimicrobial Stewardship Strategies

Due to concern over MDROs and the push to improve patient outcomes, attention has increasingly turned to antimicrobial stewardship. Many professional organizations have weighed in, and in recent years the US government held a summit to discuss the challenges and look for solutions.[40]

Global health concerns related to overuse of antibiotics include the following:

- Antimicrobial resistance threatens the effective prevention and treatment of an ever-increasing range of infections caused by bacteria, parasites, viruses, and fungi.
- Antimicrobial resistance threatens global public health and requires action across all government sectors and societies.
- Antimicrobial resistance is present in all parts of the world. New resistant organisms emerge and spread globally.

Stewardship programs have been shown to help decrease infection rates and the incidence of resistant organisms. These programs can also have a positive cost benefit for a health care organization, often saving money that can be used elsewhere.

Core elements of the CDC antimicrobial stewardship program include the following:[41]

- Leadership commitment
- Accountability
- Drug expertise
- Action
- Tracking
- Reporting
- Education

Depending on the structure of the organization, the IPs may have varying responsibilities related to antimicrobial stewardship. At minimum, the IP should play an important role by providing accurate HAI data. Preventing infections is the first step in limiting the need for and use of antibiotics.

IPs can function as an integral part of the antimicrobial stewardship team by collecting data that are relevant to the stewardship program. Penn Medicine's Antimicrobial Stewardship Checklist is helpful for reviewing medical records and collecting data. The chart-review checklist includes an assessment of culture results, indications for antimicrobials, and days of anticipated antimicrobial therapy.[42] The checklist also provides a comprehensive list of topics and data points that should be gathered during the review. Using a uniform, consistent process for each chart or antibiotic ensures reliable data are collected in a standardized format, which is a key feature of surveillance.

Additional guidance is included in the Joint Commission standards for antimicrobial stewardship in the "Medication Management" (MM) chapter: Standard MM.09.01.01 for domestic hospitals, critical access hospitals, and nursing care centers and Standard MM.09.01.03 for the ambulatory health care setting.[43] JCI Standard MMU.1.1 for medication management covers antimicrobial stewardship for hospitals, including academic medical center hospitals, as well as ambulatory care settings.

The CDC offers the guide Implementation of Antibiotic Stewardship Core Elements in Small and Critical Access Hospitals at https://www.cdc.gov/antibiotic-use/core-elements/small-critical.html.

Also, antimicrobial stewardship information is available from the SHEA website,[44,45] https://www.shea-online.org/index.php/practice-resources/priority-topics/antimicrobial-stewardship.

Antimicrobial prophylaxis in surgery guidelines have also been published and serve as a reference when evaluating preoperative antimicrobial prophylaxis.[46] The guidelines cover antimicrobial selection, dosing and re-dosing, and critical information to evaluate practice.

For additional resources related to antimicrobial stewardship, see the "Key Infection Prevention Documents" and "Antimicrobial Stewardship Resources" sections at the end of this chapter.

TIP | ## Five Things Providers and Patients Should Question about Antibiotic Use

A useful educational handout about appropriate use of antibiotics has been published by SHEA under the title of Choosing Wisely®.[45]

Key points include the following:

1. Do not continue antibiotics beyond 72 hours in a hospitalized patient unless the patient has clear evidence of infection.

2. Avoid invasive devices (including central venous catheters, endotracheal tubes, and urinary catheters) and, if required, use them no longer than necessary. They pose a major risk for infection.

3. Do not perform urinalyses, blood, or urine cultures or *Clostridioides/Clostridium difficile* (*C. difficile*) testing unless patients have signs or symptoms of infection. Tests can be falsely positive, leading to overdiagnosis and overtreatment.

4. Do not use antibiotics in patients with recent *C. difficile* infection without convincing evidence of need. Antibiotics pose a high risk of *C. difficile* recurrence.

5. Do not continue surgical prophylactic antibiotics after the patient has left the operating room.

Source: Society for Healthcare Epidemiology of America. Choosing Wisely: Five Things Providers and Patients Should Question. Oct 1, 2015. Accessed Mar 11, 2020. https://www.shea-online.org/images/docs/SHEA_Choosing_Wisely_List_of_5.pdf

Implementing Evidence-Based Practices (IC.02.05.01 and IPSG.5.1)

An IP should assemble a comprehensive portfolio of established guidelines and recommendations for the prevention and control strategies being planned and should consider ways to incorporate improvement strategies into ongoing practice standards. With these insights, the IP can develop teams and implementation strategies based on established guidelines and recommendations. One goal of an IPC program is to identify ways of embedding recommended IPC strategies into daily routine practices. A key collaboration to ensure a safe environment is the partnership between the IP and the construction, maintenance and repair, and renovation staff.

This section provides ideas and resources for implementing these strategies.[47,48] (In addition to the resources mentioned in this section, refer to the references, resources, and websites listed at the end of this chapter.) *See also* Table 6-4 and Sidebar 6-2 on page 150.

Table 6-4. Human Factors Engineering: Challenges for IPC

Challenges	Effect	Potential Solutions
Delayed feedback	<ul><li>No observable outcome of action from a less-than-desirable IPC action.</li><li>May be observed later by persons not involved.</li><li>Cause and effect are unclear.</li></ul>	Improve feedback using products that provide information. Examples include the following:<ul><li>Product that glows when hand hygiene is inadequate</li><li>Environmental markers for cleaning</li><li>Volume and use of alcohol-based hand rub for hand hygiene measurements</li><li>Electronic badges to monitor hand hygiene</li></ul>
Lack of connection with a positive outcome for preventing infection	<ul><li>Tangible positive result is not generally apparent to the staff who performed an IPC procedure correctly because of time differences.<ul><li>May reduce motivation to perform correctly again.</li><li>Disconnection intensifies between the staff action and the patient outcome.</li></ul></li><li>Surveillance data are not available "in time," so not as effective for behavior change.</li><li>Positive deviance is not always considered.</li><li>Training does not always provide immediate feedback of positive performance.</li></ul>	<ul><li>Supplement standard surveillance procedures with data reported monthly, biannually, or yearly to immediate real-time analysis of each infection identified. This helps staff remember circumstances, can involve more people, and provides more immediate feedback for action.</li><li>Consider positive deviance; that is, observe successful providers and spread their techniques and methods to other providers. Focus on successful providers; for example, those who reduce *C. difficile* with presumptive isolation or redesign the workspace and supplies to enable more prompt isolation.</li><li>Provide simulation training, such as practice techniques, through a virtual medium that provides immediate feedback— for example, how to properly insert a urinary catheter or central line (see Tool 6-3).</li></ul>

(continued)

Table 6-4. Human Factors Engineering: Challenges for IPC (continued)

Challenges	Effect	Potential Solutions
Complexity and inefficiency	• IPC tasks that are not supported with human factors engineering, such as placement of supplies, time to complete the task, or number of steps in a procedure, may delay the process or cause staff to forget it or eliminate it from their practice.	Reduce complexity and inefficiency with product redesign and human factors considerations. Examples include the following: • Infusion pumps that do not allow incorrect settings • Antimicrobial stewardship programs requiring approval before administering certain drugs • Time-limited orders to remind the provider to take action such as removal of a urinary catheter • Intravenous connectors that do not allow incorrect connections
Time pressure and workload	• When time pressure is in place, tasks other than infection prevention may take priority, provide immediate feedback, and are more connected with positive results.	Use task observation and analysis to identify process flow and gaps. Examples include the following: • Observe health care workers gather supplies for central catheter placement, demonstrating steps. • Bundle supplies to help reduce inefficiency. • Reduce interruptions during central line placement by posting large sign saying "Do Not Disturb." • Observe whether more staff or equipment are needed. • Identify deficiencies in the layout of the room that may lead to cross-contamination. • Use checklists for directing and evaluating tasks.
Few IPC cues to guide staff	• Few embedded cues for IPC indicate to staff when to stop or change procedure—for example, if central line is placed in wrong location or if antiseptic is applied using incorrect technique or not allowed to dry.	• Use badges or flashing lights to provide a clue to behavior such as hand hygiene. • Pictures, stickers, and color-coding are all examples. *(continued)*

Table 6-4. Human Factors Engineering: Challenges for IPC (continued)

Challenges	Effect	Potential Solutions
Inconsistent ergonomic design for the work environment	• Inconsistent/inappropriate placement of resources needed by caregivers leads to failure to follow proper IPC practices (for example, hand hygiene dispensers inaccessible or absent leading to lack of hand hygiene). • Poor visibility, difficulty of access, wrong heights, and separation of tools used in sequence are issues.	• Include and use ergonomic design principles when designing workplace layout—for example, the placement of alcohol-based hand rub dispensers in visible and accessible locations. • Provide signage to indicate location of supplies and store them at reasonable heights in easily accessible locations.
Need additional problem-solving tools for IPC	• Examine broader systems issues when analyzing challenges that may allow gaps or breaches of care to occur—for example, badly designed patient care space, mixing clean and dirty, poor environmental cleaning, lack of appropriate timing of preoperative antimicrobial prophylaxis, or understaffing of caregivers.	• Use effective problem-solving techniques that address system issues—for example, root-cause analysis to include the team involved, observations of the workflow and the environment, policies and procedures, training, and so forth.

Source: Adapted from Anderson J, et al. Using human factors engineering to improve the effectiveness of infection prevention and control. *Crit Care Med.* 2010 Aug;38(8 Suppl):S269–S281. © International Federation of Infection Control. Used with permission.

The IP has an obligation and responsibility to ensure that patients and residents receive high-quality care through incorporation of evidence-based guidelines in direct care practices. A critical step in implementation is to assess the current state of an organization's IPC program. The CDC provides several tools to assist in this effort and guidelines that should help organizations reach their goal of zero HAIs.[1,49]

When considering evidence-based practices, an IP may refer to the guidelines from the HICPAC of the CDC and other CDC documents that provide science-based IPC recommendations across the health care continuum. These recommendations are ranked by category, according to the scientific evidence associated with each recommendation, thus providing guidance to the health care provider to assess the minimal and optimal standards that should be met. For example, Category IA,

IB, or IC recommendations should be implemented across an organization because they are based on scientific, epidemiological data, or expert consensus or are required by regulations or law.

In April 2017, HICPAC formed a workgroup to update recommendation categories. Its charge was "to update the categorization recommendations to reflect evolving methodology, provide options for incorporating opinions into guideline development, and to increase transparency regarding the rationale for decisions on the strength of recommendations."[50] Table 1 in the HICPAC document discusses strength of recommendations and has three categories: recommendation, conditional recommendation, and no recommendation. Table 2 addresses justification for choice of recommendation strength with the components supporting evidence, level of confidence in the evidence, benefits, risk and harms, resource use, benefit/harms

Sidebar 6-2. Successfully Implementing IPC Strategies

Infection prevention and control (IPC) programs that have achieved success in reducing risks for health care–associated infections have used common approaches to implementation, including the following:

1. Team-driven, staff-empowered activities
2. Commitment from administration
3. Involvement of practice leaders as champions
4. Use of consistent and evidenced-based policies and procedures
5. Assurance that needed supplies are readily available to facilitate adherence to recommended practice
6. Requirements for education and competency verification
7. Monitoring and measurement of practices and outcomes via surveillance
8. Effective communication, including feedback of surveillance findings to staff
9. Ongoing evaluation of interventions and continuous improvement activity
10. Interventions hardwired into culture to maintain the gain
11. Celebrations of success

Developing and implementing strategies to reduce infection risks is a great challenge for IPC programs. Bidirectional communication with all health care providers will help the IPC team to achieve and sustain effective IPC practices. More information on communication can be found in Chapter 9.

TIP **CDC Toolkits for Assessment**

- Infection Prevention and Control Assessment Tool for Acute Care Hospitals. Accessed Mar 13, 2020. https://www.cdc.gov/infectioncontrol/pdf/ICAR/Hospital.pdf

- Infection Prevention and Control Assessment Tool for Long-Term Care Facilities. Accessed Mar 13, 2020. https://www.cdc.gov/infectioncontrol/pdf/ICAR/LTCF.pdf

- Infection Prevention and Control Assessment Tool for Outpatient Settings. Accessed Mar 13, 2020. https://www.cdc.gov/infectioncontrol/pdf/ICAR/Outpatient.pdf

- Infection Prevention and Control Assessment Tool for Hemodialysis Facilities. Accessed Mar 13, 2020. https://www.cdc.gov/infectioncontrol/pdf/ICAR/Dialysis.pdf

assessment, value judgements, intentional vagueness, and exceptions. Finally, Table 3 addresses the aggregate level of confidence in effect estimate. The topics are the level of confidence (high, medium, low) and description. Future guidelines will refer to this schema. Refer to the HICPAC website for details.[50]

HICPAC guidelines include performance measures to assist an IP when validating an IPC program's compliance. These guidelines serve as a valuable resource when developing performance measures for the IPC plan, as do the Joint Commission standards listed here:

- Prevention of Intravascular Catheter-Related Infections (IC.02.05.01, PI.02.01.01, IPSG.5.1)
- Prevention of Catheter-Associated Urinary Tract Infections (IC.02.05.01, IPSG.5.1)
- Prevention and Control of Norovirus Gastroenteritis Outbreaks in Healthcare Settings
- Public Reporting of Healthcare-Associated Infections
- Infection Control in Hospital Personnel
- Prevention of Surgical Site Infection (IC.02.05.01, PI.02.01.01, IPSG.5.1)
- Environmental Infection Control in Health-Care Facilities

- Management of Multidrug-Resistant Organisms in Healthcare Settings (IC.02.05.01, PI.02.01.01, IPSG.5.1)
- Isolation Precautions: Preventing Transmission of Infectious Agents in Healthcare Settings
- Disinfection and Sterilization in Healthcare Facilities

All these documents are available on the CDC/HICPAC webpage at https://www.cdc.gov/infectioncontrol/guidelines/index.html.[51] (*See also* the "Key Infection Prevention Documents" section at the end of of this chapter.)

The CDC updated its guidelines for preventing catheter-associated urinary tract infections in 2017.[52] The document may be viewed at https://www.cdc.gov/infectioncontrol/guidelines/cauti/index.html.

Additional recommendations and guidelines produced by HICPAC are listed below:
- Antibiotic Stewardship Statement for Antibiotic Guidelines—Recommendations of HICPAC. 2016. https://www.cdc.gov/hicpac/pdf/antibiotic-stewardship-statement.pdf
- Essential Elements of Reprocessing Program for Flexible Endoscopes—Recommendations of the HICPAC. 2016. Updated Jan 25, 2017. https://www.cdc.gov/hicpac/recommendations/flexible-endoscope-reprocessing.html
- A Process for Assessing Products for Infection Prevention in Healthcare Settings. Jul 2017–Nov 2018. https://www.cdc.gov/hicpac/workgroup/product-assessment.html
- *Clostridioides difficile* in Neonatal Intensive Care Unit Patients: A Systemic Review. Centers for Disease Control and Prevention, National Center for Emerging and Zoonotic Infectious Diseases, Division of Healthcare Quality and Promotion, Atlanta, GA. Aug 30, 2018. https://www.cdc.gov/hicpac/pdf/cdiff-nicu-H.pdf

Professional organizations, such as APIC, SHEA, and the Infectious Diseases Society of America (IDSA), have championed evidence-based prevention strategies. Multiple publications are available to assist IPs in guiding and directing the implementation of their organizations' IPC programs. For example, APIC's series of implementation guides (https://apic.org/Professional-Practice/Implementation-guides/) covers topics such as *C. difficile*, catheter-associated urinary tract infections

(CAUTIs), and central line–associated bloodstream infections (CLABSIs).[53] Likewise, the SHEA/IDSA *Compendium of Strategies to Prevent Healthcare-Associated Infections in Acute Care Hospitals*[54] received support from multiple organizations, including APIC and The Joint Commission, and offers many tools and strategies to help with implementation efforts. It simplifies the CDC guidelines and emphasizes the practical aspects of prevention. The implementation guides are available for download at https://www.APIC.org.

Practice Bundles

The Institute for Healthcare Improvement (IHI) has raised the standard for patient safety with initiatives aimed at reducing HAIs and has garnered the attention of health care providers, administrators, and the public. Scientific partners with IHI include APIC and SHEA as well as many other professional organizations. Targeted prevention modules can be found on the IHI website that provide improvement strategies for preventing CLABSI, CAUTI, MDROs, and surgical site infections (SSIs).[55]

TIP **The Institute for Healthcare Improvement (IHI) Prevention Modules**

IHI prevention modules (see https://www.ihi.org) address the following:
- Central line–associated bloodstream infection (CLABSI)
- Ventilator-associated pneumonia (VAP)
- Catheter-associated urinary tract infection (CAUTI)
- Methicillin-resistant *Staphylococcus aureus* (MRSA)
- Surgical site infection and pediatric surgical site infection
- Hand hygiene improvement

The IHI, as well as other health care stakeholders, has adopted practice bundles proven to decrease infection risk when all elements of a bundle are applied consistently to each patient.[56] Specific recommendations from HICPAC and APIC guidelines, as well as other IPC literature, are chosen for a bundle. Each element of a bundle is an evidence-based practice supported by research or expert consensus. It is important to note that some Category IA and IB HICPAC recommendations are not included. For instance, the IHI ventilator-associated pneumonia (VAP) bundle assumes that the standard practices recommended by HICPAC are already in place (that is, the handling of tubing, water reservoirs, nebulizers, and other recommendations).[13] It is important for each organization to consider other recommendations, such as those from the AHRQ, American Hospital Association (AHA), Hospital Engagement Network (HEN), and Health Research and Educational Trust (HRET), and how they can be used when designing prevention strategies based on the IHI bundles. Measuring compliance with bundle implementation is necessary to determine if the bundles are making a difference in patient outcomes.

In addition to the bundles for CAUTI, CLABSI, VAP, MRSA, and SSI, a procedure bundle developed by Rahman et al. is available for external ventricular drain placement.[57] Depending on the facility type and specialty area coverage, the ventriculostomy device bundle may prove useful in your care setting. Tool 6-2 includes a ventriculostomy placement bundle checklist as well as others.

TRY THIS TOOL

Tool 6-2. Assessment for Compliance with Prevention Bundles

Suggested steps for preventing device-associated infections include the following:

1. Use a device only when medically necessary, according to established criteria.
2. Remove a device when it is no longer clinically needed.
3. Implement a "bundled care" approach, including daily evaluation of whether a patient still needs the device.
4. Use a checklist specific for each procedure to ensure compliance with all key bundle components.
5. Monitor practice, assess compliance, and provide feedback to all involved in care.
6. Educate health care providers about their role in prevention and use return demonstration to establish competency.
7. Educate patients and families about practices they can use to reduce infection risk.
8. Observe and monitor insertion of all devices and other critical activities.

9. Obtain commitments from all health care providers to do their part in reducing device-related infections and stress their accountability for adherence to prevention practices.
10. Standardize contents and availability of supplies and kits to facilitate compliance.
11. Perform outcome surveillance for device-associated infections. Report findings to frontline staff, managers, medical staff, and administrators.
12. Promote good hand hygiene and proper sterile and/ or aseptic technique.

The AHA and HEN have been successful partners for prevention with tools and educational programs. The American Recovery and Reinvestment Act of 2009 made funds available through the CDC for states to obtain grants for projects and IPC collaboratives. Each state website houses its HAI prevention initiative's tools. IPs seeking examples of state-sponsored CLABSI projects should check with their state health department and the CDC.

The AHA, HRET, and AHRQ have had significant impacts on prevention initiatives. The plethora of tools and education materials can be found at the website http://www.ahrq.gov/professionals/index.html.

One of the early—and successful—infection prevention programs is the Comprehensive Unit-Based Safety Program (CUSP).[58,59] CUSP uses an evidence-based framework for multidisciplinary teams that integrate TeamSTEPPS® communication tools and quality-improvement methods.

The main components of the CUSP framework are listed below:
- Culture of safety
- Sciences of safety education
- Staff identification of safety concerns
- Senior executive adoption of a unit
- Improvement implemented from safety concerns
- Efforts documented and analyzed
- Results shared
- Culture reassessment

TeamSTEPPS® is a teamwork system designed for health care professionals. It is scientifically rooted in more than 20 years of research and was developed by the Department of Defense Patient Safety Program in collaboration with the AHRQ. It is a great source for ready-to-use materials and a training curriculum. The system has been shown to produce highly effective medical teams.[60] For more information, visit https://www.ahrq.gov/teamstepps/index.html.

More information on TeamSTEPPS® is available on its website. Core curriculum tools address hospital settings as well as long term care, office-based settings, and dental programs, and assist with project implementation and sustainability. The site also provides educational tools for the team to develop simulation programs to enhance patient safety.[61] For more information on simulation training and its potential role in infection prevention and control, download Tool 6-3.

The team can also delve into several AHRQ tools for prevention initiatives. A few examples include the following:
- CLABSI: https://www.ahrq.gov/hai/clabsi-tools/index.html
- CAUTI: https://www.ahrq.gov/hai/tools/cauti-hospitals/modules.html
- Patient and Family Engagement: https://www.ahrq.gov/patient-safety/resources/patient-family-engagement/index.html

The IP and the unit team can use these methodologies to identify performance gaps and workflow issues such as supply accessibility and staff knowledge. The assessment process helps to identify clear and agreed-upon goals. HRET and TeamSTEPPS® have been successful in creating a culture of accountability and continuous improvement.[61]

Factors for Successful Implementation of Patient Safety and IPC Initiatives

A combination of factors help ensure successful implementation of IPC initiatives, including understanding organizational culture, identifying and using human factors, communicating throughout the organization, and engaging personal commitment from all health care workers and staff.

Checklists allow implementation of the bundled strategies to be aligned with detailed institutional policies, procedures, and specific resources. In 2013, the IHI named bundles that include checklists to prevent CLABSI as one of the top 10 "strongly encouraged patient safety practices."[64]

TIP Health Protection Scotland (HPS) has developed a compendium containing a wide variety of infection control tools. The HPS website in the United Kingdom provides multiple prevention tools[68]:
https://hpspubsrepo.blob.core.windows.net/hps-website/nss/1513/documents/1_hai-compendium.pdf

The HPS compendium provides information on the following:
- Preventing Catheter Associated Urinary Tract Infections: Acute Care Setting
- Preventing Catheter Associated Urinary Tract Infections: Community care
- Preventing Infections When Inserting and Maintaining a Central Vascular Catheter (CVC)
- Preventing Surgical Site Infections (SSI)

The page https://www.nipcm.hps.scot.nhs.uk/appendices/ provides multiple tools. Of special interest are two for outbreaks:
- Healthcare Infection, Incident and Outbreak Reporting Template (HIIORT)
- Healthcare Infection Incident Assessment Tool (HIIAT)

You can also find the mobile app Preventing Homecare Infections[69] on the Scotland HAI Education for Prevention and Control site.

Checklists are both effective and popular; they are championed by international experts, such as Atul Gawande, MD, author of the bestselling book *The Checklist Manifesto: How to Get Things Right* (2009),[65] and Peter Pronovost, MD, coauthor of *Safe Patients, Smart Hospitals: How One Doctor's Checklist Can Help Us Change Health Care from the Inside Out* (2010).[66] Their work repeatedly demonstrates that checklists can lead to substantial improvements in patient outcomes—but only when integrated with enhanced organizational safety culture, an invigorated sense of teamwork, and regular open communication and feedback.[64,67] The Joint Commission Big Book of Checklists for Infection Prevention and Control provides checklists from a broad overview of the IPC program to topics such as standard and transmission-based precautions, HAIs, and occupational health and worker safety.

> **TIP** Reminders improve bundle compliance. Checklists, posters, and reminders are all important tools to facilitate compliance with IPC practices. For instance, Saint et al. developed a urinary catheter reminder that was attached to the physician's notes of the chart of each patient who had an indwelling catheter in place for 48 hours.[70] This reminder significantly reduced the catheterization time in the intervention group compared to the control group, which did not have a reminder. Incorporating this type of reminder into the management of other devices, besides urinary catheters can be helpful in decreasing device utilization and associated exposure risks.

Patient and Family Education

A helpful resource for patient and family education is provided on the SHEA website. SHEA patient education handouts can be downloaded and adapted for the organization and printed to distribute to patients and their families.[71] Education handouts are available on the following topics:

- SSI
- CLABSI
- CAUTI
- VAP

- *Clostridium difficile*
- VRE
- MRSA

Also, depending on the facility's scope of patient care, IPs may find useful screening forms and guidelines for family-centered residential facilities, such as Ronald McDonald House. See https://www.shea-online.org/images/patients/RMHC-Patient-Guides.pdf for more information.

Assigning Responsibility for Implementing Infection Prevention and Control Strategies

As discussed in Chapter 1, an organization must assign responsibility for IPC efforts, including responsibility for implementing IPC strategies. Although designating oversight responsibility is critical, many collaborating groups have recommended that successful strategies also require a personal commitment to implementation from each person involved in prevention initiatives.[63] Commitment of each and every health care provider is critical for the efforts to be incorporated into daily practices and for sustainability. The IP can have a variety of roles in improvement initiatives: content expert, leader, team member, coordinator, cheerleader, communicator, data provider, and data analyst. The goals of IPs are prevention and control of infections and patient, visitor, and health care worker safety.

Animals in the Health Care Setting

If an organization uses pet therapy or service animals in its facility, it must assess and respond to the risks associated with those animals. The therapeutic value of contact with animals is undeniable, and the risks can be minimized with the proper precautions. Animals that enter a health care organization fall into three categories:
1. Service animals
2. Pet therapy animals
3. Personal pets that are brought in to visit their owners

Regardless of the category into which an animal falls, guidelines must be in place to ensure patient, resident, personnel, and visitor safety.

The SHEA expert guidance on animals in health care facilities[6] provides comprehensive information on creating policies and procedures for safe practices. Key areas include animal-assisted activities, service animals, animals in research, and personal pet visitations, as well as recommendations for leeches, aquariums, larvae, and zoo animals. It is important to recognize that the Americans with Disabilities Act of 1990 (ADA) governs service animals that assist their owners. Each health care setting should have a policy that addresses service animals, is consistent with the ADA, and outlines expectations such as grooming, handling, and care provisions for the service animals.[72]

Therapy animals and personal pet visitations are not covered under the ADA but serve important functions in health care settings. See Table 6-5, below, for the issues to consider when establishing an animal visitation policy. It is particularly important to delineate specific rules and limitations for personal pets that may visit. It may also be prudent to limit personal pets to interactions only with their owners because behavior screening prior to visitation may not be possible.

Table 6-5. Key Considerations for Reducing Risk Associated with Animals in the Health Care Setting

People Factors	Animal Factors
Education • Handler • Staff • Patient • Family	Animal types • Dogs • Cats • Miniature horses • Other

Hand hygiene and personal protective equipment
• After animal encounter
• Wear gloves to clean up and clean hands after removing gloves when cleaning up animal excreta
	Animal health
	• Vaccinations
	• Flea and tick control
	• Grooming
	• Routine care
	  ○ Feeding
	  ○ Walking
	• Zoonotic diseases

Identification of high-risk patients • Physician approval • Immunosuppressed patients • Intensive care units and high-risk areas	Animal behavior • Animal temperament ○ Predictability of animal type • Transportation • Leash • Crate
Environmental factors • Patient room assignment • Allergies • Hallways • Waiting rooms/lounges	Animal identification • License • Special garb/kerchief
Policy and procedures • Clear delineation of responsibilities and acceptable practices	Cleanup and disposal • Excreta • Hair shedding, etc.

This table shows both animal- and people-related considerations for reducing risks associated with animals in the health care setting.

Source: Loretta Litz Fauerbach, MS, FSHEA, FAPIC, CIC. Used with permission.

Optimizing Use of Personal Protective Equipment (PPE)

Now that the basics of the requirements for implementing clinical strategies to reduce infection risks have been discussed, the following scenario provides one approach that may be taken in a given facility to implement optimal use of PPE.

The infection preventionist is concerned about having enough PPE, alcohol-based hand rubs, and Environmental Protection Agency–registered hospital disinfectants. She discusses her concerns with the hospital epidemiologist and the administrator. She suggests that a multidisciplinary team be created to address PPE and other supplies. Suggested steps that the team should take are included below.

Goal: Develop a plan with an algorithm for optimization of PPE and other critical infection prevention–related supplies.

- Form a multidisciplinary team to evaluate the use of and access to specific PPE.
    - Individuals should be chosen from those who have responsibilities for the following:
        - Using the product and being part of the health care staff
        (Select a variety of positions to ensure this is met.)
        - Stocking the product on a patient care unit
        - Ordering the product for the unit and facility
        - Budgeting the product and associated resources
- Provide the optimization scenarios developed by the CDC.
- Develop strategies for routine use, increased use such as during flu season, and use during crises or epidemics such as Ebola or COVID-19.
    - Identify steps for how to safely implement extended use.
    - Develop procedures for how to clean and store for the same individual and how to reprocess for safe use by other health care staff.
- Present plan to administration for approval.
- Develop a communication plan to inform the organization of the new plan and methods to provide timely updates.
    - Develop an educational plan and strategies for dissemination of the education.
- Monitor supplies and analyze to determine the effectiveness of the program.
- Review and modify recommendations based on the assessment.

Summary

A critical aspect of any successful IPC program is implementation of clinical strategies to reduce identified risk of infection. Organizations must ensure that their interventions are based on their IPC plans; address risks in the environment; comply with local, state, and federal laws and regulations; address manufacturers' instructions for use; and follow evidence-based practices and standards as well as consensus documents. This chapter provides many resources for IPs to consult when designing implementation efforts, including efforts related to medical equipment, animal safety, standard and transmission-based precautions, safe injection and medication handling practices, and outbreak management.

Resources

The following sections provide further information on this topic and can serve as valuable references when implementing a comprehensive IPC program.

Tools to Try

Tool 6-1. Compliance Check Sheet for Isolation Precautions

Tool 6-2. Assessment for Compliance with Prevention Bundles

Tool 6-3. Simulation-Based Training (SBT) Fact Sheet and Checklist

Key Infection Prevention Documents

APIC Resources

APIC's Implementation Guides. Accessed Mar 11, 2020. https://apic.org/Professional-Practice/Implementation-guides. This site will host all future implementation guides, as well as those listed here:

- Infection Preventionist's Guide to the OR. 2018. Accessed Mar 11, 2020. https://apic.org/Professional-Practice/Implementation-guides/#implementaion-guide-7463

- Guide to Preventing Central Line–Associated Bloodstream Infections. 2015. Accessed Mar 11, 2020. https://apic.org/Professional-Practice/Implementation-guides/#implementaion-guide-7464

- Guide to Hand Hygiene Programs for Infection Prevention. 2015. Accessed Mar 11, 2020. https://apic.org/Professional-Practice/Implementation-guides/#implementaion-guide-7467

- Guide to Preventing Catheter-Associated Urinary Tract Infections. 2014. Accessed Mar 11, 2020. https://apic.org/Professional-Practice/Implementation-guides/#implementaion-guide-7454

- Guide to Preventing *Clostridium difficile* Infections. 2013. Accessed Mar 11, 2020. https://apic.org/Professional-Practice/Implementation-guides/#implementaion-guide-7455

- Guide for the Prevention of Mediastinitis Surgical Site Infections Following Cardiac Surgery. 2008. Accessed Mar 11, 2020. https://apic.org/Professional-Practice/Implementation-guides/#implementaion-guide-7459

- Guide to the Elimination of Methicillin-Resistant *Staphylococcus aureus* (MRSA) Transmission in Hospital Settings, 2nd ed. 2010. Accessed Mar 11, 2020. https://apic.org/Professional-Practice/Implementation-guides/#implementaion-guide-7461

- Guide to the Elimination of Methicillin-Resistant *Staphylococcus aureus* (MRSA) Transmission in Hospital Settings—California Supplement. 2009. Accessed Mar 11, 2020. https://apic.org/Professional-Practice/Implementation-guides/#implementaion-guide-7457

- Guide to Infection Prevention in Emergency Medical Services. 2013. Accessed Mar 13, 2020. https://apic.org/Professional-Practice/Implementation-guides/#implementaion-guide-7466

- APIC. Healthcare Personnel Immunization Toolkit. 2012. Accessed Apr 18, 2020. https://www.apic.org/Resource_/TinyMceFileManager/Practice_Guidance/HCW_Immunization_Toolkit_122012.pdf

- APIC. Public Policy and Emergency Preparedness Committees: APIC Position Paper: Reuse of Respiratory Protection in Prevention and Control of Epidemic- and Pandemic-prone Acute Respiratory Diseases (ARD) in Healthcare. 2008. Accessed Apr 2, 2020. https://www.apic.org/Resource_/TinyMceFileManager/Advocacy-PDFs/Reuse_of_Respiratory_Proctection_archive_1209.pdf

- Bartley JM. The 1997, 1998, and 1999 APIC Guidelines Committees. APIC State-of-the-Art Report: The role of infection control during construction in health care facilities. *Am J Infect Control.* 2000 Apr;28(2):156–169.

- Friedman C, et al. APIC/CHICA-Canada infection prevention, control, and epidemiology: Professional and practice standards. *Am J Infect Control.* 2000 Aug;36(6):385–389.

- Greene LR, et al. APIC Position Paper: Influenza vaccination should be a condition of employment for health care personnel, unless medically contraindicated. Oct 2008. Accessed Apr 18, 2020. https://www.apic.org/Resource_/TinyMceFileManager/Advocacy-PDFs/APIC_Influenza_Immunization_of_HCP_12711.pdf

- The Writing Panel of the Working Group, Lefebvre SL, et al. Guidelines for animal-assisted interventions in health care facilities. *Am J Infect Control.* 2008 Mar;36(2):78–85.

- Dolan SA, et al. APIC position paper: Safe injection, infusion, and medication vial practices in health care. *Am J Infect Control.* 2016 Jul;44(7):750–757.

- The Do's and Don'ts for Wearing Gowns in Non-surgical Healthcare Settings. 2017. Accessed Mar 15, 2020. https://infectionpreventionandyou.org/wp-content/uploads/2017/09/APIC_DosDonts_GOWNS.pdf

- Do's and Don'ts for Wearing Procedure Masks in Non-surgical Healthcare Settings. 2015. Accessed Mar 15, 2020. https://www.apic.org/Resource_/TinyMceFileManager/consumers_professionals/APIC_DosDontsofMasks_hiq.pdf

SHEA/IDSA Resources

- Outbreak Response Training Program (ORTP). Accessed Mar 13, 2020. http://ortp.shea-online.org/

- Outbreak Response Tool Kits. Implementing COVID-19 Prevention Practices. Accessed Aug 24, 2020. https://ortp.guidelinecentral.com/covid-19/

- Family-Centered Residential Facility: Guest Health Screening Questions. 2017. Accessed Mar 11, 2020. https://www.shea-online.org/images/patients/RMHC-Patient-Guides.pdf

- Smith PW, et al. SHEA/APIC Guideline: Infection prevention and control in the long-term care facility. *Infect Control Hosp Epidemiol.* 2008 Sep;29(9):785–814.

- Yokoe DS, et al. A compendium of strategies to prevent health care-associated infections in acute care hospitals: 2014 updates. *Infect Control Hosp Epidemiol.* 2014 Sep;35(Suppl 2):S21–S31.

- World Alliance Against Antibiotic Resistance: (Alliance Contre le Développement des Bactéries Multi-Résistantes). The WAAAR Declaration Against Antibiotic Resistance. Accessed Apr 18, 2020. https://www.shea-online.org/images/position-statements/DECLARATION_WAAAR.pdf

- Carlet J. The world alliance against antibiotic resistance: Consensus for a declaration. *Clin Infect Dis.* 2015 Jun;60(12):1837–1841.

- All of the following are available at https://www.jstor.org/stable/10.1086/593984 in the table of contents. Accessed Apr 18, 2020.
  - SHEA/IDSA Practice Recommendation: Central Line–Associated Bloodstream Infection
  - SHEA/IDSA Practice Recommendation: Ventilator-Associated Pneumonia
  - SHEA/IDSA Practice Recommendation: Catheter-Associated Urinary Tract Infections
  - SHEA/IDSA Practice Recommendation: Surgical Site Infection
  - SHEA/IDSA Practice Recommendation: Methicillin-Resistant *Staphylococcus aureus*
  - SHEA/IDSA Practice Recommendation: *Clostridium difficile*

Joint Commission

Home page. Accessed Mar 13, 2020. https://www.jointcommission.org.

- Measuring Hand Hygiene Adherence: Overcoming the Challenges. 2009. Accessed Mar 13, 2020. https://www.jointcommission.org/assets/1/18/hh_monograph.pdf

- National Patient Safety Goals. Accessed Mar 13, 2020. https://www.jointcommission.org/PatientSafety/NationalPatientSafetyGoals

- Joint Commission Center for Transforming Healthcare. Home page. Accessed Mar 13, 2021. https://www.centerfortransforminghealthcare.org

- The Joint Commission Big Book of Checklists for Infection Prevention and Control. 2020. Oak Brook, IL: Joint Commission Resources. https://store.jcrinc.com/the-joint-commission-big-book-of-checklists-for-infection-prevention-and-control-/

IHI Resources

- How-to Guide: Pediatric Supplement: Reduce Methicillin-Resistant *Staphylococcus aureus* (MRSA) Infection. Accessed Mar 11, 2020. http://www.ihi.org/resources/Pages/Tools/HowtoGuideReduceMRSAInfection.aspx

- How-to Guide: Prevent Central Line–Associated Bloodstream Infection. Accessed Mar 11, 2020. https://www.ihi.org/resources/Pages/Tools/HowtoGuidePreventCentralLineAssociatedBloodstreamInfection.aspx

- How-to Guide: Prevent Ventilator-Associated Pneumonia. Accessed Mar 11, 2020. https://www.ihi.org/resources/Pages/Tools/HowtoGuidePreventVAP.aspx

CDC and HICPAC Resources

- CDC Guidelines Library. Accessed Jul 16, 2020. https://www.cdc.gov/infectioncontrol/guidelines/index.html

- Catheter-Associated Urinary Tract Infections (CAUTI). Accessed Jul 16, 2020. https://www.cdc.gov/infectioncontrol/guidelines/cauti/index.html

- CDC. Guideline for hand hygiene in health-care settings: Recommendations of the Healthcare Infection Control Practices Advisory Committee and the HICPAC/SHEA/APIC/IDSA Hand Hygiene Task Force. *MMWR Recomm Rep.* 2002 Oct;51(RR-16):1–45.

- CDC. Guidelines for preventing the transmission of Mycobacterium tuberculosis in health-care settings, 2005. *MMWR Recomm Rep.* 2005 Dec;54(RR-17):1–141.

- Tablan OC, et al. Guidelines for preventing health care-associated pneumonia, 2003. *MMWR Recomm Rep.* 2004 Mar;53(RR-3):1–36.

- Sehulster L, Chinn RY., CDC, HICPAC. Guidelines for environmental infection control in health-care facilities: Recommendations of CDC and the Healthcare Infection Control Practice Advisory Committee (HICPAC). *MMWR Recomm Rep.* 2003 Jun;52(RR-10):1–42.

- CDC/HICPAC. Guidelines for infection control in health care personnel, 1998. *Am J Infect Control.* 1998 Jun;26(3):289–354.

- Infection Control in Long-Term Care Facilities. Accessed Mar 11, 2020. https://www.cdc.gov/longtermcare/

- Poster on PPE. Accessed Mar 13, 2020. https://www.cdc.gov/hai/pdfs/ppe/PPE-Sequence.pdf

- Sequencing of Gowns and Gloves. Accessed Mar 13, 2020. http://www.cdc.gov/HAI/pdfs/ppe/ppeposter148.pdf

- Fiore AE, et al. Prevention and control of influenza: Recommendations of the Advisory Committee on Immunization Practices (ACIP), 2008. *MMWR Recomm Rep.* 2008 Aug;57(RR-7):1–60.

- Sharps Safety for Healthcare Settings. Accessed Apr 2, 2020. https://www.cdc.gov/sharpssafety/

- Workbook for Designing, Implementing, and Evaluating a Sharps Injury Prevention Program. Accessed Apr 2, 2020. https://www.cdc.gov/sharpssafety/pdf/sharpsworkbook_2008.pdf

- Standard Precautions. Accessed Mar 22, 2020. https://www.cdc.gov/hai/

- Berríos-Torres SI, et al. Centers for disease control and prevention guideline for the prevention of surgical site infection, 2017. *JAMA Surg.* 2017 Aug;152(8):784–791. doi:10.1001/jamasurg.2017.0904

- Rutala WA, Weber DJ, HICPAC. Guideline for Disinfection and Sterilization in Healthcare Facilities, 2008. Updated May 2019. Accessed Mar 13, 2020. https://www.cdc.gov/infectioncontrol/pdf/guidelines/disinfection-guidelines-H.pdf

- Siegel JD, Rhinehart E, Jackson M, Chiarello L. 2007 Guideline for isolation precautions: Preventing transmission of infectious agents in health care settings. *Am J Infect Control*. 2007 Dec;35(10):S65–S164.

- Siegel JD, Rhinehart E, Jackson M, Chiarello L, HICPAC. Management of multidrug-resistant organisms in health care settings, 2006. *Am J Infect Control*. 2007 Dec;35(10 Suppl 2):S165–193.

- HICPAC. Update to the CDC and the HICPAC Recommendation Categorization Scheme for Infection Control and Prevention Guideline Recommendations. 2019. Accessed Mar 27, 2020. https://www.cdc.gov/hicpac/workgroup/recommendation-scheme-update.html

- Chopra V, et al. A process for assessing products for infection prevention in health care settings: A framework from the Healthcare Infection Control Practices Advisory Committee of the Centers for Disease Control and Prevention. *Ann Intern Med*. 2020;172(1):30–34.

- Systematic Review Documents. Accessed Apr 18, 2020. https://www.cdc.gov/hicpac/reviews/index.html

- Essential Elements of a Reprocessing Program for Flexible Endoscopes—Recommendations of the Healthcare Infection Control Practices Advisory Committee. Accessed Apr 18, 2020. https://www.cdc.gov/hicpac/pdf/flexible-endoscope-reprocessing.pdf

- Antibiotic Stewardship Statement for Antibiotic Guidelines—Recommendations of the Healthcare Infection Control Practices Advisory Committee. Accessed Apr 18, 2020. https://www.cdc.gov/hicpac/pdf/antibiotic-stewardship-statement.pdf

- Optimizing Personal Protective Equipment (PPE) Supplies. Accessed Aug 20, 2020. https://www.cdc.gov/coronavirus/2019-ncov/hcp/ppe-strategy/index.html

- Use Masks to Slow the Spread of COVID-19. Accessed Aug 20, 2020. https://www.cdc.gov/coronavirus/2019-ncov/prevent-getting-sick/diy-cloth-face-coverings.html

- Fisher KA, et al. Factors Associated with Cloth Face Covering Use Among Adults During the COVID-19 Pandemic—United States, April and May 2020. *MMWR Morb Mortal Wkly Rep*. 2020;69(28):933–937. Accessed Aug 20, 2020. https://www.cdc.gov/mmwr/volumes/69/wr/mm6928e3.htm?s_cid=mm6928e3_w

- CDC/NIOSH. Infographic – Understanding the Difference, Surgical Mask, N95 Respirator. Accessed Apr 8, 2020. https://www.cdc.gov/niosh/npptl/pdfs/UnderstandDifferenceInfographic-508.pdf

- Respiratory Hygiene and Cough Etiquette in Healthcare Settings. Accessed Mar 14, 2020. https://www.cdc.gov/flu/professionals/infectioncontrol/resphygiene.htm

- Guide to Infection Prevention for Outpatient Settings: Minimum Expectations for Safe Care. 2016. Accessed Jul 16, 2020. https://www.cdc.gov/infectioncontrol/pdf/outpatient/guide.pdf

- Interim Infection Prevention and Control Recommendations to Prevent SARS-CoV-2 Spread in Nursing Homes. Accessed Aug 17, 2020. https://www.cdc.gov/coronavirus/2019-ncov/hcp/long-term-care.html

- Strategies for Optimizing the Supply of Eye Protection. Accessed Aug 21, 2020. https://www.cdc.gov/coronavirus/2019-ncov/hcp/ppe-strategy/eye-protection.html

- Investigating Outbreaks. Using Data to Link Foodborne Disease Outbreaks to a Contaminated Source. May 25, 2016. Accessed Apr 1, 2020. https://www.cdc.gov/foodsafety/outbreaks/investigating-outbreaks/index.html

- Steps in a Foodborne Outbreak Investigation. Accessed Apr 1, 2020. https://www.cdc.gov/foodsafety/outbreaks/investigating-outbreaks/investigations/index.html

- A Process for Assessing Products for Infection Prevention in Healthcare Settings. Jul 2017–Nov 2018. Accessed Mar 28, 2020. https://www.cdc.gov/hicpac/workgroup/product-assessment.html

- *Clostridioides difficile* in Neonatal Intensive Care Unit Patients: A Systemic Review. Aug 30, 2018. Accessed Mar 28, 2020. https://www.cdc.gov/hicpac/pdf/cdiff-nicu-H.pdf

Agency for Healthcare Research and Quality (AHRQ) Resources

- Making Health Care Safer II: An Updated Critical Analysis of the Evidence for Patient Safety Practices—Executive Summary. 2013. Accessed Mar 13, 2020. https://www.ahrq.gov/research/findings/evidence-based-reports/ptsafetysum.html

- Carbapenem-Resistant *Enterobacteriaceae* (CRE) Control and Prevention Toolkit. Accessed Apr 18, 2020. https://www.ahrq.gov/sites/default/files/publications/files/cretoolkit.pdf

- Agency for Healthcare Research and Quality (AHRQ) Prevention Initiatives. Accessed Mar 13, 2020. http://www.ahrq.gov/professionals/index.html
  - CLABSI. Accessed Mar 13, 2020. https://www.ahrq.gov/hai/clabsi-tools/index.html
  - CAUTI. Accessed Mar 13, 2020. https://www.ahrq.gov/hai/tools/cauti-hospitals/modules.html
  - Engaging Patients and Families in Their Health Care. Accessed May 25, 2021. https://www.ahrq.gov/patient-safety/resources/patient-family-engagement/index.html

- TeamSTEPPS®: Strategies and Tools to Enhance Performance and Patient Safety. 2020. Accessed Mar 13, 2020. https://www.ahrq.gov/teamstepps/index.html

Dialysis Resources

- The CDC provides several checklists and tools for dialysis facilities, including the following (*see* https://www.cdc.gov/dialysis/prevention-tools/:
  - Core Approach to BSI Prevention in Dialysis Facilities (that is, the Core Interventions for Dialysis Bloodstream Infection [BSI] Prevention)
  - Staff Competencies
  - Key Areas for Patient Education

- CDC Approach to BSI Prevention in Dialysis Facilities. Accessed Mar 13, 2020. https://www.cdc.gov/dialysis/PDFs/Dialysis-Core-Interventions-5_10_13.pdf

- Audit Tool: Hemodialysis Hand Hygiene Observations. Accessed Mar 13, 2020. https://www.cdc.gov/dialysis/PDFs/collaborative/Hemodialysis-Hand-Hygiene-Observations.pdf

- Audit Tools and Checklists. Accessed Mar 13, 2020. https://www.cdc.gov/dialysis/prevention-tools/audit-tools.html

CDC Safe Injection and Medication Practices Resources

- The One & Only Campaign. Accessed Mar 13, 2020. https://www.oneandonlycampaign.org

- The One & Only Campaign Print Materials. Accessed Mar 13, 2020. https://www.oneandonlycampaign.org/content/print-materials

- Dolan SA, et al. APIC position paper: Safe injection, infusion, and medication vial practices in health care. *Am J Infect Control.* 2016;44(7):750–757.

World Health Organization (WHO) Resources

- Clean Care Is Safer Care. Accessed Mar 13, 2020. https://www.who.int/gpsc/en/

- Five Moments for Hand Hygiene Poster. Accessed Mar 13, 2020. https://www.who.int/gpsc/tools/Five_moments/en/

- WHO Surgical Safety Checklist. Accessed Mar 13, 2020. https://apps.who.int/iris/bitstream/10665/44186/2/9789241598590_eng_Checklist.pdf

- Implementation Manual: WHO Surgical Safety Checklist. Accessed Mar 13, 2020. https://apps.who.int/iris/bitstream/10665/44186/1/9789241598590_eng.pdf

- WHO Guidelines on Hand Hygiene in Health Care. First Global Patient Safety Challenge: Clean Care Is Safer Care. Accessed Mar 13, 2020. https://apps.who.int/iris/bitstream/10665/44102/1/9789241597906_eng.pdf

- WHO Prevention of Hospital-Acquired Infections: A Practical Guide, 2nd ed. Accessed Mar 13, 2020. https://www.who.int/csr/resources/publications/whocdscsreph200212.pdf

- Steps to Put on Personal Protective Equipment (PPE) Including Gown. 2015. Accessed Sep 20, 2020. https://apps.who.int/iris/bitstream/handle/10665/150115/WHO_HIS_SDS_2015.1_eng.pdf%3Bjsessionid=1DFA8E0F32D206E59A6484342DA25B04?sequence=1

- Steps to Take Off Personal Protective Equipment (PPE) Including Gown. 2015. Accessed Sep 20, 2020. https://apps.who.int/iris/bitstream/handle/10665/150117/WHO_HIS_SDS_2015.3_eng.pdf?sequence=1

Other Government Sites

- US Centers for Medicare & Medicaid Services. Home page. Accessed Mar 13, 2020. https://www.cms.hhs.gov/home/medicare.asp

- US National Institute for Occupational Safety and Health (NIOSH). Recommendations for the Selection and Use of Respirators and Protective Clothing for Protection Against Biological Agents. NIOSH Publication No. 2009-132, Apr 2009. Accessed Mar 13, 2020. https://www.cdc.gov/niosh/docs/2009-132/

- US Department of Veterans Affairs, Office of Public Health and Environmental Hazards. Infection: Don't Pass It On. Accessed Mar 13, 2020. https://www.publichealth.va.gov/infectiondontpassiton/

- US Centers for Medicare & Medicaid Services. Toolkit on State Actions to Mitigate COVID-19 Prevalence in Nursing Homes. Accessed Sep 20, 2020. https://www.cms.gov/files/document/covid-toolkit-states-mitigate-covid-19-nursing-homes.pdf

Antimicrobial Stewardship Resources

- American Nurses Association/Centers for Disease Control and Prevention (ANA/CDC). Redefining the antibiotic stewardship team: Recommendations from the American Nurses Association/Centers for Disease Control and Prevention Workgroup on the role of registered nurses in hospital antibiotic stewardship practices. *JAC-Antimicrobial Resistance*. 2019;1(2). doi:10.1093/jacamr/dlz037

- CDC. Redefining the Antibiotic Stewardship Team: Recommendations from the American Nurses Association/Centers for Disease Control and Prevention Workgroup on the Role of Registered Nurses in Hospital Antibiotic Stewardship Practices. Effective Date: 2017. Executive Summary. Accessed Apr 13, 2020. https://www.cdc.gov/antibiotic-use/healthcare/pdfs/ANA-CDC-whitepaper.pdf

- Stewardship Program Examples. Accessed Apr 13, 2020. https://www.cdc.gov/antibiotic-use/healthcare/programs.html

- Carlet J. The world alliance against antibiotic resistance: Consensus for a declaration. *Clin Infect Dis*. 2015 Jun;60(12):1837–1841.

- World Alliance Against Antibiotic Resistance (Alliance Contre le Développement des Bactéries Multi-Résistantes). The WAAAR Declaration Against Antibiotic Resistance. Accessed Apr 13, 2020. https://www.shea-online.org/images/position-statements/DECLARATION_WAAAR.pdf

- CDC. Core Elements of Antibiotic Stewardship. Accessed Mar 23, 2020. https://www.cdc.gov/antibiotic-use/core-elements/index.html

- CDC. Core Elements of Hospital Antibiotic Stewardship Programs. Accessed Mar 13, 2020. https://www.cdc.gov/antibiotic-use/healthcare/pdfs/core-elements.pdf

- CDC. Checklist for Core Elements of Hospital Antibiotic Stewardship Programs. Accessed Mar 13, 2020. https://www.cdc.gov/antibiotic-use/healthcare/pdfs/checklist.pdf

- CDC. IHI and CDC Antibiotic Stewardship Driver Diagram and Change Package. Accessed Jan 1, 2017. https://www.cdc.gov/antibiotic-use/healthcare/pdfs/Antibiotic_Stewardship_Change_Package.pdf

- CDC. Antibiotic Stewardship Measurement Framework. Accessed Mar 13, 2020. https://www.cdc.gov/antibiotic-use/healthcare/pdfs/Antibiotic_Stewardship_Measurement_Framework.pdf

- Penn Medicine. Penn Epicenter Antimicrobial Stewardship Checklist. Accessed Mar 23, 2020. https://www.pennmedicine.org/~/media/documents%20and%20audio/patient%20forms/infectious%20diseases/antibiotic%20flowsheet%20final%20check%20list.ashx?la=en

- SHEA. Antimicrobial Stewardship: Implementation Tools & Resources. Accessed Mar 14, 2020. https://www.shea-online.org/index.php/practice-resources/priority-topics/antimicrobial-stewardship/implementation-tools-resources

- Five Things Providers and Patients Should Question. Accessed Mar 14, 2020. https://www.shea-online.org/images/docs/SHEA_Choosing_Wisely_List_of_5.pdf

Other Society and Initiative Resources

- Health Protection Scotland. Guidance. Accessed Mar 13, 2020. https://www.hps.scot.nhs.uk/guidance/

- American Academy of Pediatrics Committee on Infectious Diseases. Infection prevention and control in pediatric ambulatory settings. *Pediatrics*. 2007 Sep;120(3):650–655.

- American Association for Gastrointestinal Endoscopy. Multi-society guideline on reprocessing flexible gastrointestinal endoscopes: 2011. Accessed Mar 13, 2020. https://www.asge.org/uploadedFiles/Public_E-Blast_PDFs/ReprocessingEndoscopes.pdf

Regional and State Organization Resources

- Bartley J. Michigan Society for Infection Control. Guidelines for Prevention and Control of Antimicrobial Resistant Organisms (ARO). Focus on: Methicillin-Resistant *Staphylococcus aureus* (MRSA) and Vancomycin Resistant *Enterococcus* (VRE). 2002. Accessed Mar 13, 2020. https://www.msic-online.org/resource_sections/aro_guidelines.html

- Sirio CA, et al. Pittsburgh Regional Healthcare Initiative: A systems approach for achieving perfect patient care. *Health Affairs*. 2003 Sep;22(5):157–165.

- Grunden N. PRHI Executive Summary. Pittsburgh Regional Health care Initiative, Oct 2004. Accessed Jul 16, 2020. https://www.prhi.org/resources/resources-article/archives/2005-earlier/222-executive-summary-10/file

References

1. Grunden N. PRHI Executive Summary Report. Pittsburgh Regional Healthcare Initiative. 2004. Accessed Jul 16, 2020. https://www.jhf.org/publications-videos/pub-and-vids/archives/2005-and-earlier/222-executive-summary-10/file

2. Pittsburgh Regional Healthcare Initiative puts new spin on improving healthcare quality. *Qual Lett Healthc Lead*. 2002;14(11):2–11.

3. Sirio CA, et al. Pittsburgh Regional Healthcare Initiative: A systems approach for achieving perfect patient care. *Health Affairs*. 2003;22(5):157–165.

4. National Health Safety Network (NHSN). Resources by Facility. 2020. Accessed Apr 14, 2020. https://www.cdc.gov/nhsn/enrolled-facilities/index.html

5. Moir T. Why is implementation science important for intervention design and evaluation within educational settings? *Front Educ*. 2018;3(61).

6. Siegel JD, et al. Guideline for isolation precautions: Preventing transmission of infectious agents in health care settings. *Am J Infect Control*. 2007;35(10 Suppl 2):S65-164.

7. Dolan SA, et al. APIC position paper: Safe injection, infusion, and medication vial practices in health care. *Am J Infect Control*. 2016;44(7):750–757.

8. Centers for Disease Control and Prevention (CDC). Sharps Safety for Healthcare Settings. 2018. Accessed Apr 2, 2020. https://www.cdc.gov/sharpssafety

9. Association for Professionals in Infection Control and Epidemiology (APIC). Do's and Don'ts for Wearing Gowns in Non-Surgical Healthcare Settings. 2017. Accessed Mar 15, 2020. http://professionals.site.apic.org/files/2017/09/APIC_DosDonts_GOWNS.pdf

10. Association for Professionals in Infection Control and Epidemiology (APIC). Do's and Don'ts for Wearing Procedure Masks in Non-Surgical Healthcare Settings. 2015. Accessed Mar 15, 2020. http://www.apic.org/Resource_/TinyMceFileManager/consumers_professionals/APIC_DosDontsofMasks_hiq.pdf

11. Centers for Disease Control and Prevention (CDC). Guide to Infection Prevention for Outpatient Settings: Minimum Expectations for Safe Care. 2016. Accessed Jul 16, 2020. https://www.cdc.gov/infectioncontrol/pdf/outpatient/guide.pdf

12. Bertin ML, et al. Outbreak of methicillin-resistant *Staphylococcus aureus* colonization and infection in a neonatal intensive care unit epidemiologically linked to a healthcare worker with chronic otitis. *Infect Control Hosp Epidemiol.* 2006;27(6):581–585.

13. Tablan OC, et al. Guidelines for preventing health-care–associated pneumonia, 2003: Recommendations of CDC and the Healthcare Infection Control Practices Advisory Committee. *MMWR Recomm Rep.* 2004;53(RR-3):1–36.

14. Centers for Disease Control and Prevention (CDC). Healthcare Facilities: Information about CRE. 2019. http://www.cdc.gov/hai/organisms/CRE/CRE-toolkit/index.html

15. Agency for Healthcare Research and Quality (AHRQ). Carbapenem-Resistant *Enterobacteriaceae* (CRE) Control and Prevention Toolkit. Apr 2014. Accessed Mar 23, 2020. https://www.ahrq.gov/sites/default/files/publications/files/cretoolkit.pdf

16. McGoldrick M, Rhinehart E. Managing multidrug-resistant organisms in home care and hospice: surveillance, prevention, and control. *Home Healthc Nurse.* 2007;25(9):580–586; quiz 587–588.

17. Jenkins TC, et al. Epidemiology of healthcare-associated bloodstream infection caused by USA300 strains of methicillin-resistant *Staphylococcus aureus* in 3 affiliated hospitals. *Infect Control Hosp Epidemiol.* 2009;30(3):233–241.

18. Gravel D, et al. Infection control practices related to *Clostridium difficile* infection in acute care hospitals in Canada. *Am J Infect Control.* 2009;37(1):9–14.

19. Cohen AL, et al. Recommendations for metrics for multidrug-resistant organisms in healthcare settings: SHEA/HICPAC Position paper. *Infect Control Hosp Epidemiol.* 2008;29(10):901–913.

20. Septimus E, et al. Approaches for preventing healthcare-associated infections: Go long or go wide? *Infect Control Hosp Epidemiol.* 2014;35(7):797–801.

21. Bearman GM, et al. A controlled trial of universal gloving versus contact precautions for preventing the transmission of multidrug-resistant organisms. *Am J Infect Control.* 2007;35(10):650–655.

22. Centers for Disease Control and Prevention. Use Personal Protective Equipment (PPE) When Caring for Patients with Confirmed or Suspected COVID-19. 2020. Accessed Nov 23, 2020. https://www.cdc.gov/coronavirus/2019-ncov/downloads/A_FS_HCP_COVID19_PPE.pdf

23. Centers for Medicare & Medicaid Services (CMS). Toolkit on State Actions to Mitigate COVID-19 Prevalence in Nursing Homes. 2020. Accessed Sep 20, 2020. https://www.cms.gov/files/document/covid-toolkit-states-mitigate-covid-19-nursing-homes.pdf

24. Ellison AM, Kotelchuck M, Bauchner H. Standard precautions in the pediatric emergency department: Knowledge, attitudes, and behaviors of pediatric and emergency medicine residents. *Pediatr Emerg Care.* 2007;23(12):877–880.

25. Centers for Disease Control and Prevention (CDC). Sequence for Donning Personal Protective Equipment. Accessed Mar 13, 2020. http://www.cdc.gov/HAI/pdfs/ppe/ppeposter148.pdf

26. Fisher KA, et al. Factors Associated with Cloth Face Covering Use Among Adults During the COVID-19 Pandemic—United States, April and May 2020. *MMWR Morb Mortal Wkly Rep.* 2020;69(28):933–937.

27. Centers for Disease Control and Prevention (CDC). Use Masks to Slow the Spread. 2020. Accessed Aug 20, 2020. https://www.cdc.gov/coronavirus/2019-ncov/prevent-getting-sick/diy-cloth-face-coverings.html

28. CDC Calls on Americans to Wear Masks to Prevent COVID-19 Spread. Jul 14, 2020. Accessed Aug 20, 2020. https://www.cdc.gov/media/releases/2020/p0714-americans-to-wear-masks.html

29. Brooks JT, Butler JC, Redfield RR. Universal masking to prevent SARS-CoV-2 transmission—The time is now. *JAMA.* 2020;324(7):635–637.

30. Hendrix MJ, et al. Absence of Apparent Transmission of SARS-CoV-2 from Two Stylists After Exposure at a Hair Salon with a Universal Face Covering Policy—Springfield, Missouri, May 2020. *MMWR Morb Mortal Wkly Rep.* 2020;69(28):930–932.

31. WHO. When and How to Use Masks. 2020. Accessed Nov 22, 2020. https://www.who.int/emergencies/diseases/novel-coronavirus-2019/advice-for-public/when-and-how-to-use-masks

32. WHO. Coronavirus Disease (COVID-19): Masks. 2020. Accessed Nov 22, 2020. https://www.who.int/emergencies/diseases/novel-coronavirus-2019/question-and-answers-hub/q-a-detail/coronavirus-disease-covid-19-masks

33. Centers for Disease Control and Prevention (CDC). Understanding the Difference. 2020. Accessed Apr 8, 2020. https://www.cdc.gov/niosh/npptl/pdfs/UnderstandDifferenceInfographic-508.pdf

34. Centers for Disease Control and Prevention (CDC). Stop the Spread of Germs. 2020. Accessed Sep 20, 2020. https://www.cdc.gov/coronavirus/2019-ncov/downloads/stop-the-spread-of-germs.pdf

35. McGarry BE, Grabowski DC, Barnett ML. Severe staffing and personal protective equipment shortages faced by nursing homes during the COVID-19 pandemic. *Health Aff* (Millwood). 2020:101377hlthaff202001269.

36. Centers for Disease Control and Prevention (CDC). Summary for Healthcare Facilities: Strategies for Optimizing the Supply of PPE During Shortages. 2020. Accessed Sep 20, 2020. https://www.cdc.gov/coronavirus/2019-ncov/hcp/ppe-strategy/strategies-optimize-ppe-shortages.html

37. Banach DB, et al. Outbreak response and incident management: SHEA guidance and resources for healthcare epidemiologists in United States acute-care hospitals. *Infect Control Hosp Epidemiol.* 2017;38(12):1393–1419.

38. Chopra V, et al. How Should U.S. Hospitals Prepare for Coronavirus Disease 2019 (COVID-19)? *Ann Intern Med.* 2020;172(9):621–622.

39. US Environmental Protection Agency (EPA). About List N: Disinfectants for Coronavirus (COVID-19). US EPA 2020. Accessed Aug 24, 2020. https://www.epa.gov/pesticide-registration/list-n-disinfectants-use-against-sars-cov-2-covid-19

40. The Joint Commission. APPROVED: New antimicrobial stewardship standard. *Jt Comm Perspect.* 2016;36(7):1,3–4,8.

41. American Nurses Association/Centers for Disease Control and Prevention (ANA/CDC). Redefining the antibiotic stewardship team: Recommendations from the American Nurses Association/Centers for Disease Control and Prevention Workgroup on the role of registered nurses in hospital antibiotic stewardship practices. *JAC-Antimicrobial Resistance.* 2019;1(2).

42. Penn Medicine. Antimicrobial Stewardship Checklist. 2016. Accessed Sep 20, 2020. https://www.pennmedicine.org/~/media/documents%20and%20audio/patient%20forms/infectious%20diseases/antibiotic%20flowsheet%20final%20check%20list.ashx?la=en

43. The Joint Commission. New Antimicrobial Stewardship Standard. 2016. Accessed Apr 4, 2020. https://www.jointcommission.org/assets/1/6/HAP-CAH_Antimicrobial_Prepub.pdf

44. Society for Healthcare Epidemiology of America (SHEA). Antimicrobial Stewardship. Accessed Apr 4, 2020. https://www.shea-online.org/index.php/practice-resources/priority-topics/antimicrobial-stewardship

45. Society for Healthcare Epidemiology of America (SHEA). Five Things Providers and Patients Should Question. 2015. Accessed Apr 4, 2020. https://www.shea-online.org/images/docs/SHEA_Choosing_Wisely_List_of_5.pdf

46. Bratzler DW, et al. Clinical practice guidelines for antimicrobial prophylaxis in surgery. *Am J Health Syst Pharm.* 2013;70(3):195–283.

47. Soule, BM. Table 1.2: Human factors engineering: Challenges for IPC. In Friedman C, editor: *International Federation of Infection Control: Basic Concepts of Infection Control*, 3rd edition. Craigavon, County Armagh: IFIC, 2016.

48. Pennathur PR, Herwaldt LA. Role of human factors engineering in infection prevention: Gaps and opportunities. *Curr Treat Options Infect Dis.* 2017;9(2):230–249.

49. Warye K, Granato J. Target: Zero hospital-acquired infections. *Healthc Financ Manage.* 2009;63(1):86–91.

50. HICPAC. Update to the CDC and the HICPAC Recommendation Categorization Scheme for Infection Control and Prevention Guideline Recommendations. 2019. Accessed Mar 27, 2020. https://www.cdc.gov/hicpac/workgroup/recommendation-scheme-update.html

51. Centers for Disease Control and Prevention (CDC). Guidelines & Guidance Library. 2020. Accessed Jul 16, 2020. https://www.cdc.gov/infectioncontrol/guidelines/index.html

52. Lo E, et al. Strategies to prevent catheter-associated urinary tract infections in acute care hospitals: 2014 update. *Infect Control Hosp Epidemiol.* 2014;35(5):464–479.

53. Association for Professionals in Infection Control and Epidemiology (APIC). Implementation Guides. 2020. Accessed Mar 11, 2020. https://apic.org/Professional-Practice/Implementation-guides

54. Yokoe DS, et al. A compendium of strategies to prevent healthcare-associated infections in acute care hospitals: 2014 updates. *Infect Control Hosp Epidemiol.* 2014;35(8):967–977.

55. Institute for Healthcare Improvement (IHI). How-to Guide: Improving Hand Hygiene. 2006 Apr. Accessed Mar 11, 2020. http://www.ihi.org/resources/Pages/Tools/HowtoGuideImprovingHandHygiene.aspx

56. Centers for Disease Control and Prevention (CDC). 2019 National and State Healthcare-Associated Infections Progress Report. 2018. Accessed Jul 16, 2020. https://www.cdc.gov/hai/data/portal/progress-report.html

57. Rahman M, et al. Reducing ventriculostomy-related infections to near zero: The eliminating ventriculostomy infection study. *Jt Comm J Qual Patient Saf.* 2012;38(10):459–464.

58. Pronovost PJ, et al. Sustaining reductions in catheter related bloodstream infections in Michigan intensive care units: Observational study. *Bmj.* 2010;340:c309.

59. Agency for Healthcare Research and Quality (AHRQ). Eliminating CLABSI, A National Patient Safety Imperative: Final Report on the National On the CUSP: Stop BSI Project. Oct 2012. Accessed Mar 22, 2020. https://www.ahrq.gov/sites/default/files/publications/files/clabsifinal.pdf

60. Agency for Healthcare Research and Quality (AHRQ). TeamSTEPPS®: Strategies and Tools to Enhance Performance and Patient Safety. 2020. Accessed Mar 13, 2020. https://www.ahrq.gov/teamstepps/index.html

61. Agency for Healthcare Research and Quality (AHRQ). Training Guide: Using Simulation in TeamSTEPPS® Training: Classroom Slides. 2019 Jun. Accessed Mar 22, 2020. https://www.ahrq.gov/teamstepps/simulation/simulationslides/simslides.html

62. Timmel J, et al. Impact of the Comprehensive Unit-based Safety Program (CUSP) on safety culture in a surgical inpatient unit. *Jt Comm J Qual Patient Saf.* 2010;36(6):252–260.

63. Cohen PM, Ptaskiewicz M, Mipos D. The case for unit-based teams: A model for front-line engagement and performance improvement. *Perm J.* 2010;14(2):70–75.

64. Resar R, et al. Using care bundles to improve health care quality. IHI Innovation Series white paper. Cambridge, MA: IHI, 2012.

65. Gawande A. *The Checklist Manifesto: How to Get Things Right.* New York: Metropolitan Books, 2009.

66. Pronovost P, Vohr E. *How One Doctor's Checklist Can Help Us Change Health Care from the Inside Out.* New York: Penguin, 2010.

67. Agency for Healthcare Research and Quality (AHRQ). Making Health Care Safer II: An Updated Critical Analysis of the Evidence for Patient Safety Practices—Executive Summary. 2013. Accessed Mar 13, 2020. https://www.ahrq.gov/research/findings/evidence-based-reports/ptsafetysum.html

68. Health Protection Scotland (HPS). Compendium of HAI Guidance. 2020. Accessed Jul 19, 2020. https://hpspubsrepo.blob.core.windows.net/hps-website/nss/1513/documents/1_hai-compendium.pdf

69. Health Protection Scotland (HPS). National Infection Prevention and Control Manual. Accessed Jul 19, 2020. http://www.nipcm.hps.scot.nhs.uk/

70. Saint S, et al. A reminder reduces urinary catheterization in hospitalized patients. *Jt Comm J Qual Patient Saf.* 2005;31(8):455–462.

71. Society for Healthcare Epidemiology of America (SHEA). Family-Centered Residential Facility: Guest Health Screening Questions. 2017. Accessed Mar 11, 2020. https://www.shea-online.org/images/patients/RMHC-Patient-Guides.pdf

72. Murthy R, et al. Animals in healthcare facilities: Recommendations to minimize potential risks. *Infect Control Hosp Epidemiol.* 2015;36(5):495–516.

Chapter 7

Maintaining a Safe Environment of Care

By Kathleen Meehan Arias, MS, MT(ASCP), SM(AAM), CIC, FAPIC

Disclaimer: Strategies, tools, and examples discussed in this book do not necessarily reflect Joint Commission or Joint Commission International requirements for all settings. Always refer to the most current standards applicable to your health care setting to ensure compliance.

Introduction

The Joint Commission's Infection Prevention and Control (IC) standards and Environment of Care (EC) standards as well as Joint Commission International (JCI) Prevention and Control of Infection and Facility Management and Safety standards aim to promote a safe, functional, and supportive environment. They stress the importance of providing a proactive, systematic approach to managing infection prevention and control (IPC) risks in the environment. The standards require that organizations identify and manage risks related to the following:

- Medical equipment, devices, and supplies (discussed in detail in Chapter 8)
- Utility systems
- Infectious waste
- Building design, construction, and renovation
- Environment of care/facility management and safety (FMS)

Organizations are expected to engage in ongoing efforts to provide a safe environment and to ensure immediate intervention when conditions result in a threat to life or health. This chapter examines the relationship between the environment of care/facility management and the IPC program and provides suggestions and best practices for ensuring a safe, functional, and supportive environment that effectively reduces IPC risks.

Relevant Joint Commission Standards Addressed in This Chapter

Note: These standards were in effect at the time of publication. They refer to Joint Commission standards effective January 1, 2021. Always consult the most recent version of Joint Commission standards for the most accurate requirements for your setting.

IC.02.01.01 The [organization] implements its infection prevention and control plan.

EP 6 The [organization] minimizes the risk of infection when storing and disposing of infectious waste. (*See also* EC.02.02.01, EPs 1 and 12)

EC.02.05.01 The [organization] manages risks associated with its utility systems.

EP 14 The [organization] minimizes pathogenic biological agents in cooling towers, domestic hot- and cold-water systems, and other aerosolizing water systems.

(continued)

(continued)

EC.02.06.01 The [organization] establishes and maintains a safe, functional environment.

EC.02.06.05 The [organization] manages its environment during demolition, renovation, or new construction to reduce risks to those in the organization.

EP 1 When planning for new, altered, or renovated space, the [organization] uses one of the following design criteria:
- State and local rules and regulations
- *Guidelines for Design and Construction of Hospitals and Outpatient Facilities*, 2018 edition, administered by the Facility Guidelines Institute and published by the American Society for Healthcare Engineering (ASHE)

When the above rules, regulations, and guidelines do not meet specific design needs, use other reputable standards and guidelines that provide equivalent design criteria.

EP 2 When planning for demolition, construction, renovation, or general maintenance, the [organization] conducts a preconstruction risk assessment for air quality requirements, infection control, utility requirements, noise, vibration, and other hazards that affect care, treatment, and services. **Note:** See *LS.01.02.01 for information on fire safety procedures to implement during construction or renovation*.

EP 3 The [organization] takes action based on its assessment to minimize risks during demolition, construction, renovation or general maintenance.

EC.04.01.01 The [organization] collects information to monitor conditions in the environment.

EP 1 The [organization] establishes a process(es) for continually monitoring, internally reporting, and investigating the following:
- Injuries to patients or others within the hospital's facilities
- Occupational illnesses and staff injuries
- Incidents of damage to its property or the property of others
- Security incidents involving patients, staff, or others within its facilities
- Hazardous materials and waste spills and exposures
- Fire safety management problems, deficiencies, and failures
- Medical or laboratory equipment management problems, failures, and use errors
- Utility systems management problems, failures, or use errors

Note 1: *All the incidents and issues listed above may be reported to staff in quality assessment, improvement, or other functions. A summary of such incidents may also be shared with the person designated to coordinate safety management activities.*

Note 2: *Review of incident reports often requires that legal processes be followed to preserve confidentiality. Opportunities to improve care, treatment, or services, or to prevent similar incidents, are not lost as a result of following the legal process.*

EC.04.01.05 The [organization] improves its environment of care.

Relevant Joint Commission International (JCI) Standards Addressed in This Chapter

Note: These standards were in effect at the time of publication. They refer to the *Joint Commission International Accreditation Standards for Hospitals, seventh edition,* ©2020. Always consult the most recent version of Joint Commission International standards for the most accurate requirements for your hospital or medical center setting.

FMS.4 Data are collected and analyzed from each of the facility management and safety programs to reduce risks in the environment, track progress on goals and improvements, and support planning for replacing and upgrading facilities, systems, and equipment.

ME 1 Monitoring data are collected and analyzed for each of the facility management and safety programs and used to reduce risks in the environment and support planning for replacing or upgrading facilities, systems, and equipment.

ME 2 Monitoring data for the facility management and safety programs are documented and integrated into the hospital's quality and patient safety program.

FMS.5 The hospital develops and implements a program to provide a safe physical facility through inspection and planning to reduce risks.

FMS.7 The hospital develops and implements a program for the management of hazardous materials and waste.

ME 1 The hospital develops and implements a written program for the management of hazardous materials and waste.

FMS.7.1 The hospital's program for the management of hazardous materials and waste includes the inventory, handling, storage, and use of hazardous materials.

ME 2 The hazardous materials and waste program establishes and implements procedures for safe handling, storage, and use of hazardous materials.

ME 3 The hazardous materials and waste program establishes and implements the proper protective equipment required during handling and use of hazardous materials.

FMS.7.2 The hospital's program for the management of hazardous materials and waste includes the types, handling, storage, and disposal of hazardous waste.

ME 2 The hazardous materials and waste program establishes and implements procedures and the proper protective equipment required for safe handling and storage of hazardous waste.

FMS.10.2 The hospital utility systems program ensures that essential utilities, including power, water, and medical gases, are available at all times and alternative sources for essential utilities are established and tested.

ME 1 The hospital identifies the areas and services at greatest risk when essential utilities (including power, water, and medical gas) become unavailable.

ME 2 The hospital ensures backup availability/ continuity of essential utilities (including power, water, and medical gas) 24 hours a day, 7 days a week.

ME 3 The hospital assesses for and reduces the risks of interruption, contamination, and failure of essential utilities (including power, water, and medical gas).

FMS.12, ME 1 When planning for construction, renovation, or demolition projects, or maintenance activities that affect patient care, the hospital conducts a preconstruction risk assessment (PCRA) for
- air quality;
- infection prevention and control;
- utilities;
- noise;

(continued)

(continued)

- vibration;
- hazardous materials and waste;
- fire safety;
- security;
- emergency procedures, including alternate pathways/exits and access to emergency services; and
- other hazards that affect care, treatment, and services.

ME 2 The hospital takes action based on its assessment to minimize risks during construction, renovation, and demolition projects, and maintenance activities that affect patient care.

PCI.7 The infection prevention and control program identifies and implements standards from recognized infection prevention and control programs to address cleaning and disinfection of the environment and environmental surfaces.

PCI.8 The hospital reduces the risk of infections through proper disposal of waste, proper management of human tissues, and safe handling and disposal of sharps and needles.

ME 1 The handling and disposal of infectious waste, blood and blood components, body fluids, and body tissues is managed to minimize infection transmission risk.

ME 2 The hospital identifies and implements practices to reduce the risk of injury and infection from the handling and management of sharps and needles.

PCI.11, ME 1 The hospital has a program that uses risk criteria to assess the impact of renovation or new construction and implements the program when demolition, construction, or renovation take place.

ME 2 The hospital assesses the risks and impact of demolition, renovation, or construction activities on air quality and infection prevention and control activities throughout the hospital.

ME 3 The risks and impact of the demolition, renovation, or construction are managed to protect patients, staff, and visitors from infection.

The Impact of the Environment on Infection Prevention and Control Efforts

Because the health care environment can serve as a source of pathogenic organisms—particularly contaminated air, water, surfaces, and medical devices—an organization's IPC program risk assessment should address the role that the environment contributes to IPC risk in its setting. Based on the risk assessment, the IPC program should identify and implement measures that will reduce the risk of transmission or acquisition of organisms to patients, residents, staff, or visitors from environmental sources and monitor compliance with those measures.

TIP Organizations are expected to engage in ongoing efforts to provide a safe environment and to ensure immediate interventions when conditions result in a threat to life or health.

One aspect of the environment that should receive attention from the IPC program is the role of environmental surfaces in transmitting disease. Studies in the 1970s and 1980s suggested that environmental surface contamination played a negligible role in the transmission of health care–associated infections (HAIs).

However, there is now much evidence that both hard and soft contaminated surfaces contribute to the transmission of pathogenic organisms, including well-known organisms such as *Clostridium difficile* (also known as *Clostridioides difficile* or *C. difficile*), vancomycin-resistant *Enterococci*, methicillin-resistant *Staphylococcus aureus*, *Acinetobacter baumannii*, *Pseudomonas aeruginosa*, and norovirus and new and emerging pathogens such as Ebola, carbapenem-resistant *Enterobacteriaceae*, and *Candida auris*.[1-3] Some of these agents, such as norovirus and *C. auris*, are not readily killed by disinfectants commonly used in health care facilities for environmental cleaning and disinfection.[3]

Infectious agents can be transmitted from person to person via direct contact with skin and body fluids (urine, saliva, feces, vomit, breast milk, and semen) and by respiratory droplets; via indirect contact with contaminated environmental surfaces and fomites; and by the airborne route.[2] Because pathogens can remain infective on environmental surfaces for prolonged periods, organizations should ensure that protocols for cleaning and disinfecting environmental surfaces and furnishings and for handling linens and waste are integral components of the IPC program.[2,4]

HAIs remain a major cause of morbidity and mortality. Most often related to the patient's endogenous flora, HAIs have also been attributed to cross-infection from the hands of health care workers who have become contaminated either from direct contact with the patient or indirect contact, by touching contaminated environmental surfaces.[2,4] Organisms also may be transmitted directly to a patient who comes in contact with a contaminated surface.[1] Studies have shown that many of the organisms that have caused HAIs associated with contaminated environmental surfaces possess the following characteristics:

- Have the ability to survive and remain virulent for prolonged periods of time on environmental surfaces
- Have the ability to colonize patients and staff
- Have the capacity to transiently colonize the hands of health care workers and be subsequently transmitted to other persons and surfaces
- Are powerful in small infectious doses
- Show relative resistance to disinfectants used on environmental surfaces

Because many pathogens can be transmitted following contact with contaminated environmental surfaces, staff in health care facilities must pay close attention to cleaning and disinfecting the environment.

In addition to environmental surfaces, the following factors have contributed to serious outbreaks in health care settings and have been well documented in the literature:[2,5]

- Construction, renovation, and alteration of the physical facility
- Contamination of the water supply
- Inadequate ventilation

Outbreaks in a variety of health care settings have been associated with the transmission of pathogenic organisms spread via the airborne route, including those causing measles, influenza, chickenpox, tuberculosis, Legionnaire's disease, and aspergillosis.[2] The rapid worldwide spread and the multiple outbreaks of Novel Coronavirus 2019 (COVID-19) in health care settings have called attention to the potential for human pathogens to be transmitted from person to person through contaminated air and surfaces.[6]

Regardless of the setting, health care organizations should implement and monitor the use of evidence-based practices that can effectively reduce the risk of transmission of organisms from environmental sources to patients, residents, personnel, visitors, and others who enter the facility.

Exploring the Infection Prevention and Control and Environment of Care Standards

This chapter focuses on the IC/PCI and EC/FMS standards related to the following:

- Infectious waste
- Utility systems
  - Water
  - Heating, ventilating, and air conditioning (HVAC)
- Environmental services and housekeeping
- Demolition, renovation, and construction
- Monitoring and improving conditions in the environment

The following sections address these topics and provide practical strategies and interventions to help organizations and infection preventionists (IPs) provide a safe environment and prevent infections.

Infectious Waste

Requirements related to infectious waste are designed to ensure that health care organizations have developed and implemented safe systems and processes to handle infectious waste from the time it is generated, such as at the bedside or during a procedure, to the time it leaves the facility and to final disposal. In addition, the organization should appropriately handle any medical waste spills in a manner that minimizes IPC risks to staff, patients, and visitors. The IP can help ensure that this requirement is met by assessing the organization's practices and policies for collecting, storing, and disposing of infectious waste (also called regulated medical waste) and by ensuring that these policies are in compliance with local, state, and federal requirements. This evaluation can be done when performing the annual risk assessment. The IP may also evaluate staff compliance with accepted practices by performing environmental rounds, documenting findings, and sending a report to the units surveyed.

Most regulations related to infectious or regulated medical waste (including sharps and needles) are defined at the state or local level, usually by the state or local health department. These requirements typically address the following:

- Treatment
- Storage
- Transportation
- Transfer facilities
- Packaging and labeling of potentially infectious waste

The IP may collaborate with staff members in the organization who generate and manage infectious waste to identify the applicable requirements and to ensure compliance with those requirements.

Information on some state requirements can be found on the US Environmental Protection Agency (EPA) website.[7] The US Occupational Safety and Health Administration also addresses the issue of infectious waste and specifies certain features of regulated waste containers—including appropriate tagging—to protect staff against exposure to bloodborne pathogens as well as personal protective equipment (PPE) to use when exposed to medical waste and management of exposures.[8]

The IP may collaborate with other disciplines to clearly define what constitutes regulated waste versus regular waste. The organization should post signs at disposal sites to ensure proper placement of waste. This practice can prevent infectious waste (for example, blood or body fluids) from being placed with regular waste, which could possibly result in an exposure to waste handlers or fines for placing infectious waste in regular containers. The ultimate disposal method (landfilling, incinerating, and so forth) for infectious waste falls under the purview of the EPA and state and local agencies.[7]

The IP may obtain current information on infectious waste handling and disposal by joining health department mailing lists, linking to the websites in the Resources section at the end of this chapter, and maintaining a close relationship with others in the organization who may receive this information on a regular basis.

A written procedure, including use of PPE and precautions to take for managing medical waste spills, is recommended. Staff responsible for cleaning up these spills should be appropriately trained in the organization's spill management procedure.

Another recommended practice is that environmental service staff, IPs, and other personnel, as appropriate, observe practices for waste disposal and cleanup during scheduled environmental rounding or daily rounding to help ensure that infectious waste is handled properly.

Utility Systems

An organization's utility systems can present opportunities for pathogenic growth and transmission. The following sections discuss these aspects of utility systems and strategies for addressing them.

Water, aqueous solutions, water systems, and moist environments can serve as sources and reservoirs for pathogenic agents. Environmental reservoirs and sources for microbial pathogens include the following[2,9,10]:

- Cooling towers and evaporative condensers
- Potable water system (for example, aerators, shower hoses/heads)
- Dialysis water and equipment
- Ice machines and ice
- Hydrotherapy tanks and pools
- Heating and cooling equipment
- Equipment connected to main water systems (such as endoscope reprocessors and dental unit water lines)
- Indoor water features

Because of the potential for pathogens associated with water in the environment, IPs should be familiar with the basic components of water systems in their health care facilities, the types and modes of transmission of waterborne infectious diseases in health care facilities, and strategies for preventing and controlling waterborne microbial transmission, acquisition, and contamination.[2] Strategies for preventing and controlling the transmission and acquisition of waterborne agents include the following[2,9-12]:

- Contingency plans for providing potable water during periods of contamination or disruption
- Management of water systems during construction/renovation projects
- A surveillance program to detect health care–associated infections resulting from *Legionella* spp. and other waterborne organisms
- A program for maintaining and monitoring dialysis system water and dialysate quality
- Adherence to the Association for the Advancement of Medical Instrumentation standards for hemodialysis[12]

In 2017, the US Centers for Medicare & Medicaid Services announced that Medicare-certified health care facilities must develop and maintain water management policies and procedures to reduce the risk of growth and the spread of *Legionella* and other opportunistic pathogens in building water systems.[13] This directive applies to hospitals, critical access hospitals, and long term care facilities, but it also is intended to provide general awareness to other health care settings.

The directive states that organizations should do the following:

- Conduct a risk assessment to identify potential areas of growth and spread of *Legionella* and other pathogens associated with water supply systems
- Include high-risk patient groups and facets of health care (for example, patient care devices and medical equipment) in the risk assessment
- Implement a water management program that considers the American Society of Heating, Refrigerating and Air-Conditioning Engineers industry standard and Centers for Disease Control and Prevention (CDC) toolkits and includes the following components:
  - Establishes a water management program team
  - Describes the building water systems using diagrams and schematics
  - Identifies areas where *Legionella* and other waterborne pathogens could grow and spread
  - Defines control measures (such as physical controls, temperature management, disinfectant

level control, visual inspections, and environmental testing)
  - Describes where and how control measures should be applied and how they are monitored
  - Identifies acceptable ranges for control measures and describes intervention processes to follow when control limits are not maintained
  - Describes intervention processes to follow when control limits are not met
  - Defines a process for evaluating the water management program's effectiveness
  - Documents results of testing and corrective actions to take when limits are not maintained

IPs may collaborate with the building's facilities management staff to ensure that the organization has a water management program. The organization should consider convening a team to ensure that the water management program meets all relevant regulations and requirements related to water systems in health care facilities. Consider including staff from facilities management, environmental services, IPC, and quality and risk management staff. The CDC developed a toolkit to assist organizations in setting up a team and implementing and maintaining a water management program. A link to the toolkit is in the Resources section at the end of this chapter.

Dental unit water lines are often not considered in the facility infection control risk assessment. However, they are connected to main water systems and could transmit infection if not properly maintained. An organization can use the following strategies to reduce the risk of transmission of infection related to dental water lines[14,15]:

- Use water that meets local or EPA regulatory standards for drinking water.
- Consult with dental unit manufacturer for appropriate methods and equipment needed to maintain the recommended quality of dental water.
- Adhere to recommendations for monitoring water quality provided by the manufacturer of the unit and the water line treatment product.
- Discharge water and air for a minimum of 20–30 seconds after each patient use from any device connected to the dental water system that enters the patient's mouth, such as headpieces, ultrasonic scalers, and air/water syringes.
- Consult with the dental unit manufacturer on the need for periodic maintenance of anti-retraction mechanisms.

TIP Because of the potential for pathogens associated with water in the environment, infection preventionists should be familiar with the basic components of water systems in their health care facilities, the types and modes of transmission of waterborne infectious diseases in health care facilities, and strategies for preventing and controlling waterborne microbial contamination, transmission, and acquisition.

HVAC systems have long been recognized as reservoirs and sources of pathogenic organisms and have been involved in disease transmission in health care facilities.[2,16-18] The COVID-19 pandemic focused attention on indoor air quality and recirculation in all types of buildings, including health care settings.[18] IPs should become familiar with the airborne infectious diseases transmitted in health care facilities and the basic components and operations of HVAC systems. They may consider reviewing publications about HVAC systems and infectious diseases associated with these systems,[2,16-18] attending educational programs, and working with their organization's facilities and maintenance staff.

Some recommended strategies for complying with Joint Commission and JCI requirements for HVAC systems include the following:

- Developing and implementing evidence-based policies and procedures for ensuring the proper maintenance and functioning of HVAC systems in the facility.
- Documenting routine monitoring of the functioning of air-handling systems in special care areas—such as airborne infection isolation rooms, protective environments, and operating rooms.
- Documenting steps taken if the system is not functioning according to established criteria.
- Ensuring that strategies for IPC are implemented during demolition, construction, and renovation, as discussed later in this chapter.

Strategies that can be used to help ensure that an organization provides both safe water and HVAC systems are listed in Sidebar 7-1.[16,17]

As previously discussed, contaminated environmental surfaces—such as floors, bedrails, furnishings, sinks, and

---

Sidebar 7-1. Safe Water and Heating, Ventilating, and Air Conditioning (HVAC) Systems

Strategies to help ensure that an organization provides safe water and HVAC systems include the following:

- Periodically invite facilities staff to infection prevention and control (IPC) committee or other applicable meetings to discuss their IPC programs and how they monitor compliance with them.
- Develop and adhere to preventive maintenance schedules.
- Monitor and distribute quality assurance testing results to the appropriate staff in the organization (for example, administration, IPC, quality assurance/performance improvement).
- Implement a protocol to notify the infection preventionist about HVAC system failures and potable water interruptions and concerns in the organization.
- Base policies and practices for maintaining indoor air quality—including ventilation rates, temperatures, humidity levels, pressure relationships, and minimum air changes per hour—on the Facility Guidelines Institute's *Guidelines for Design and Construction of Hospitals and Outpatient Facilities*.[17]

---

curtains—have been increasingly recognized as playing a role in transmitting infection, in particular when cleaning and disinfection of surfaces are not adequate and consistent.[1-4,19] The higher the bioburden on surfaces, the greater the chance that organisms will be transferred to hands or supplies used in patient care. Therefore, careful attention should be given to environmental cleaning and disinfection.

Organizations should provide written, clearly defined cleaning and disinfection policies and procedures, use evidence-based monitoring protocols, and ensure compliance with environmental services and housekeeping protocols. Adherence to these practices should effectively reduce the bioburden on environmental

Environmental services and housekeeping protocols should effectively reduce the bioburden on environmental surfaces to lessen the likelihood that they could serve as a source for pathogenic agents. Such protocols should also ensure an aesthetically pleasing environment for patients, residents, health care staff, and others.

surfaces, lessen the likelihood that they could serve as a source for pathogenic agents, and provide an aesthetic environment for patients, residents, visitors, health care staff, and others.

Selecting and Using Cleaners and Disinfectants

One important function of the IP is to provide evidence-based information that can help the organization choose appropriate cleaners and disinfectants for the facility.[20] There are many types and manufacturers of cleaners and disinfectants.[2,4,20,21] The organization should have written policies and protocols for the following:

- Selecting, trialing, and evaluating cleaners and disinfectants
- Using cleaners and disinfectants appropriately and following manufacturers' instructions for use
- Training and testing competency of staff who use cleaners and disinfectants
- Monitoring and evaluating cleaning and disinfection practices
- Standardizing products
- Approving new products through a multidisciplinary organizational committee, including IPC and environmental services staff, when applicable
- Using appropriate tools for cleaning

Several studies have reported that liquid disinfectants are not always effective at killing all bioburden on surfaces or destroying spores. However, the types of liquid disinfectant products and newer technologies for improving cleaning and disinfection of health care environmental surfaces are continuously evolving.[4,22-24]

Because studies have shown that manual cleaning and disinfection practices often are inadequate in successfully removing and killing pathogens on environmental surfaces, several "no touch" room decontamination technologies have been developed in recent years. These include ultraviolet light systems, vaporized hydrogen peroxide, and continuous room decontamination technologies, such as self-disinfecting surfaces.[22-24] It is important to recognize that these technologies can supplement manual cleaning and disinfection but should not replace them. This is because surfaces must first be physically cleaned to remove soil before they can be disinfected.[4] Because these systems and technologies have advantages and limitations, the IP must carefully evaluate their effective use and applications in health care settings as well as the time needed to implement them.[4,25]

An in-depth discussion of selecting and using cleaners, disinfectants, and decontamination technologies is beyond the scope of this book; however, additional information can be found in several references and in the Resources section at the end of this chapter.

Evaluating and Monitoring Environmental Cleaning

Options for evaluating environmental cleaning are provided by the CDC.[26] These options are divided into two levels, both of which stress the need for collaboration among the IP, hospital epidemiologist (when available), and environmental services staff. The CDC recommends that the monitoring program be jointly developed but internally coordinated and maintained through environmental services management–level participation. The CDC strategies include the following[26]:

- Develop and implement policies and procedures for cleaning and disinfecting environmental surfaces and handling laundry and medical waste (including sharps and needles).
- Conduct a risk assessment to identify and focus on appropriate cleaning and disinfection of high-touch surfaces—such as bedrails and the area around toilets in a patient's or resident's room.
- Clearly define high-touch areas by area or department. (For example, operating room high-touch areas are clearly different than patient rooms.)
- Ensure that policies define who is responsible for cleaning and disinfecting areas, environmental surfaces, and objects.
- Ensure that appropriate cleaning and disinfecting agents and equipment are used and that they do not damage the surfaces on which they are used.

- Ensure that cleaning and disinfection practices comply with evidence-based recommendations, regulations, and other requirements.
- Provide ongoing training and monitoring of environmental services staff to ensure that they use appropriate practices and types and concentrations of cleaners and disinfectants. Include training on processes such as washing hands, changing gloves, and safe handling of linen and trash.
- Use a multidisciplinary team approach for conducting routine rounds to evaluate environment of care issues such as cleanliness, supply storage, eating and drinking on care units, and management of medical devices and equipment. Members of a multidisciplinary rounds team may include staff from IPC, environmental services, nursing services, the area being evaluated, facilities management, safety, and quality and performance improvement. Use an environmental rounds tool to guide the review and document findings and recommendations. Tool 7-1 is a sample environmental rounds tool for a hospital that can be customized for use.
- Share audit findings with staff from environmental services, the area surveyed, IPC, and leadership. Be sure to applaud success.
- Reiterate the importance of what is being done to prevent and control infection.
- Assess the competence of environmental services and housekeeping personnel, including use of return demonstration for cleaning and disinfection practices per organizational policy.
- Reward and recognize staff for their accomplishments.

TRY THIS TOOL

Tool 7-1. Environmental Rounds for Infection Control Template

Monitoring the Efficacy of Cleaning and Disinfection Practices

Often visual assessment is not a reliable indicator of surface decontamination. An objective method for evaluating environmental cleanliness may be indicated.[22,26] There are several options for monitoring the efficacy of cleaning and disinfection practices, including but not limited to the following:

- Direct observation
- Swab cultures
- Agar slide plates
- Fluorescent markers
- Adenosine triphosphate (ATP) bioluminescence

Each of the above practices has pros and cons. ATP measures only organic debris; however, it can assess how well things are cleaned. Microbiological cultures are costly, and the results are generally poor indicators for assessing disinfection practices. Fluorescent markers are easily applied and can be a very useful tool to educate staff and evaluate cleaning processes. Organizations need to determine what method or methods are appropriate for their use.

More information on options for evaluating and monitoring environmental cleaning and disinfection practices can be found in the CDC's *Options for Evaluating Environmental Cleaning*[26] and in the References section at the end of this chapter.

TIP When observing cleaning and disinfection practices, focus on tools, disinfectants, and equipment. Ensure that the cleaners and disinfectants are those approved by the organization and are properly diluted, labeled, and used according to the manufacturer's instructions for use. Improper practices can lead to inadequate disinfection and damaged surfaces.

Collaboration Is Key

Collaboration between infection prevention and environmental services staff is essential for success in providing a clean, safe, and functional environment. Environmental service personnel play a critical role in efforts to decrease rates of *C. difficile* infection and other HAIs. The case on page 179, provides an example of a collaborative effort that led to the reduction of *C. difficile* infection rates in hospitals in Maryland.[27]

Reducing Surface Contamination in Health Care

In 2016 the Maryland Patient Safety Center initiated the Clean Collaborative, involving 17 acute care hospitals, 3 long term care facilities, and 4 ambulatory surgical centers.[27] Reducing Environmental Surface Contamination in Health Care Settings: A Statewide Collaborative focused on improving environmental surface cleaning with the goal of reducing rates of *Clostridium difficile* infections (CDIs), which were selected as a proxy for health care–associated infections (HAIs). The goals of the collaborative were "to achieve a minimum of 10% improvement in cleanliness and to simultaneously decrease CDI rates." Facilities collected and reported data between April 2016 and March 2017.

Collaborative facilities implemented the following infection prevention and control (IPC) practices:
- Used an adenosine triphosphate (ATP) validation technology system to measure cleaning effectiveness.
- Conducted training sessions on topics such as surface cleaning, surface disinfection and product selection, and using ATP monitoring validation technology.
- Used a web-based portal for distributing forms and educational materials and for inputting participant data.
- Identified areas to be sampled and developed protocols for collecting samples.
- Created an advisory board consisting of representatives from the Maryland health department, Maryland hospital systems, and industry.
- Used National Healthcare Safety Network definitions to identify CDI and reported ATP monitoring results as relative light units (RLUs) to measure cleanliness of surfaces.

The results were clear: Of the 24 participating facilities, 21 (88%) achieved a 10% reduction in RLUs from the baseline month to the last month of collecting data. Seventy-five percent of participating facilities exceeded the goal by reducing average RLUs by more than 50%.

When the team did a comparison of the CDI rates of participating acute care facilities with the CDI rates of Maryland facilities that did not participate in the project, they found that participants in the collaborative achieved a 14.2% decrease in CDI rates compared to a 5.9% decrease in nonparticipating facilities. Many of the participating facilities found that the IPC activities put in place by the collaborative not only improved cleanliness in an effort to reduce the rates of the targeted HAI but also fostered teamwork between environmental services and IPC staff.

Demolition, Renovation, and Construction

Some recommended strategies and practices for providing a safe environment of care during facility design, demolition, construction, and renovation include the following:
- Form a multidisciplinary, collaborative team to identify and proactively mitigate the effects of demolition, construction, and renovation activities on air quality, water, and HVAC systems, environmental cleanliness, and traffic flow. The team may include the IP (or person responsible for IPC), experts in facility design and ventilation, safety officers, epidemiologists, building engineers, managers and staff in the area involved in the new construction, renovation, or demolition, direct care supervisors, risk managers, and building contractors.
- Document when IPs are actively involved in a health care facility's planning, design, demolition,

construction, and renovation activities. Proof of involvement could include documentation of attendance at meetings and sign-off on planning and design documents or IPC construction permits.

- Identify and use applicable state and local regulations and other relevant requirements when designing, renovating, and constructing new health care facilities.
- Use the Facility Guidelines Institute's *Guidelines for Design and Construction of Hospitals and Outpatient Facilities* when designing and planning new spaces and renovating existing ones.[17]
- Complete a preconstruction risk assessment, including an infection control risk assessment (ICRA) that incorporates risk criteria for evaluating the type of activity that will occur and the types of patients who will be affected during construction and renovation projects.[2,17] See the tools listed in the box at right for several examples of ICRA tools that can be customized for use or for reference and refer to Chapter 3. Issues to assess during a preconstruction risk assessment include the following:
    ◦ Disruption of essential services
    ◦ Relocation or placement of patients
    ◦ Barrier placements to control airborne contaminants
    ◦ Debris cleanup and removal
    ◦ Traffic flow
    ◦ Utility disruption
- Use an infection control permit for demolition, construction, and renovation activities. This tool documents and communicates with contractors about their responsibilities regarding the preconstruction risk assessment and documents follow-up visits by the IP or safety manager. A sample IC permit (Tool 7-4) can be downloaded for reference.
- Use barriers, high-efficiency particulate air units, and other measures to create negative pressure in the construction space and prevent the dispersion of airborne organisms and dust particles produced by construction and renovation activities into occupied areas, if indicated.

- Monitor and document daily the presence of negative airflow in the construction zone or renovation area.[2]
- Develop and implement a comprehensive IPC program prior to, during, and upon completion of maintenance, demolition, construction, and renovation projects.
- Implement a multidisciplinary program for training, monitoring, and promoting adherence to IPC practices during construction and renovation—and documenting these practices.

TRY THESE TOOLS

Tool 7-2. Pre-Construction Risk Assessment Checklist

Tool 7-3. Infection Control Risk Assessment (ICRA) Matrix of Precautions for Construction and Renovation

Tool 7-4. Sample Infection Control Construction Permit

Tool 7-5. Construction and Renovation Infection Control Checklist

Tool 7-6. Infection Control and Safety Construction Compliance Monitor

---

In addition to these strategies and guidelines, an organization should address the construction design and function considerations in Sidebar 7-2 on page 181 and the IPC measures for internal construction and repair projects in Table 7-1 on pages 182 and 183.

Sidebar 7-2. Construction Design and Function Considerations for Environmental Infection Control

- Location of sinks and dispensers for hand-washing products and hand hygiene products
- Types of faucets (for example, aerated vs. nonaerated)
- Air-handling systems engineered for optimal performance, easy maintenance, and repair
- Air changes per hour and pressure differentials to accommodate special patient care areas
- Location of fixed sharps containers
- Types of surface finishes (for example, porous vs. nonporous)
- Well-caulked walls with minimal seams
- Location of adequate storage and supply areas
- Appropriate location of medicine preparations areas (for example, greater than 3 feet from a sink)
- Appropriate location and type of ice machines (for example, preferably ice dispensers rather than ice bins)
- Appropriate materials for sinks and wall coverings
- Appropriate traffic flow (for example, no "dirty" movement through "clean" areas)
- Isolation rooms with anterooms, as appropriate
- Appropriate flooring (for example, seamless floors in dialysis units)
- Sensible-use carpeting (for example, no carpeting in special care areas or areas likely to become wet)
- Convenient location of soiled utility areas
- Properly engineered areas for linen services and solid waste management
- Location of main generator to minimize the risk of system failure from flooding or other emergency
- Installation guidelines for drywall

Source: US Centers for Disease Control and Prevention (CDC). *Guidelines for Environmental Infection Control in Health-Care Facilities*. Healthcare Infection Control Practices Advisory Committee (HICPAC). 2003.

Table 7-1. Infection Prevention and Control Measures for Internal Construction and Repair Projects

Infection Control Measure	Steps for Implementation
Prepare for the project.	1. Use a multidisciplinary team approach to incorporate infection prevention and control (IPC) into the project. 2. Conduct the risk assessment and a preliminary walk-through with project managers and staff.
Educate staff and construction workers.	1. Educate staff and construction workers about the importance of adhering to IPC measures during the project. 2. Provide educational materials in the language of the workers. 3. Include language in the construction contract requiring construction workers and subcontractors to participate in IPC training.
Issue hazard and warning notices.	1. Post signs to identify construction areas and potential hazards. 2. Mark detours requiring pedestrians to avoid the work area.
Relocate high-risk patients as needed, particularly if the construction is in or adjacent to a protective environment area.	1. Identify target patient populations for relocation based on the risk assessment. 2. Arrange for the transfer in advance to avoid delays. 3. Ensure that at-risk patients wear protective respiratory equipment (e.g., a high-efficiency or N95 mask) when outside their protective environment rooms.
Establish alternative traffic patterns for staff, patients, visitors, and construction workers.	1. Use the risk assessment to determine appropriate alternate routes 2. Designate areas (e.g., hallways, elevators, restrooms, and entrances/exits) for construction worker use. 3. Do not transport patients on the same elevator with construction materials and debris.
Erect appropriate barrier containment.	1. Use prefabricated plastic units or plastic sheeting for short-term projects that will generate minimal dust. 2. Use durable rigid barriers for ongoing, long-term projects.
Establish proper ventilation.	1. Shut off return air vents in the construction zone, if possible, and seal around grilles. 2. Exhaust air and dust to the outside, if possible. 3. If recirculated air from the construction zone is unavoidable, use a prefilter and a high-efficiency particulate air (HEPA) filter before the air returns to the heating, ventilating, and air conditioning (HVAC) system. 4. When vibration-related work is being done that may dislodge dust in the ventilation system or when modifications are made to ductwork serving occupied spaces, install filters on the supply air grilles temporarily. 5. Set pressure differentials so that the contained work area is under negative pressure. 6. Use air flow monitoring devices to verify the direction of the air pattern. 7. Exhaust air and dust to the outside, if possible. 8. Monitor temperature, air changes per hour (ACH), and humidity levels (humidity levels should be < 65%). 9. Use portable, industrial-grade HEPA filters in the adjacent area and/or the construction zone for additional ACH. 10. Keep windows closed, if possible.

(continued)

Table 7-1. Infection Prevention and Control Measures for Internal Construction and Repair Projects (continued)

Infection Control Measure	Steps for Implementation
Control solid debris.	1. When replacing filters, place the old filter in a bag prior to transport and dispose as a routine solid waste. 2. Clean the construction zone daily or more often, as needed. 3. Designate a removal route for small quantities of solid debris. 4. Mist debris and cover disposal carts before transport (i.e., before leaving the construction zone). 5. Designate an elevator for construction crew use. 6. Use window chutes and negative-pressure equipment for removal of larger pieces of debris while maintaining pressure differentials in the construction zone. 7. Schedule debris removal for periods when patient exposure to dust is minimal.
Control water damage	1. Make provisions for dry storage of building materials. 2. Do not install wet, porous building materials (for example, drywall). 3. Replace water-damaged porous building materials if they cannot be completely dried out within 72 hours.
Control dust in air and on surfaces.	1. Monitor the construction area daily for compliance with the IPC plan. 2. Ensure that construction workers remove protective outer clothing before entering clean areas. 3. Use mats with tacky surfaces within the construction zone at the entry; cover sufficient area so that both feet make contact with the mat while walking through the entry. 4. Construct an anteroom, as needed, where coveralls can be donned and removed. 5. Clean the construction zone and all areas used by construction workers with a wet mop. 6. If the area is carpeted, vacuum daily with a HEPA filter–equipped vacuum. 7. Provide temporary essential services (e.g., toilets) and worker conveniences (e.g., vending machines) in the construction zone, as appropriate. 8. Damp-wipe tools if removed from the construction zone or left in the area. 9. Ensure that construction barriers remain well sealed; use particle sampling, as needed. 10. Ensure that the clinical laboratory is free from dust contamination.
Complete the project.	1. Flush the main water system to clear dust-contaminated lines. 2. Terminally clean the construction zone before the construction barriers are removed. 3. Check for visible mold and mildew and eliminate it (i.e., decontaminate and remove), if present. 4. Verify appropriate ventilation parameters for the new area, as needed. 5. Do not accept ventilation deficiencies, particularly in special care areas. 6. Clean or replace HVAC filters using proper dust-containment procedures. 7. Remove the barriers and clean the area of any dust generated during this work. 8. Ensure that the designated air balances in the operating rooms (ORs) and protective environments (PEs) are achieved before occupancy. 9. Commission the space as indicated, particularly in the OR and PE, ensuring that the room's required engineering specifications are met.

Source: CDC. Guidelines & Guidance Library. Accessed Nov 25, 2020. http://www.cdc.gov/hicpac/pdf/guidelines/eic_in_HCF_03.pdf

Monitoring and Improving Conditions in the Environment

The Joint Commission and JCI require organizations to monitor conditions in the environment, identify areas that need improvement, and implement measures to improve performance.

To demonstrate compliance, organizations may develop a monitoring and improvement program that includes the following:

- Environmental tours or rounds, which are among the most useful tools for assessing infection risks and evaluating IPC practices in a variety of health care settings. Tours should be conducted by a multidisciplinary team and documented using a standardized form. The team should consist of IPC personnel, supervisory and nonsupervisory staff from the area being surveyed, housekeeping, facilities, maintenance, safety, and other areas, as needed. Tours should be conducted following a defined schedule and in both patient care and non-patient care areas.
- A process for reporting both findings and recommendations for corrective measures or performance improvement, as revealed by the environmental rounds. Reports should be sent to the multidisciplinary team members and those in the organization who are able to approve the needed corrections or desired improvements.
- A process for recording and documenting daily the negative airflow in airborne infection isolation rooms and positive airflow in protective environments, particularly when patients requiring isolation precautions are in these rooms, as recommended by the CDC.
- A process for showing that the information collected to monitor conditions in the environment is used to improve the environment of care. Examples of how an organization can do this include:
  - The ability to show that recommendations for improving performance, such as those documented in environmental rounds reports, are used by each area to identify and implement practices that lead to improvement
  - Documentation that environmental service staff actively participate on a performance improvement or products selection and standardization committee
  - Documentation that actions are taken to respond to problems identified during renovation and construction activities or positive Legionella cultures from the potable water system
  - Documentation that actions are taken to correct malfunctions in the facility's HVAC system, such as out-of-range temperature readings

---

TRY THESE TOOLS

Tool 7-7. Sample Physician Office or Clinic Infection Control Checklist

Tool 7-8. Infection Prevention Checklist for a Hospital Unit

Tool 7-9. Infection Prevention Guidelines for the Operating Room

---

Summary

The health care environment—particularly contaminated air, water, and surfaces—can serve as a source of pathogenic organisms. The rapid worldwide spread and multiple outbreaks of COVID-19 in health care settings have called attention to the potential for human pathogens to be transmitted from person to person through contaminated air and surfaces. To ensure a safe environment, a health care organization must continuously assess the role of its environment in potential IPC risks. Based on its risk assessment, the organization must identify and implement measures that will reduce the risk of transmission or acquisition of organisms to patients, residents, staff, and visitors from environmental sources. In addition, the organization must monitor and ensure compliance with these measures. This chapter discusses a variety of strategies for organizations to provide a safe health care environment and monitor their IPC activities related to the environment of care or facility management and safety.

Resources

The following sections provide more information on this topic and can serve as a valuable reference in implementing measures to ensure a safe health care environment.

Tools to Try

Tool 7-1. Environmental Rounds for Infection Control Template

Tool 7-2. Pre-Construction Risk Assessment Checklist

Tool 7-3. Infection Control Risk Assessment Matrix of Precautions for Construction and Renovation

Tool 7-4. Sample Infection Control Construction Permit

Tool 7-5. Construction and Renovation Infection Control Checklist

Tool 7-6. Infection Control and Safety Construction Compliance Monitor

Tool 7-7. Sample Physician Office or Clinic Infection Control Checklist

Tool 7-8. Infection Prevention Checklist for a Hospital Unit

Tool 7-9. Infection Prevention Guidelines for the Operating Room

Additional Tools

These tools are available from a variety of sources. Because these tools may be periodically updated, users are advised to check the provider's website to determine that they have the most recent version.

- World Health Organization. Health Care Waste Management Rapid Assessment Tool. https://www.who.int/water_sanitation_health/medicalwaste/ratupd05.pdf

- US Centers for Disease Control and Prevention. Worksheet to Identify Buildings at Increased Risk for *Legionella* Growth and Spread. Accessed Nov 27, 2020. http://www.cdc.gov/legionella/maintenance/wmp-risk.html

- US Centers for Disease Control and Prevention. Toolkit: Developing a Water Management Program to Reduce *Legionella* Growth and Spread in Buildings. Accessed Nov 25, 2020. https://www.cdc.gov/legionella/wmp/toolkit/index.html

- US Centers for Disease Control and Prevention. Options for Evaluating Environmental Cleaning Toolkit. Accessed Nov 27, 2020. https://www.cdc.gov/hai/toolkits/Evaluating-Environmental-Cleaning.html

- State Government of Victoria, Australia, Department of Health. Environmental Health Topics. Accessed Nov 27, 2020. https://www2.health.vic.gov.au/public-health/environmental-health

- Association of periOperative Registered Nurses. Implementing AORN Recommended Practices for Environmental Cleaning. Accessed Nov 27, 2020. https://www.guidelinecentral.com/summaries/recommended-practices-for-environmental-cleaning/#section-society

- Association of periOperative Registered Nurses. Guideline for Environmental Cleaning, 2019. Accessed Nov. 27, 2020. https://aornguidelines.org/guidelines/content?sectionId=173715702

- Premier Medical. EOC Rounds Checklist. Accessed Nov. 27, 2020. https://www.premiermedicalhv.com/wp-content/uploads/2013/01/EOC-Checklist.pdf

- Premier Medical. Infection Control Risk Assessment Matrix (ICRA). Accessed Nov 27, 2020. https://www.premiersafetyinstitute.org/safety-topics-az/building-design/infection-control-risk-assessment-icra/

Websites

- American Society of Heating, Refrigeration and Air-Conditioning Engineers. Accessed Dec 9, 2020. http://www.ashrae.org

- American Society for Health Care Engineering of the American Hospital Association. Accessed Nov. 27, 2020. https://www.ashe.org/

- US Centers for Disease Control and Prevention (CDC).
  - CDC. Infection Control. Accessed Dec 6, 2020. https://www.cdc.gov/infectioncontrol/index.html
  - CDC. *Legionella* (Legionnaires' Disease and Pontiac Fever). Healthcare Water Management Program Frequently Asked Questions. Accessed Dec 2, 2020. https://www.cdc.gov/legionella/wmp/healthcare-facilities/healthcare-wmp-faq.html
  - CDC. Infection Prevention and Control in Dental Settings. Accessed Dec 6, 2020. http://www.cdc.gov/oralhealth/infectioncontrol/

- Legionella.org. Publications and Guidelines Related to *Legionella*. Accessed Dec 6, 2020. https://legionella.org/

Supplemental Resources

- Association for Professionals in Infection Control and Epidemiology. Infection Prevention Manual for Construction and Renovation. 2015. Accessed Nov 27, 2020. https://apic.org/apic-releases-manual-for-construction-and-renovation-projects-in-healthcare-facilities/

- Sehulster L, Chinn RY, Centers for Disease Control and Prevention, HICPAC. Guidelines for environmental infection control in health-care facilities: Recommendations of CDC and the Healthcare Infection Control Practice Advisory Committee (HICPAC). Accessed Nov. 27, 2020. *MMWR Recomm Rep.* 2003;52:1–42 https://www.cdc.gov/infectioncontrol/pdf/guidelines/environmental-guidelines-P.pdf

- Grota P. *APIC Text of Infection Control and Epidemiology*, 4th ed. Washington, DC: Association for Professionals in Infection Control and Epidemiology, 2014.
  - Chapter 109: Environmental Services
  - Chapter 113: Healthcare Textile Services
  - Chapter 114: Maintenance and Engineering
  - Chapter 115: Waste Management
  - Chapter 116: Heating, Ventilation, and Air Conditioning
  - Chapter 117: Water Systems Issues and Prevention of Waterborne Infectious Diseases in Healthcare Facilities
  - Chapter 118: Construction and Renovation

- The Joint Commission. *Planning, Design, and Construction of Health Care Facilities*, 4th ed. Oakbrook, IL: Joint Commission Resources, 2019.

- The Joint Commission. *Infection Prevention and Control Issues in the Environment of Care*, 4th ed. Oakbrook, IL: Joint Commission Resources, 2019.

Facility Guidelines Institute (FGI) Guidelines for Design and Construction of Health Care Facilities

Although the FGI *Guidelines* were updated in 2018, some states still require compliance with the 2010 edition of the FGI *Guidelines*. To ensure compliance with state requirements for design, construction, and renovation of health care facilities, organizations must identify which guidelines edition their state(s) uses.

- Facility Guidelines Institute (FGI). 2010 FGI *Guidelines for Design and Construction of Health Care Facilities*. Accessed Dec 6, 2020. https://fgiguidelines.org/guidelines/earlier-editions//

- Facility Guidelines Institute (FGI). FGI 2014 *Guidelines for Design and Construction of Hospitals and Outpatient Facilities*. Provides minimum standards for clinical and support areas of hospitals, rehabilitation facilities, and ambulatory health care facilities. Accessed Dec 6, 2020 . https://fgiguidelines.org/guidelines/2014-fgi-guidelines/

- Facility Guidelines Institute (FGI). FGI 2014 *Guidelines for Design and Construction of Residential Health, Care, and Support Facilities*. Provides minimum standards for design and construction of residential health, care, and support facilities for long term care. Accessed Dec 6, 2020. https://fgiguidelines.org/guidelines/2014-fgi-guidelines/

American Society for Health Care Engineering (ASHE)

- ASHE. Using the Health Care Physical Environment to Prevent and Control Infection: A Best Practice Guide to Help Health Care Organizations Create Safe, Healing Environments. Accessed Nov 27, 2020. https://www.ashe.org/infectionprevention

- ASHE. ASHE Quick Guides. Accessed Nov 27, 2020. https://www.ashe.org/infectionprevention

References

1. Chen LF, et al. A prospective study of transmission of multidrug-resistant organisms (MDROs) between environmental sites and hospitalized patients—The TransFER study. *Infect Control Hosp Epidemiol*. 2019 Jan;40(1):47–52.

2. Sehulster L, et al., HICPAC. Guidelines for Environmental Infection Control in Health-Care Facilities: Recommendations of CDC and the Healthcare Infection Control Practices Advisory Committee (HICPAC), 2003. Updated July 2019 . Accessed Nov 30, 2020. https://www.cdc.gov/infectioncontrol/guidelines/environmental/index.html

3. Weber DJ, et al. New and emerging infectious diseases (Ebola, Middle Eastern Respiratory Syndrome, coronavirus, carbapenem-resistant *Enterobacteriaceae, Candida auris*): Focus on environmental survival and germicide susceptibility. *Am J Infect Control.* 2019;47(Suppl):S29–S38.

4. Rutala WA, Weber DJ. Best practices for disinfection of noncritical environmental surfaces and equipment in health care facilities: A bundle approach. *Am J Infect Control.* 2019;47(Suppl):S96–S105.

5. Mousavi ES, et al. Renovation in hospitals: Training construction crews to work in healthcare facilities. *Am J Infect Control.* 2020;48:403–409.

6. Noorimotlagh Z, et al. A systematic review of emerging human coronavirus (SARS-CoV-2) outbreak: Focus on disinfection methods, environmental survival, and control and prevention strategies. *Environ Sci Pollut Res.* 2020 Oct;2:1–15 https://doi.org/10.1007/s11356-020-11060-z

7. US Environmental Protection Agency. Medical Waste. Accessed Dec 2, 2020. https://www.epa.gov/rcra/medical-waste

8. US Department of Labor, Occupational Safety and Health Administration. OSHA Standard 29 CFR 1910.1030. Bloodborne Pathogens. Accessed Dec 2, 2020. https://www.osha.gov/laws-regs/regulations/standardnumber/1910/1910.1030

9. US Centers for Disease Control and Prevention. *Legionella* (Legionnaires' Disease and Pontiac Fever). Accessed Dec 9, 2020. https://www.cdc.gov/legionella/index.html

10. American Society of Heating, Refrigerating and Air-Conditioning Engineers. ANSI/ASHRAE Standard 188-2015. Legionellosis: Risk Management for Building Water Systems. 2018. Accessed Dec 9, 2020. https://www.ashrae.org/technical-resources/bookstore/ansi-ashrae-standard-188-2018-legionellosis-risk-management-for-building-water-systems

11. Kanamori H, et al. Healthcare outbreaks associated with a water reservoir and infection prevention strategies. *Clin Infect Dis.* 2016 Jun;62(11):1423–1435.

12. Association for the Advancement of Medical Instrumentation. Complete Dialysis Collection 2020. Accessed Dec 9, 2020. https://www.aami.org/news-resources/publications/complete-dialysis-collection-2020

13. Centers for Medicare & Medicaid Services. Requirement to Reduce *Legionella* Risk in Healthcare Facility Water Systems to Prevent Cases and Outbreaks of Legionnaires' Disease (LD). Accessed Dec 2, 2020. https://www.cms.gov/Medicare/Provider-Enrollment-and-Certification/SurveyCertificationGenInfo/Downloads/QSO17-30-HospitalCAH-NH-REVISED-.pdf

14. Kohn WG, et al. Centers for Disease Control and Prevention (CDC). Guidelines for infection control in dental health-care settings—2003. *MMWR Recomm Rep.* 2003 Dec 19;52(RR-17):1–61. Accessed Dec 9, 2020. https://pubmed.ncbi.nlm.nih.gov/14685139/

15. Sebastiani FR, et al. Infection control in the dental office. *Dent Clin North Am.* 2017 Apr;61(2):435–457.

16. American Society of Heating, Refrigerating and Air-Conditioning Engineers. Standards 62.1 & 62.2: The Standards for Ventilation and Indoor Air Quality. 2019. Accessed Dec 9, 2020. https://www.ashrae.org/technical-resources/bookstore/standards-62-1-62-26

17. Facility Guidelines Institute. Guidelines for Design and Construction of Hospitals and Outpatient Facilities. Accessed Dec 6, 2020. https://fgiguidelines.org/guidelines-main/

18. Mousavi ES, et al. COVID-19 Outbreak and hospital air quality: A systematic review of evidence on air filtration and recirculation. *Environ Sci Technol.* 2021;55(7):4134–4147. https://dx.doi.org/10.1021/acs.est.0c03247?ref=pdf

19. Donskey CJ. Beyond high-touch surfaces: Portable equipment and floors as potential sources of transmission of health care–associated pathogens. *Am J Infect Control.* 2019;47(Suppl):S90–S95.

20. Rutala WA, Weber DJ. Selection of the ideal disinfectant. *Infect Control Hosp Epidemiol.* 2014 Jul;35(7):855–865.

21. Rutala WA, Weber DJ, Healthcare Infection Control Practices Advisory Committee (HICPAC). Guideline for Disinfection and Sterilization in Healthcare Facilities, 2008. Accessed Dec 9, 2020. https://www.cdc.gov/infectioncontrol/guidelines/Disinfection/index.html

22. Boyce JM. Modern technologies for improving cleaning and disinfection of environmental surfaces in hospitals. *Antimicrob Resist Infect Control*. 2016 Apr;5:10.

23. Weber DJ, et al. Effectiveness of ultraviolet devices and hydrogen peroxide systems for terminal room decontamination: Focus on clinical trials. *Am J Infect Control*. 2016 May;44(5 Suppl):e77–e84.

24. Weber DJ, et al. Continuous room decontamination technologies. *Am J Infect Control*. 2019;47(Suppl):S72–S78.

25. Donsky CJ. Decontamination devices in health care facilities: Practical issues and emerging applications. *Am J Infect Control*. 2019;47(Suppl):S23–S28.

26. US Centers for Disease Control and Prevention. Options for Evaluating Environmental Cleaning. Accessed Dec 9, 2020. http://www.cdc.gov/hai/toolkits/Evaluating-Environmental-Cleaning.html

27. Solomon SL, et al. Reducing environmental surface contamination in healthcare settings: A statewide collaborative. *Am J Infect Control*. 2018;48(208):e71–e73.

Chapter 8

Cleaning, Disinfection, and Sterilization of Medical Devices and Equipment

By Sylvia Garcia-Houchins, RN, MBA, CIC

Disclaimer: Strategies, tools, and examples discussed in this book do not necessarily reflect Joint Commission or Joint Commission International requirements for all settings. Always refer to the most current standards applicable to your health care setting to ensure compliance.

Introduction

Cleaning, disinfection, and sterilization of medical devices and equipment has emerged as a serious, widespread challenge for many health care organizations. These organizations include inpatient settings, such as acute care and long term care facilities, and outpatient settings, such as ambulatory surgery centers, endoscopy centers, outpatient clinics, pain clinics, hemodialysis centers, and dental and physician offices. Inadequate cleaning of devices between patients can result in the retention of blood, tissue, and other biological debris in certain types of reusable medical devices. Inadequate reprocessing may lead to adverse patient outcomes such as tissue irritation from reprocessing materials, including chemical disinfectant. Poor management of medical devices and equipment has led to outbreaks of infection, causing morbidity and mortality among patients.[1-7] As a result, each step of cleaning, disinfection, and sterilization is critical to reducing the risk of infection. Infection transmission risks related to use, cleaning, disinfection, and sterilization failures include the following[8-11]:

- Reprocessing in a manner inconsistent with the intended use of the instrument or equipment
- Not following manufacturers' instructions for use
- Inadequate or ineffective manufacturers' instructions for use
- Lack of adequate training and competency of staff responsible for using or reprocessing medical devices and equipment
- Not following standard reprocessing procedures

- Use of expired detergents, disinfectants, or sterilants
- Continued use of devices, despite integrity, maintenance, and mechanical issues
- Design flaws in the device or equipment

According to the US Food and Drug Administration (FDA), the number of health care–associated infections (HAIs) in the United States that can be attributed to inadequate reusable medical device reprocessing is unknown, primarily because it is not often investigated as a cause of HAIs, and infections from inadequately reprocessed devices are often not reported. However, given the large number of such devices in use, the potential for infections associated with them remains an important public health concern.[7]

HAIs can be prevented when facilities do the following:

- Use instruments as intended by the manufacturer.
- Explicitly follow manufacturers' instructions.
- Implement clear policies and procedures that ensure that the reprocessing level (low-, intermediate-, or high-level disinfection or sterilization) is based on intended use and follows the medical device manufacturer's instructions unless they are unclear or inconsistent with intended use.
- Contact the device manufacturer when the intended use and reprocessing level specified in the manufacturer's instructions do not match to clarify instructions.
- Identify alternative devices or contact the FDA or local regulatory agencies for assistance in resolving issues with reprocessing instructions when unable to resolve these issues with the device manufacturer. (See Sidebar 8-1 on page 190.)

- Provide appropriate space as well as compatible supplies and equipment to support use and reprocessing. (Note that supplies used to perform or support medical device reprocessing are referred to as reprocessing accessories and include detergents, bushes, washers, sterilization pouches, wraps and containers, sterilizers, biological and chemical indicators, disinfectants, and so on).
- Ensure that staff are trained and competent to reprocess each instrument or medical device.
- Ensure that staff are trained and competent to use each reprocessing accessory.
- Implement stringent quality controls on use and reprocessing.

Sidebar 8-1. Resolving Issues with Reprocessing Instructions

- Check the label for date of issuance or the date of the latest revision.
- Contact the manufacturer's technical service representatives for new instructions that comply with the US Food and Drug Administration (FDA) Reprocessing Guidance or other local regulations
- Search the FDA 510(k) Premarket Notification database, at https://www.accessdata.fda.gov/scripts/cdrh/cfdocs/cfpmn/pmn.cfm
- Seek assistance from the FDA:
  ○ Contact the FDA Division of Industry and Consumer Education (DICE) via phone, 800-638-2041, or email, DICE@fda.hhs.gov.
  ○ File a voluntary report of a medical device problem: https://www.fda.gov/medical-devices/medical-device-safety/medical-device-reporting-mdr-how-report-medical-device-problems
  ○ Report allegations of regulatory misconduct: https://www.fda.gov/medical-devices/medical-device-safety/reporting-allegations-regulatory-misconduct
  ○ Report to the appropriate agency complaints such as for misleading or incomplete instructions after attempting to resolve issue with device manufacturer.

The US Centers for Medicare & Medicaid Services (CMS), The Joint Commission, and Joint Commission International (JCI) have recognized problems with cleaning, disinfection, and sterilization of medical devices and have intensified survey processes to better address and improve care involving reprocessed medical devices and equipment. Requirements for managing medical equipment, devices, and supplies are included in both the "Infection Prevention and Control" (IC) and "Environment of Care" (EC) chapters of The Joint Commission *Comprehensive Accreditation Manuals* standards manual. Similar requirements are included in the "Prevention and Control of Infections" (PCI) chapter of the JCI accreditation manual. The Joint Commission also enforces standards that meet CMS requirements (for example, Conditions of Participation [CoPs]) and as such has been granted "deeming authority" to survey organizations on behalf of CMS. During surveys of organizations that use their Joint Commission accreditation for deemed status purposes, surveyors must ensure that the minimum CMS requirements are met; therefore, current CMS references are included for related discussions. Infection preventionists (IPs) and others responsible for device reprocessing should review the most current CMS CoPs, Conditions for Coverage (CfCs), and the CMS surveyors' infection control worksheets for hospitals and ambulatory surgical centers.

This chapter explains key concepts and proposed strategies for meeting Joint Commission, CMS, and JCI requirements related to reprocessing of medical devices. The Joint Commission and JCI standards related to cleaning and disinfection of the environment are covered in Chapter 7.

Requirements Versus Recommendations

A key issue that organizations face when ensuring compliance with Joint Commission or JCI standards is knowing the difference between a requirement (that is, what must be done to ensure compliance) and a recommendation (what should be considered, if applicable, as a best practice). Organizations that undergo a survey, regardless of whether it is a government or an accrediting organization survey, must follow laws, rules, and regulations. These are requirements. When surveys are conducted to evaluate whether a health care provider meets applicable requirements for participation in the CMS-eligible programs, organizations being surveyed

Relevant Joint Commission Standards Addressed in This Chapter

Note: These standards were in effect at the time of publication. They refer to Joint Commission standards effective January 1, 2021. Always consult the most recent version of Joint Commission standards for the most accurate requirements for your setting.

IC.02.02.01 The [organization] reduces the risk of infection associated with medical equipment, devices, and supplies.

EP 1 The [organization] implements infection prevention and control activities when doing the following: Cleaning and performing low-level disinfection of medical equipment, devices, and supplies.

Note: *Low-level disinfection is used for items such as stethoscopes and blood glucose meters. Additional cleaning and disinfecting is required for medical equipment, devices, and supplies used by patients or residents who are isolated as part of implementing transmission-based precautions.*

EP 2 The [organization] implements infection prevention and control activities when doing the following: Performing intermediate and high-level disinfection and sterilization of medical equipment, devices, and supplies. (*See also* EC.02.04.03, EP 4)

Note: *Sterilization is used for items such as implants and surgical instruments. High-level*

disinfection may also be used if sterilization is not possible, as is the case with flexible endoscopes.

EP 3 The [organization] implements infection prevention and control activities when doing the following: Disposing of medical equipment, devices, and supplies.

EP 4 The [organization] implements infection prevention and control activities when doing the following: Storing medical equipment, devices, and supplies.

EP 5 When reprocessing single-use devices, the [organization] implements infection prevention and control activities that are consistent with regulatory and professional standards.

EC.02.04.03 The [organization] inspects, tests, and maintains medical equipment.

EP 4 The [organization] conducts performance testing of and maintains all sterilizers. These activities are documented. (*See also* IC.02.02.01, EP 2)

Relevant Joint Commission International (JCI) Standards Addressed in This Chapter

---

Note: These standards were in effect at the time of publication. They refer to the *Joint Commission International Accreditation Standards for Hospitals, seventh edition,* ©2020. Always consult the most recent version of Joint Commission International standards for the most accurate requirements for your hospital or medical center setting.

PCI.6 The hospital reduces the risk of infections associated with medical/surgical equipment, devices, and supplies by ensuring adequate cleaning, disinfection, sterilization, and storage.

ME 1 The hospital follows professional practice guidelines and manufacturer guidelines for sterilization techniques that best fit the type of situations for sterilization and devices and supplies being sterilized.

ME 2 The hospital follows professional practice guidelines and manufacturer guidelines for low- and high-level disinfection that best fit the type of devices and equipment being disinfected.

ME 3 Staff processing medical/surgical equipment, devices, and supplies are oriented to, trained in, and demonstrate competency in cleaning, disinfection, and sterilization, and they receive proper supervision.

ME 4 Methods for medical/surgical cleaning, disinfection, and sterilization are coordinated and uniformly applied throughout the hospital.

ME 5 Clean and sterile supplies are properly stored in designated storage areas that are clean and dry and protected from dust, moisture, and temperature extremes.

PCI.6.1 The hospital identifies and implements a process for managing the reuse of single-use devices consistent with regional and local laws and regulations and implements a process for managing expired supplies.

ME 1 The hospital identifies single-use devices and materials that may be reused in accordance with local and national laws and regulations and implements a process for managing expired supplies.

ME 2 The hospital utilizes a standardized process for identifying when a single-use device is no longer safe or suitable for reuse.

ME 3 The hospital has a clear protocol for the cleaning, disinfecting, and sterilization as appropriate, for each reusable, single-use device.

ME 4 The cleaning process for each device is followed as per protocol.

ME 5 The hospital identifies patients on whom reusable medical devices have been used.

ME 6 When adverse events resulting from reuse of single-use devices occur, patients using these devices are tracked and an analysis is performed, with results used to identify and implement improvements.

must also show compliance with the minimum health and safety standards established by the Social Security Act. Set requirements for each type of health care entity are provided in the CoPs, CfCs, and requirements for skilled nursing facilities and nursing facilities. Conditions or requirements can be found in the CMS State Operations Manual. International health care organizations must meet local or national laws and regulations such as those required by ministries of health.

Quality standards associated with the condition or requirement are expressed in the State Operations Manual in a summary lead sentence or paragraph characterizing the quality or result of operations to which all the subsidiary standards are directed. Interpretive guidelines are provided to clarify the condition (or requirement). The purpose of interpretive guidelines is to define or explain the relevant statute and regulations, not to impose any requirements that are not otherwise set forth in statute or regulation. Organizations should be aware that when they are surveyed for deemed status purposes, The Joint Commission uses a crosswalk for its standards to CMS standards to ensure CMS requirements are covered.

Organizations also should be aware that The Joint Commission does not survey to law and regulations related to disinfection and sterilization by using regulatory compliance documents, such as the US Occupational Safety and Health Administration (OSHA) document OSHA Instruction Directive Number CPL 02-02-069, "Enforcement Procedures for the Occupational Exposure to Bloodborne Pathogens" (available at https://www.osha.gov/sites/default/files/enforcement/directives/CPL_02-02-069.pdf) to evaluate compliance with measures required to protect workers from exposure to bloodborne pathogens and other potentially infectious materials (OPIM).

However, surveyors are trained to identify noncompliance with regulations and will cite noncompliance with a law or regulation, when identified. For example, if the organization has not performed a hazard assessment that includes risks of exposure to bloodborne pathogens in central sterile processing, and if staff members are not wearing appropriate personal protective equipment (PPE) to protect from exposure to blood, Joint Commission surveyors could cite the organization for noncompliance with OSHA requirements.

The Joint Commission and JCI standards require that organizations comply with standard precautions. Applicable elements of standard precautions are

identified in Section 5f of the US Centers for Disease Control and Prevention (CDC) document Core Infection Prevention and Control Practices for Safe Healthcare Delivery in All Settings—Recommendations of the Healthcare Infection Control Practices Advisory Committee and include the following core practices related to reprocessing:

- Follow manufacturers' instructions for proper use of cleaning and disinfecting products (for example, dilution, contact time, material compatibility, storage, shelf life, safe use, and disposal).
- Consult and adhere to manufacturers' instructions for reprocessing.

If a manufacturer's instructions for equipment or device cleaning do not meet the required processing level outlined in the Spaulding classification—which categorizes instruments and other items for patient care as critical, semicritical, or noncritical, according to the degree of infection risk—the device should not be used unless the level of disinfection or sterilization associated with its intended use can be achieved. (The Spaulding classification is discussed in more detail later in this chapter.) In addition, if the instructions are unclear or in conflict, organizations are required to resolve those conflicts. Sidebar 8-2 on page 194 outlines The Joint Commission's guidance on addressing conflicts in reprocessing instructions.

Requirements that must be met include federal laws and regulations issued by agencies such OSHA and CMS; state public health, licensing, or certification requirements and directives; local rules and regulations; Joint Commission or JCI standards; and standard precautions, such as the CDC or World Health Organization hand hygiene guidelines. In contrast, evidence-based guidelines (for example, those issued by the CDC or the Association of periOperative Registered Nurses [AORN]), practice guidelines, national standards (such as those issued by the Association for the Advancement of Medical Instrumentation [AAMI]), and consensus documents such as those created by professional organizations are not requirements. They are recommendations, which organizations should consider for implementation when developing their cleaning, disinfection, and sterilization processes, protocols, policies, and procedures. Organizations may choose to adopt all or a portion of chosen evidence-based guidelines. A list of resources that can assist with developing cleaning, disinfection, and sterilization policies and procedures is provided in the Resources section at the end of this chapter.

Sidebar 8-2. Addressing Conflicts Among Instructions for Use (IFUs) for Different Equipment and Products

Reprocessing medical devices and equipment may involve use of several products and devices. Manufacturers are the experts on their products and, for certain devices or products, are required to submit IFUs to the US Food and Drug Administration or the US Environmental Protection Agency for approval. When an organization identifies a conflict with the manufacturer's recommended instructions or products, The Joint Commission expects the organization to contact the manufacturer's technical services to resolve these conflicts.

This resolution should also include contacting manufacturers of the alternative products, if applicable, to determine if they can provide additional information regarding compatibility. When contacting a manufacture to determine if alternative products may be used, organizations should include a discussion of biological, chemical, and functional compatibilities. Organizations may also consider the impact of their decision on liability, warranty, and long-term maintenance of the item. If clear compatibility information is not obtainable, the organization should clearly identify the risks and strategies to mitigate those risks and implement a risk mitigation plan.

All Joint Commission–accredited organizations are responsible for meeting the minimum reprocessing requirement, based on how the device is used. (For example, per the Spaulding classification system, a device that enters the vascular system must be sterilized.)

Source: The Joint Commission. Manufacturers Instructions for Use—Addressing Conflicts Amongst IFUs for Different Equipment and Products. Apr 15, 2020. Accessed Feb 5, 2021. https://www.jointcommission.org/standards/standard-faqs/ambulatory/infection-prevention-and-control-ic/000002252/

The Hierarchical Approach to Reprocessing Standards

Ensuring Compliance with Infection Prevention and Control Standards

Joint Commission standards and elements of performance (EPs) and JCI standards and measurable elements (MEs) are written to allow each health care organization to determine the best methods and practices for its facility. This is because infection prevention and control requirements vary across states and countries. Although there are common federal rules and regulations, there are different state and local regulations, a variety of devices and equipment used, and a spectrum of acceptable patient care practices. Many health care organizations develop policies and procedures based on evidence-based guidelines alone; however, The Joint Commission requires that organizations adhere to applicable federal, state, and local laws and regulations. In addition, deemed organizations must meet applicable CMS requirements, and international health care organizations should always comply with their local or national laws and regulations.

When establishing policies that ensure compliance with Joint Commission requirements related to cleaning, disinfection, and sterilization, organizations in the United States should follow the hierarchical approach illustrated in Figure 8-1 on page 195. This figure was introduced in Chapter 3 and is presented again here to reinforce how the framework can also be used to help ensure compliance when developing cleaning, disinfection, and sterilization policies. The hierarchical approach includes the following steps:

1. Identify and review applicable rules and regulations.
2. If applicable, review CMS requirements (CoPs for hospitals, CfCs for ambulatory care organizations, and Requirements for Participation for long term care and hospice organizations).
3. Review and comply with manufacturer instructions for use—as long as they comply with the intended use of the device. If reprocessing instructions are not clear or do not follow FDA requirements related to the Spaulding classification (with reprocessing level based on intended use), organizations must seek clarification from the manufacturer to ensure patient safety.
4. Use evidence-based guidelines, practice guidelines, and national standards, as applicable. In some cases,

Figure 8-1. A Hierarchical Approach to Developing an IPC Policy

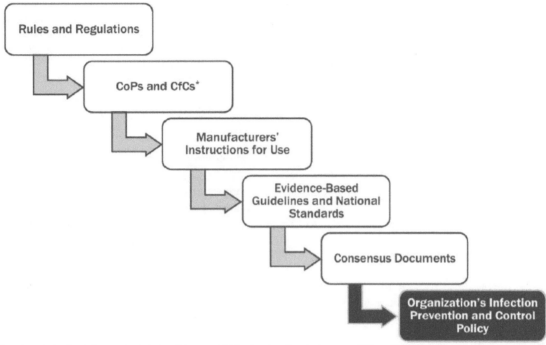

* For organizations that use Joint Commission accreditation for deemed status purposes or that are required by state regulation or directive, Conditions of Participation (CoPs) and/or Conditions for Coverage (CfCs) should be reviewed for applicable mandatory requirements.

the choice of evidence-based guidelines and/or standards is dictated by state regulation, government directive (for example, the US military and Veterans Administration), or Joint Commission requirements (for example, use of standard precautions as documented in the CDC's Core Practices). If not dictated by regulation, directive, or The Joint Commission, organizations should determine which evidence-based guidelines and national standards are needed to provide additional direction for staff performing cleaning, disinfection, and sterilization. Organizations may choose to use all or part of their chosen guidelines or standards but should also be able to describe their process for determining applicability of optional guidelines and standards.

5. When additional guidance or direction is needed on a particular issue, health care organizations may choose to follow consensus documents to reduce patient risk or to enhance IPC practices. For example, some disinfection and sterilization guidelines do not

address actions to protect patients from toxic anterior segment syndrome following cataract surgery. The American Society of Cataract and Refractive Surgery and the American Society of Ophthalmic Registered Nurses developed recommended guidelines for cleaning and sterilizing intraocular surgical instruments in ambulatory surgery centers.

Key Concepts Related to Disinfection and Sterilization

The Spaulding Classification

The most common approach to disinfection and sterilization was described by Earle H. Spaulding more than 60 years ago—and with some exceptions for more recent discoveries, such as prion disease, it still applies today.[12] Spaulding classified medical devices to be reprocessed as critical, semicritical, and noncritical, according to risk of infection, as described in Table 8-1.

Table 8-1. Categorization of Items to Be Reprocessed Based on Risk of Infection*

Level	Risk of Infection	Description (Intended Use)	Examples of Items	Reprocessing Methods
Critical	High	Item comes in contact with or enters sterile tissue, sterile body cavity, or the vascular system	Surgical and dental instruments, inner surfaces of hemodialyzers, urinary catheters, biopsy forceps, implants, intravascular devices, and needles, ultrasound probes used in sterile body cavities	Sterilization
Semicritical	Moderate	Item comes in contact with mucous membrane or nonintact skin	Respiratory therapy and anesthesia equipment, some endoscopes, laryngoscope blades, esophageal manometry probes, vaginal ultrasound probes and specula, and diaphragm fitting rings	Minimum: high-level disinfection (when practical, sterilization preferred)
Noncritical	Low	Item comes in contact with intact skin	Patient care items: bedpans, blood pressure cuffs, crutches, incubators, and computers Environmental surfaces: bed rails, bedside tables, patient furniture, counters, and floor	Low or intermediate disinfection*

* Because of new developments in disinfection and sterilization technologies, some changes to the Spaulding classification are being considered by experts in the field.

- **Critical.** Items that enter the vascular system or have contact with sterile tissues or fluids create a high risk of infection and are categorized as critical. These items require sterilization.
- **Semicritical.** Mucous membranes such as those of the gastrointestinal tract and nonintact skin are generally more resistant to infection by common bacteria. Therefore, items that come in contact with mucous membranes (for example, eyes, mouth, nose, vagina, gastrointestinal tract) and nonintact skin are categorized as semicritical. These items require at least high-level disinfection.
- **Noncritical.** Items that come in contact with intact skin are categorized as noncritical and require cleaning with or without low- or intermediate-level disinfection, depending on intended use.

Manufacturer's Instructions for Use

Manufacturers should provide cleaning, disinfection, and sterilization instructions, as appropriate, for reusable medical devices, equipment, and supplies used in health care facilities or on patients if cleared by the FDA[14] or local regulators. Particular care should be taken to follow manufacturers' instructions, as failure to do so could cause damage to the devices or result in increased infection risk to the patient or staff.[15,16]

Organizations must confirm that a manufacturer's instructions achieve the level of cleaning, disinfection, or sterilization outlined by the Spaulding classification. As stated previously, if a manufacturer's instructions for equipment or device cleaning does not meet the required processing level outlined in the Spaulding classification, it should not be used unless the level of disinfection or sterilization associated with its intended use can be achieved.

Tool 8-1 can be used as a basis for ensuring assessment of equipment. It can assist users in taking into account the item's intended use, the manufacturer's instructions for use, and the facility's ability to perform disinfection and sterilization. Failure to follow manufacturers' instructions or apply the Spaulding classification is a frequent reason for noncompliance with Joint Commission, JCI, and CMS requirements.

TRY THIS TOOL

Tool 8-1. Assessment of Item for Reprocessing Form

TIP Facilities should evaluate each item that they reprocess to ensure that the appropriate level of reprocessing is being performed and that instructions for reprocessing can and are being followed.

Evidence-based guidelines, such as the CDC's Guideline for Disinfection and Sterilization in Healthcare Facilities, can assist the IP in evaluating cleaning, disinfection, and sterilization issues to be considered. For example, this guideline notes that despite the CDC's recommendation *prior* to 2008 to use 3% hydrogen peroxide and 70% isopropyl alcohol to disinfect tonometer tips (used to measure intraocular pressure), updated information indicates that these disinfectants are not effective against adenovirus and similar viruses that can cause epidemic keratoconjunctivitis, and they should not be used for disinfecting applanation tonometers. In May 2019, The Joint Commission issued a *Quick Safety* newsletter on disinfecting tonometers and other ophthalmology devices.

Compatible cleaning, disinfection, and sterilization accessories (for example, products and equipment) must be available to reprocessing staff to implement the instructions. A recommended best practice is for the purchasing process to include a formal review of the intended use of a medical device as well as the manufacturer's cleaning, disinfection, and sterilization instructions for the device. This can help ensure that the device can be reprocessed and that compatible

---

TIP The US Centers for Disease Control and Prevention Disinfection and Sterilization Guideline can assist the infection preventionist in addressing cleaning, disinfection, and sterilization issues and provides an excellent overview of the following:
- Active ingredients used in disinfectants and their spectrum of effectiveness in killing specific organisms that have been linked to outbreaks.
- Evidence-based cleaning, disinfection, and sterilization methods, including mode of action and potential uses and recommended practices.

---

accessories are available. If the cleanser or disinfectant manufacturer's instructions indicate that a product is compatible, but the equipment or device manufacturer's instructions do not indicate compatibility, the organization should contact the device manufacturer for clarification or confirmation so the items can safely be reprocessed. Accreditation and regulatory agencies and other surveyors may ask how the organization resolves conflicts among manufacturers' instructions for use.

Cleaning and disinfection chemicals can create health hazards to employees. Organizations should evaluate each product to ensure that it can be used safely and include a review of dilutions, storage, shelf life, PPE needed, and disposal and ventilation requirements to ensure that OSHA, Environmental Protection Agency (EPA), or local requirements are met. For example, some products can cause blindness if splashed in an eye or cause a fire if improperly disposed of. Organizations should have processes in place to prevent or mitigate those risks. Steps to consider when evaluating instruments and tools for reprocessing are listed in Tool 8-2.

TRY THIS TOOL

Tool 8-2. Evaluation Steps for Medical Devices and Supplies Reprocessing

---

During cleaning, staff must wear appropriate PPE to prevent exposure to infectious agents or chemicals.[13]

The OSHA Bloodborne Pathogens Standard and Personal Protective Equipment Standard, as well as material safety data sheets, provide requirements and guidance for selection and use of PPE to be worn to protect health care workers.

Low-Level and Intermediate-Level Disinfection

The risk of infection from medical equipment and devices that have contact with intact skin, such as stethoscopes, pulse oximetry sensors, and blood pressure cuffs, is low.[12] However, because these items become contaminated during use and are potential sources for transmission, organizations should implement cleaning and disinfecting procedures that follow the equipment or the device's manufacturer instructions for these reusable items. The CDC recommends a low-level disinfectant for "noncritical patient-care surfaces (for example, bedrails, over-the-bed table) and equipment (for example, blood pressure cuff) that touch intact skin."[12]

When decontaminating surfaces following spills of blood or other OPIM, the CDC recommends using an EPA–registered "tuberculocidal agent (intermediate-level disinfectant), a registered germicide on the EPA Lists D and E (i.e., products with specific label claims for HIV or HBV or freshly diluted hypochlorite solution)."[12] However, 70% isopropyl alcohol is frequently recommended by manufacturers to clean patient equipment that could become contaminated with blood (for example, point-of-care testing devices). This concentration of isopropyl alcohol is considered fully effective against lipid-enveloped viruses such as human immunodeficiency virus and hepatitis B and C.

In general, as per standard precautions, and because a patient may have an undiagnosed infection, staff should clean and disinfect equipment and devices using a method that ensures the equipment used on any patient is rendered safe for use on the next patient. However, for those patients known or suspected of being infected or colonized with organisms that are resistant to routine disinfection methods (for example, *Clostridium/ Clostridioides difficile* or norovirus), additional cleaning or disinfection or alternative products may be necessary.[13]

Standard precautions require that organizations perform routine and targeted cleaning of environmental surfaces as indicated by the level of patient contact and degree of soiling. Surfaces in close proximity to the patient and frequently touched surfaces in the patient care environment should be cleaned and disinfected more frequently than other surfaces. Surfaces contaminated with blood or OPIM should be cleaned promptly.

The frequency of cleaning or disinfection should be based on intended use and manufacturers' instructions. If not specified in manufacturers' instruction or regulatory requirements, cleaning and disinfection of the environment should be performed on a schedule that will maintain cleanliness and ensure patient, visitor, and staff safety. It should be noted that in some instances, such as during the public health emergency that resulted from SARS-CoV-2 (COVID-19), some authorities having jurisdiction such as OSHA may issue requirements for environmental decontamination at a regular or specified frequency where one did not previously exist. There should be a clear designation of responsibility for cleaning and disinfection of reusable noncritical patient care devices.[13]

To ensure cleaning and disinfection of the environment and noncritical devices, many organizations establish and implement policies and procedures that are consistent with manufacturers' recommendations and that also address the following:

- Who (for example, environmental services, central service worker, nursing assistant, nurse) is responsible for cleaning and disinfecting items?
- What cleaning and disinfecting products should be used (for example, quaternary ammonium compound, bleach)?
- Where should cleaning and disinfecting efforts occur (for example, patient rooms, soiled utility rooms, central processing)?
- When should cleaning and disinfecting occur (for example, after each use, prior to removing from a patient room, daily)?
- How should cleaning and disinfecting be done (for example, following manufacturers' instructions for use)?

A best practice is to create a chart or table of frequently used equipment or devices that includes the item description, the job role responsible for cleaning, the product(s) that should be used, and the frequency of cleaning. An example is provided as Table 8-2 on page 199.

High-Level Disinfection and Sterilization

Medical devices that come into contact with mucous membranes or nonintact skin are known as semicritical items and must receive at least high-level disinfection.[12-14]

Table 8-2. Guideline for Cleaning Frequently Used Equipment

Item	Location	Role Responsible for Cleaning	Frequency of Cleaning	Product Used to Clean
Blood pressure machine	Clinics Inpatient units: portable	Person using machine (e.g., medical assistant, nurse, doctor)	After every patient use	Pop-up wipe (specify compatible product name)
Blood pressure machine	Inpatient units: portable	• Person removing machine from occupied room (e.g., nursing assistant, nurse) • EVS at discharge	When removing from patient room or at discharge	XYZ wipes
Blood pressure machine	Pre- and Postprocedure units	Person turning over bay (e.g., nurse or EVS)	At patient discharge from bay	XYZ wipes
Installed monitors	Inpatient units	EVS	After each discharge	XYZ wipes
Installed monitors	Pre- and postprocedure units	Person turning over bay (e.g., nurse or EVS)	After each discharge from bay	XYZ wipes
Pill crusher	Medication rooms	• EVS • Nurse (if soiled during use)	EVS every Friday, first shift, when cleaning medication room	Soap and water, per manufacturer's instructions
Procedure table: radiology	Scanning rooms	RT; EVS	Patient surface after every patient (RT), entire table every Friday evening shift (EVS)	ABC disinfectant

EVS, environmental services; **RT,** radiology technician.

Examples include endoscopes, such as colonoscopes, bronchoscopes, laryngoscopes, and endocavity probes (vaginal and rectal ultrasound probes, transesophageal echocardiography probes), vaginal and nasal specula, and some reusable portions of ventilator circuits.

Medical instruments or devices that contact, enter, or go through normally sterile areas of the body or enter the vascular system are known as critical items and must be sterilized.[12-14] These items include surgical and dental instruments, implants, and ultrasound probes or endoscopes used in sterile body cavities.

High-level disinfection results in a product that is rendered free of all microbial contamination, except for a small number of bacterial spores. Sterilization results in a product that is free of all forms of microbial life. In accordance with manufacturers' instructions for use, items to be high-level disinfected or sterilized must be thoroughly cleaned prior to disinfection because failure to clean the item could interfere with the disinfection and sterilization processes. All manufacturers' instructions for use must be followed, as cleaning and disinfection with incorrect products or use of an incorrect disinfection or sterilization process could result in disinfection or sterilization failure, damage to the equipment, equipment that is unsafe for use on a patient, and, possibly, exposure of a patient to an infectious agent with subsequent colonization or infection.

The IP must be aware that some manufacturers' instructions for use are not always consistent with the intended use and the Spaulding classification. To ensure the safety of patients, IPs, those responsible for oversight of disinfection and sterilization procedures, and those who process reusable instruments and devices must critically review and question instructions that do not conform to the Spaulding classification. If, for example, an item will enter a sterile area and the manufacturer's instruction indicates that high-level disinfection is the accepted method for disinfecting the item, the manufacturer should be contacted for corrected instructions. The item should not be used until the issues are resolved. Some risks for failures in high-level disinfection include, but are not limited to the following:

- Not following the manufacturer's instructions for use
- Improper or inadequate precleaning/cleaning procedures
- Inappropriate use or choice of detergent or disinfectant
- Lack of inspection/quality control
- Use of an untreated or contaminated water supply
- Failure to completely dry channels in the device
- Lack of routine maintenance
- Flaws in the mechanical design

> **TIP** Items to be high-level disinfected or sterilized must be thoroughly cleaned prior to disinfection because failure to clean the item could interfere with the disinfection and sterilization processes.

Information to Support Implementation of Disinfection and Sterilization Practices

To ensure compliance, Joint Commission–accredited domestic and international health care organizations must ensure access to information, resources, supplies, and equipment needed to correctly perform disinfection and sterilization. In addition, organizations should be aware that the CMS worksheets for hospitals and ambulatory surgery centers and CDC assessment tools address the management of medical devices and equipment and can be used to help monitor compliance with requirements.[13,23,27]

Transportation of Soiled Items

All items contaminated with blood or body fluids must be contained in a leak-proof container from the point of use to the decontamination area, in accordance with OSHA or local requirements to protect workers from exposure. Use of a puncture-resistant, leak-proof container with solid sides and bottom and red in color or labeled "biohazardous," in accordance with OSHA or local standards is required for items that are sharp. Additional requirements may be necessary if transporting items off-site for reprocessing, such as maintaining separation between clean and dirty items in the transport vehicle and packaging that will prevent exposure of transport staff to biohazards.

Training, Education, and Competence of Staff Performing Reprocessing

Regardless of the facility type or location, staff performing reprocessing must be trained on their job duties. Unless required by regulation (for example, if a regulation has incorporated a specific evidence-based guideline), competency requirements of staff performing reprocessing procedures are determined by the organization. Education is the process of receiving systematic instruction resulting in the acquisition of theoretical knowledge. Training differs from education in that training focuses on gaining specific—often manually performed—technical skills.

Competency requires a third attribute—ability. Ability is simply being able to do something. The ability to do something competently is based on an individual's capability to synthesize and correctly apply the knowledge and technical skills to a task. In addition, while The Joint Commission and JCI do not define required competencies that must be completed, when determining competency requirements, consideration should be given to the needs of the patient population, the types of procedures conducted, conditions or diseases treated, and the kinds of equipment used. Competency assessment then focuses on specific knowledge, technical skills, and abilities required to deliver safe, quality care. Basic infection prevention and control knowledge may be part of education; however, knowledge and skills related to sterile technique, sterilization, and high-level disinfection

To ensure that staff are properly reprocessing and handling medical devices and equipment, the following steps are recommended:

- Identify all medical devices and equipment used in the facility.
- Identify those items that require high-level disinfection or sterilization and the areas where they are used and reprocessed.
- Ensure that manufacturers' cleaning and disinfection instructions for each item are readily available to staff performing any step of the reprocessing procedures.
- Give careful attention to each step of a manufacturer's instructions to ensure that the correct environment, equipment, and supplies are available to reprocess them.
- Implement programs for training and evaluation to ensure competence of all staff who reprocess medical devices and equipment.
- Ensure consistent quality control and documentation in all areas performing high-level disinfection and sterilization so that the processes can be audited for compliance.

are competencies expected of an operating room nurse, surgical assistants, and sterile processing staff.

Recommendations regarding training content vary, but all recommendations emphasize the need for a comprehensive, intensive, and redundant training program for reprocessing staff along with a process for demonstrating specific competencies. When job roles include high-level disinfection, the Healthcare Infection Control Practices Advisory Committee (HICPAC) recommends model-specific competency for each endoscope. Model-specific competency may be required because of regulations, and most manufacturers can provide step-by-step instructions or training documents that can be used to assess competency.

High-Level Disinfection of Endoscopes

Some manufacturers provide competency checklists for their equipment and products. Figure 8.2 on page 202 shows key issues to consider for high-level disinfection of endoscopes.

A HICPAC workgroup that was formed in 2015 included key stakeholder organizations and professional societies representing users of endoscopes, sterile processing professionals, infection preventionists and hospital epidemiologists, the FDA, CMS and accrediting organizations, including The Joint Commission. This workgroup made recommendations that were finalized at the July 2016 HICPAC meeting; in keeping with other recommendations, the workgroup concluded that all endoscopes should be trackable from the reprocessing procedure through use on a patient.[15,16,21-23]

To ensure that all endoscopes can be tracked, facilities may create a master list of all endoscopes available in the facility. It is best practice that the process for taking endoscopes off the list (for example, if an endoscope is taken out of service or sent out for repair) or putting endoscopes on the list (such as loaner endoscopes) to be consistent throughout the facility, as variation may lead to inability to track all endoscopes. Tools 8-3 and 8-4 can be customized and used for tracking and auditing endoscopes. The HICPAC workgroup also developed tools that can be downloaded and modified by health care organizations. A link to the HIPAC website is provided in Resources section at the end of this chapter.

TRY THESE TOOLS

Tool 8-3. Sample Endoscope Inventory Form

Tool 8-4. Sample Endoscope Audit Form

Most manufacturers indicate that initial cleaning of flexible endoscopes should take place next to the bedside or exam table with water and an enzymatic detergent or other cleaner recommended by the manufacturer. This process is known as precleaning and should not be confused with the thorough cleaning required prior to disinfection. Some manufacturers instruct customers to perform precleaning with a brush or a sponge.

While performing precleaning, staff should be wearing PPE that is recommended by the manufacturer as well as required by their employer as part of their OSHA required hazard assessment and mitigation strategies to prevent employee exposure to potentially infectious material. After precleaning has been performed, the soiled item should be transported to the reprocessing area in a container that is leak proof, puncture resistant, and labeled as

Figure 8-2. Key Issues to Consider for High-Level Disinfection of Endoscopes

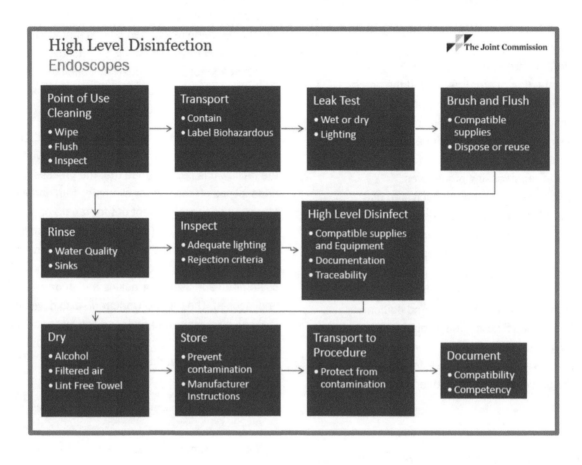

High Level Disinfection
Endoscopes
The Joint Commission

Point of Use Cleaning
• Wipe
• Flush
• Inspect

Transport
• Contain
• Label Biohazardous

Leak Test
• Wet or dry
• Lighting

Brush and Flush
• Compatible supplies
• Dispose or reuse

Rinse
• Water Quality
• Sinks

Inspect
• Adequate lighting
• Rejection criteria

High Level Disinfect
• Compatible supplies and Equipment
• Documentation
• Traceability

Dry
• Alcohol
• Filtered air
• Lint Free Towel

Store
• Prevent contamination
• Manufacturer Instructions

Transport to Procedure
• Protect from contamination

Document
• Compatibility
• Competency

biohazardous. This transport container may be a special designated box or leak-proof bag that is not contraindicated by the manufacturer.

Reprocessing instructions vary by endoscope manufacturer and should be followed to ensure safe and effective reprocessing. The routine reprocessing of flexible endoscopes normally includes the following steps[15,16,22]:

At the point of use
• Precleaning

In the reprocessing area
• Leak testing
• Manual cleaning
• Rinse after cleaning
• Visual inspection

• High-level disinfection (manual or automated)
• Rinse after high-level disinfection
• Drying (alcohol and forced air)

In storage area or location
• Storage

Staff should take care to ensure that the cleaning and disinfection process occurs within the time frame specified by the endoscope manufacturer. At least one flexible endoscope manufacturer specifies that reprocessing should occur within one hour, or an alternative reprocessing procedure that includes extended soaking may be required. In addition, manufacturers often specify a frequency for discarding or maintaining accessories used for reprocessing. Examples of issues frequently identified when assessing compliance with accessories include the following:

- **Leak testing.** Not performing leak testing or performing it incorrectly (for example, not properly testing endoscopes for leaks to detect fluid invasion)
- **Brushes.** Not using the size or type recommended by the endoscope manufacturer, reusing single-use brushes, continuing to use a damaged reusable brush
- **Sponge.** Not using the size or type recommended by the endoscope manufacturer, reusing a single-use sponge, using antiseptic scrub brushes (for example, those used for surgical scrubbing of hands)
- **Endoscope flushing devices.** Not performing routine maintenance or disinfection as recommended by the manufacturer
- **High-level disinfectant.** Using disinfectant beyond the use-by date, not checking minimal effective concentration, not performing quality control of test strips as indicated by the manufacturer's instructions, not re-dating test strip containers upon opening (see Figure 8-3)
- **Automated reprocessing machines.** Not using model specific connectors, using for reprocessing endoscopes that are not compatible, failing to install (for example, lack of air gap) or maintain (for example, changing filters, performing routine preventive maintenance)

Every channel of the endoscope must be reprocessed each time the endoscope is used, even if the channel was not used in the preceding procedure. *Each step of the appropriate process must be applied to every channel.* If an automated endoscope reprocessor is used, it is essential that the model-specific connectors are used to ensure that every channel is disinfected. After being disinfected and rinsed, channels must be dried. This usually involves injecting air through each channel, followed by an alcohol flush and then additional air to purge the alcohol. As previously stated, manufacturers' instructions should be followed. The outside of the endoscope should also be dried. Some manufacturers recommend using a clean, dry cloth, while others recommend wiping with alcohol.

Final Inspection and Storage

The flexible endoscope should undergo final inspection and be stored in accordance with the manufacturer's instructions. The Society of Gastroenterology Nurses and Associates (SGNA) recommends that unless the reprocessor has a dedicated space for accessories, such as a basket or "nook" for accessories, these items should be reprocessed separately.[21] However, AAMI Standard ST91 states that the detachable endoscope parts that are to be reused (for example, air/water and suction valves/pistons) should be processed together and stored with the specific endoscope as a unique set in order to allow traceability.[24] Each organization should determine what process it will use in accordance with the hierarchical approach to infection control standards. The IP can help guide the decision.

Many flexible endoscope manufacturers state that the endoscopes should be dried and stored in a vertical hanging position. However, horizontal forced-air drying cabinets have become very common in health care settings and may be used provided that they are not contraindicated by the flexible endoscope manufacturer. At least one leading endoscope manufacturer has provided clarification on using drying cabinets. Organizations are highly encouraged to work with their chosen vendors to clarify storage requirements.

Duration of Storage

A recent document, titled Multisociety Guideline on Reprocessing Flexible GI Endoscopes and Accessories, that was reviewed and approved by the Governing Board of the American Society for Gastrointestinal Endoscopy, echoed what the AAMI Standard ST91 has long stated: There is no data to support a requirement for reprocessing appropriately cleaned, reprocessed, dried, and stored

Figure 8-3. Testing Disinfectant with a Test Strip

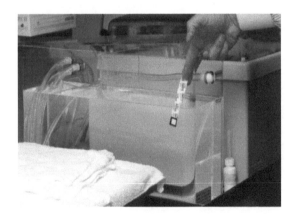

Testing the disinfectant with a test strip. **Note:** *Use of gloves is recommended to prevent chemical exposure by the manufacturer, so an organization in which staff fail to use gloves could be cited for noncompliance with manufacturers' instructions for use.* Photo by Sylvia Garcia-Houchins, RN, MBA, CIC. Used with permission.

flexible endoscopes. Unless required by regulation or manufacturer instructions, organizations may choose to evaluate the available literature and perform an assessment of the benefits and risks for developing an organizational policy that requires routine reprocessing of flexible endoscopes at specific intervals (also known as hang time). If an organizational policy specifies a required hang time, the organization will be expected to follow its stated policy.

Future Reprocessing Options for Endoscopes

Some disinfection and sterilization experts have recommended that flexible endoscopes be sterilized instead of receiving high-level disinfection. This is based on evidence that high-level disinfection does not always adequately destroy organisms in scopes (such as duodenoscopes), which has resulted in serious infections and multidrug-resistant organism outbreaks. Contamination of both duodenoscopes and flexible bronchoscopes has been found even after the manufacturer's instructions and professional guidelines were followed correctly.[8-10] IPs should follow this issue carefully and work with the reprocessing staff and others to advise their organization about which strategy is appropriate for the organization. In addition to the sources in the References list, Sidebar 8-3 lists two helpful sources. Sidebar 8-4 on page 205 lists key areas that may use semicritical devices requiring high-level disinfection.

Laryngoscopes and Other Devices That Enter the Respiratory Tract

Because they touch mucous membranes, devices such as nasal speculums and laryngoscope blades should undergo at least high-level disinfection. Some organizations find it easier to sterilize these items. Care should be taken to ensure compliance with manufacturers' instructions for reprocessing. Items that require high-level disinfection but are not required to be sterile may be removed from their sterile packaging and stored in a manner that prevents them from being contaminated. Prior to use, each item must be handled in a way that prevents contamination, (for example, not stored in a dirty drawer, which is a frequent finding in some settings). If peel pouches are used to protect laryngoscopes after high-level disinfection, care should be taken to ensure that the laryngoscope is completely dry, and the packaging label should clearly identify that the laryngoscope is high-level disinfected and not sterile.

Endocavity Probes

Many facilities use endocavity probe covers to prevent gross contamination of probes (for example, for vaginal probes). Because many probe covers have high in-use leak rates, their use does not negate the need for high-level disinfection.[25] Probes must be cleaned—following manufacturer instructions—prior to high-level disinfection. Much as with endoscopes, automated high-level disinfection is available. The choice of a high-level disinfection process should be made in accordance with the probe manufacturer's instructions.

Surface Ultrasound Transducers

There are special considerations for surface ultrasound transducers used for percutaneous procedures or if contaminated with blood or other potentially infectious material. The reprocessing of surface ultrasound transducers is based on intended use and manufacturer's instructions. If the transducer is intended to be used on non-intact skin, then it is considered a semicritical device prior to its use and should undergo high-level disinfection.

If the ultrasound transducer will only be used on intact skin, then intended use is noncritical, and regardless of whether it is contaminated with blood, the Spaulding classification would indicate a need for low-level or intermediate level disinfection. However, if the surface ultrasound transducer manufacturer's reprocessing instructions indicate that it should be high-level disinfected if used to assist with percutaneous

---

Sidebar 8-3.
Duodenoscope Resources

https://www.fda.gov/medical-devices/
reprocessing-reusable-medical-devices/
infections-associated-reprocessed-
duodenoscopes

https://www.cdc.gov/hai/organisms/cre/
cre-duodenoscope-surveillance-protocol.html

https://www.fda.gov/medical-devices/safety-
communications/fda-recommending-transition-
duodenoscopes-innovative-designs-enhance-
safety-fda-safety-communication

Sidebar 8-4. Key Areas That May Use Semicritical Devices

Key areas where devices requiring at least high-level disinfection can be found include the following:

- **Emergency department.** Endoscopes, endocavity probes, laryngoscopes, surface ultrasounds transducers*
- **OB/GYN clinic.** Endocavity probe, diaphragm fitting rings, pessaries
- **Sleep study units.** Reusable sleep study masks and tubing
- **GI or pulmonary procedure units and clinics.** Colonoscopes, duodenoscopes, bronchoscopes
- **ICUs.** Endoscopes, transesophageal echocardiography probes, surface ultrasound transducers*
- **Radiology.** Endocavity probes, surface ultrasound transducers*
- **Urology clinic.** Endoscopes, endocavity probes
- **Operating and procedure rooms.** Endoscopes, laryngoscopes, transesophageal echocardiography probes, endocavity probes, surface ultrasound transducers*
- **Ambulatory surgery centers, office-based surgery practice.** Endoscopes, laryngoscopes, transesophageal echocardiography probes, endocavity probes, surface ultrasound transducers*
- **Cardiac procedure areas.** Transesophageal echocardiography probes, surface ultrasound transducers*

*If specified by intended use or surface ultrasound IFU.

OB/GYN, obstetrics and gynecology; **GI**, gastrointestinal; **ICU**, intensive care unit; **IFU**, instructions for use.

procedures or if contaminated with blood, the expectation would be that the surface ultrasound transducer would be high-level disinfected in accordance with the manufacturer's instructions for use.

Sterilization

To ensure that devices and instruments are properly sterilized, organizations should focus on the key issues included in Figure 8-4 on page 206, which are also discussed in detail below.

Precleaning at the point of use: Start the process of cleaning instruments at the point of use (for example, in the operating or procedure room) by flushing lumens with sterile water or wiping gross tissue and blood from instruments during the procedure, as directed by the manufacturer's instructions. If instruments cannot be transported to the decontamination area for immediate reprocessing after the procedure, the manufacturer's instructions regarding the need to maintain moisture of soiled instruments and how moisture should be maintained should be followed. Options for keeping instruments and devices moist include covering used items with an enzymatic spray, gel, or foam; compatible

detergent; or a cloth moistened with water to prevent drying. Both the instrument manufacturer's and the precleaning product manufacturer's instructions should be consulted and followed. Facilities should ensure compliance with manufacturers' instructions for removal of gross debris and prevention of drying, as these procedures are needed to avoid biofilm formation.[17]

Prepare and transport the item(s) to the reprocessing area: Contain all items contaminated with blood or body fluids in a leak-proof container from the point of use to the decontamination area. Use a puncture-resistant, leak-proof, closable, and labeled container that meets OSHA or local standards for items that are sharp. Additional requirements may be necessary if transporting off-site for reprocessing.

Disassembly: Gaskets should be removed, stopcocks opened, and instruments should be completely disassembled, as specified by the instrument manufacturer's instructions, during the cleaning and sterilization process.

Cleaning and disinfection or decontamination: All items must be cleaned before they can be disinfected or sterilized. This is in addition to removal of gross contamination at

Figure 8-4. The Sterilization Process

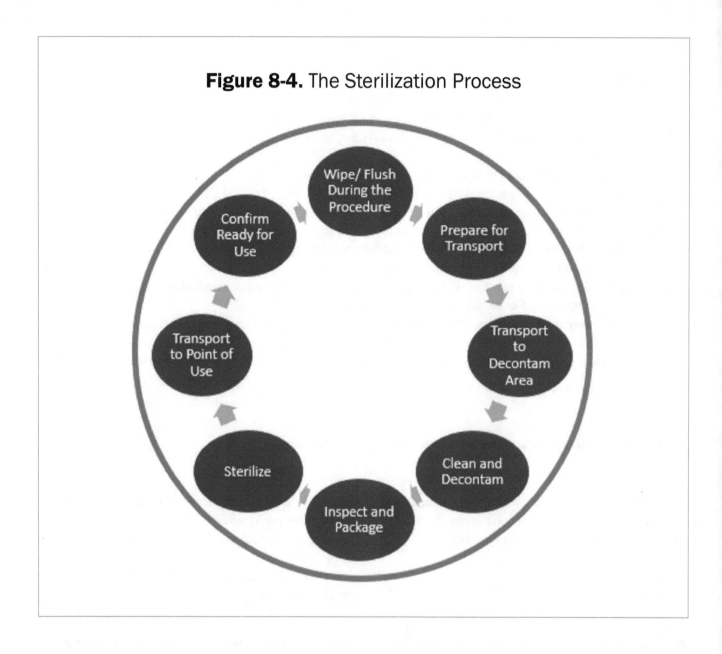

the point of use (known as precleaning). Thorough cleaning is always required prior to sterilization to remove dirt and organic matter to ensure that the sterilant can reach the surfaces of the items processed. This cleaning must be done in accordance with the manufacturer's instructions. If automated equipment is used for cleaning, it must be compatible with the item being cleaned. Automated cleaning equipment must be operated, and quality must be controlled, according to the manufacturer's instructions, regulatory requirements, and facility procedures. For example, most manufacturers of automated cleaning equipment have specific loading instructions, cleaning chemicals and rinse water requirements, and daily (for example, grate cleaning) and weekly (such as soil challenge tests) checks that

must be completed to ensure that the equipment is functioning properly.

Rinsing: Most cleaning or disinfection chemicals include specific instructions for rinsing or not rinsing between steps and the number of rinses and type of water (for example, tap, deionized, reverse osmosis) required.

Drying: Depending on the manufacturer's instructions, some items may require drying prior to further processing, while others may not. In all cases, care should be taken not to place cleaned items awaiting further processing in an area where recontamination could occur.

Physical inspection: During and after completion of the cleaning process, items should be inspected for visible soil or damage. Visual inspection can be facilitated by ensuring that there is adequate light, and a magnifier may provide additional assistance. Some state and local building codes include specific requirements for lighting and finishes in central sterile processing to facilitate the ability to perform inspections.

Lubrication: Some instruments require lubrication to prevent stains and corrosion and to keep the moving parts from rubbing and sticking. Immersion baths are generally not recommended because of the risk of microbial contamination.

Wrapping or containers: All packaging and containers must be validated for use with the sterilization process and parameters that will be used. Care should be taken to use wrapping supplies, including pouches and rigid containers, in accordance with manufacturer instructions. Cleaning recommendations and filters for rigid containers are manufacturer specific. Items and chemical indicators should be positioned in accordance with device and packaging instructions to ensure exposure to the sterilant (for example, open position for ratcheted instruments and placement of chemical indicators in corners of rigid containers directly under openings).

Labels: Labeling that allows the item to be tracked back to the sterilization load must be on the package from the time of sterilization until the item is used. Labeling should not compromise the barrier (for example, mark the plastic side of a peel pouch instead of the paper or be placed in a manner that would impede exposure to the sterilant). The label should include the contents, the date sterilized, and an identifier that allows the item to be tracked back to the sterilization load.

Sterilization: The choice of sterilant must be in compliance with the manufacturer's instructions for both the device or instrument and the sterilizer. The sterilization process must be monitored using chemical, biological, and physical indicators, as outlined by the manufacturer:

- Chemical indicators are specific to the sterilization process. Examples include the sterilization tape affixed to the outside of packs and the strips placed within the sterilization container that change color after processing. External and internal indicators should be used for every item sterilized, regardless of type of container or packaging. Indicators should be placed in the location specified by the indicator and container manufacturer. Staff who will open

packaging or containers must know what changes are expected for the indicator used at the facility.

- Biological indicators are specific to the sterilization process and should be included in at least one sterilizer load per week and in every load that includes an implant. Clear and complete documentation of the results of biological indicators and controls is required.

- Physical indicators such as time, temperature, and pressure must be monitored in accordance with the sterilizer manufacturer's instructions. Verification that parameters were met (for example, initials or signature) is required as part of the quality control process prior to removing the item from the sterilizer.

Many organizations consider the sterilization process over once the item has been sterilized and is ready for release. However, surveyors will review the entire process, including the following:

- Release from the sterilization area should be a careful and thoughtful process done by someone who is trained to ensure all necessary parameters for release have been met prior to release.
- Transportation of sterile items must be accomplished in a manner that does not compromise the integrity of the packaging or sterilized item.
- The final point to stop an unsterile or potentially unsterile item from being used on a patient is at the time that it is being opened for placement on the sterile field. Staff who are responsible for opening a sterile product must know when an item should not be considered sterile and should not be used.

Surveyors will focus on many of these issues. One example, shown in Figure 8-5 on page 208, reviews issues associated with peel pouches. If used, pouches should be sized to prevent tearing during movement or storage. Items should be packaged to ensure that sterilant can contact all surfaces and should be used in accordance with manufacturer instructions. Regardless of the container, wrap, or pouch used, the person releasing the sterilized item as well as the person opening the sterilized item must know how to identify whether an item is considered sterile prior to use. This is especially important because many organizations now use event-related sterility rather than an expiration date on items sterilized internally but have not provided clear training on what events indicate an item should not be used. The availability of an item that should be considered unsterile (for example, external or internal indicator missing,

Figure 8-5. Common Issues with Peel Pouches

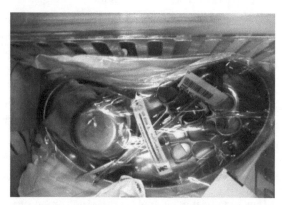

Because of instrument placement, sterilant may not be able to reach all surfaces. Photo by Sylvia Garcia-Houchins, RN, MBA, CIC. Used with permission.

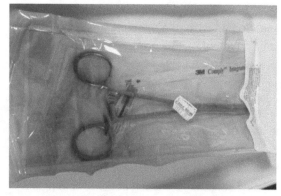

If double pouching is performed, it must be validated by the manufacturer. Photo by Sylvia Garcia-Houchins, RN, MBA, CIC. Used with permission.

folded-over or torn peel pouches, evidence of moisture damage, missing locks on rigid containers) and staff who are not knowledgeable about conditions that should result in the item not being used could result in harm to a patient and other serious situations. Some key risks for sterilization failures include the following:

Sterilant cannot reach all surfaces
- Disassembly, cleaning, and decontamination process
- Inspection and packaging
- Correct sterilization cycle

Failure of the cleaning and sterilizing equipment
- User error
- Monitoring
- Maintenance

Nonsterile product availability
- Load release
  ○ Verification of exposure to process
- Prior to use of item
  ○ Verification of exposure to the process and package integrity

Organizations can supplement applicable regulations and manufacturer's instructions with evidence-based guidelines and standards, such as those from the CDC, AAMI, SGNA, AORN, and the American Society of Cataract and Refractive Surgery, to identify other recommendations

that may add additional clarity and safety to an organization's practice.[12,17,19-24,26] These evidence-based guidelines and standards provide concrete recommendations to guide an organization's identification, development, and implementation of appropriate practices related to cleaning, disinfection, and sterilization but are not required unless they have been integrated as a requirement by regulation (for example, facility licensing) or manufacturer instructions. As previously mentioned, in some cases, accrediting organizations may require implementation of an evidence-based practice or standard through their standards; for example, use of standard precautions is required by Joint Commission standards.

The following is a summary of best practices to achieve high-level disinfection and sterilization:
- Classify all reusable medical equipment, instruments, and devices as noncritical, semicritical, or critical.
- Confirm that all single-use equipment is either discarded or reprocessed by an FDA–approved third-party reprocessing facility.
- Maintain a complete library of manufacturers' instructions for use, including reprocessing instructions, that is available to applicable staff.
- Confirm that all reusable equipment and medical devices are reprocessed according to their manufacturer's instructions for use.

- Consider use of multidisciplinary teams to develop and implement standardized policies and procedures for handling, cleaning, disinfecting, sterilizing, and disposing of or storing medical equipment, devices, and supplies.
- Ensure that cleaning, disinfection, and sterilization practices are standardized and implemented consistently throughout the organization, regardless of location.
- Provide orientation, training, and competency programs for staff involved in cleaning, disinfecting, and sterilizing medical equipment, devices, and supplies.
- Develop, implement, and monitor quality assurance protocols for high-level disinfection and sterilization processes. For example, such protocols must address the use of chemical indicators, administrative controls, and biological monitors for sterilizers and chemical test strips to evaluate the concentration of high-level disinfectants such as glutaraldehyde or peracetic acid.
- Conduct quality assurance monitoring for high-level disinfection and sterilization processes in accordance with regulatory requirements, manufacturer recommendations, and, as applicable, evidence-based guidelines and practice standards.
- Develop a recall policy and procedure that can be activated if performance monitoring or other findings indicate that the sterilization process fails.
- Ensure adequate staffing levels and supervision of staff who process medical equipment, devices, and supplies. For example, if the average time to clean an endoscope is 15–20 minutes, the average endoscope reprocessing technician can clean approximately 20 to 28 scopes if doing nothing but cleaning during an 8-hour shift (assuming standard breaks). Additional time for high-level disinfection, required documentation, storing, and so on would need to be calculated.
- Develop and implement a system for assessing staff adherence to cleaning, disinfection, and sterilization protocols and providing the findings to these staff.
- Ensure availability of policies and procedures for repair or disposal and, if indicated, replacement of damaged equipment and devices.
- Provide training, education, and competency assessment of staff who will open or use sterile products to ensure that they can identify items that have not undergone the necessary reprocessing or whose packaging or storage conditions render the products unsuitable for patient use.

An IP should work with facility staff to ensure that a risk assessment of all areas performing high-level disinfection and/or sterilization is performed and that there is consistency among all areas that perform medical device and instrument cleaning, disinfection, sterilization, and/or disposal or storage procedures. In addition, the IP should be an active participant in the quality review of all areas performing high-level disinfection and sterilization. Some key points to consider for high-level disinfection and sterilization are included in Sidebar 8-5 on page 210.

Location and Design of High-Level Disinfection and Sterilization Areas

Organizations can choose to perform centralized reprocessing (so that items to be reprocessed are brought to a central location) or decentralized reprocessing (so that items are reprocessed at or near the location of use). Regardless of the location, organizations must ensure that decentralized areas are able to meet all reprocessing requirements and should be aware that lack of qualified oversight is often found to be an issue in these areas when findings of noncompliance or an immediate threat related to high-level disinfection or sterilization are identified.

Many physical factors can affect the disinfection and sterilization process. Surveyors will expect that all areas where reprocessing occurs meet state and local building code requirements for the time the location was built or renovated or when functional use of the space was changed to reprocessing. Reprocessing areas must also meet specific requirements established by manufacturers of equipment and supplies used in these locations. These factors include the following:

- Temperature
- Humidity
- Air exchanges
- Ventilation exhaust
- Adequate space
- Finishes
- Equipment

The physical space used for reprocessing should be built to standards that make it possible for staff and equipment to be protected during decontamination, for soiled devices and equipment to be taken through a one-way flow from dirty to clean, and, as applicable, to achieve disinfection or be packaged and sterilized and held for further

Sidebar 8-5. Key Points to Consider for High-Level Disinfection and Sterilization

- Facilities should develop and implement policies and procedures for reprocessing medical devices in accordance with regulatory requirements (for example, FDA, EPA, OSHA, CMS, health care organization licensing), manufacturers' instructions for use, and required or chosen evidence-based practices (for example, AAMI, AORN, CDC, SGNA).

- Staff should be trained in the correct use, donning, removal, limitations, and indications for PPE to prevent biological and/or chemical exposure (OSHA requirement).

- Accessories necessary to follow the manufacturer's reprocessing instructions should be provided to reprocessing staff (for example, ultrasonic cleaners, brushes of the specified diameter, length, bristle type, and material).

- Organizations' processes and procedures should include following the manufacturer's instructions for all accessories used during reprocessing (for example, single versus multiple use, automated dilution systems, bushes, detergents, automated reprocessing equipment, high-level disinfectants, rinse water).

- Organizations should resolve any conflicts or discrepancies among manufacturer's instructions.

- Maintenance and validation or quality control should be performed as recommended by the manufacturer (for example, use of soil challenge tests on automated washers, validation of appropriate mixing of automated dilution systems, testing of minimal effective concentration).

AAMI, Association for the Advancement of Medical Instrumentation; **AORN,** Association of periOperative Registered Nurses; **CDC,** US Centers for Disease Control and Prevention; **CMS,** US Centers for Medicare & Medicaid Services; **EPA,** Environmental Protection Agency; **FDA,** US Food and Drug Administration; **OSHA,** US Occupational Safety and Health Administration; **PPE,** personal protective equipment; **SGNA,** Society of Gastroenterology Nurses and Associates.

distribution. Figure 8-6 demonstrates the recommended movement of equipment and staff from dirty to clean.

Water quality affects the decontamination and processing of medical devices and equipment. Treated (deionized or reverse osmosis) water must be available for rinsing medical devices and equipment, if required by manufacturer instructions. Some device manufacturers and consensus documents recommend the use of sterile water for the final rinse of ophthalmology instruments to prevent toxic anterior segment syndrome.[24]

If building code requires or is silent, hand hygiene facilities that are separate from reprocessing sinks should be provided.

Disposal of Medical Equipment, Devices, and Supplies

Health care workers must dispose of used medical equipment, devices, and supplies according to federal, state, and local requirements. Rules for managing hazardous waste can vary from state to state. In general, potentially infectious medical waste must be segregated from other waste and packaged according to applicable requirements for transportation to disposal sites. Facilities should establish clear policies and procedures to meet these requirements, educate staff, and ensure compliance.

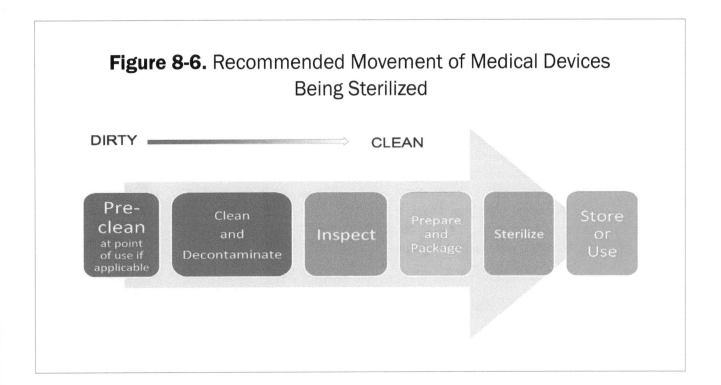

Figure 8-6. Recommended Movement of Medical Devices Being Sterilized

DIRTY ⟶ CLEAN

Pre-clean at point of use if applicable → Clean and Decontaminate → Inspect → Prepare and Package → Sterilize → Store or Use

Storage of Medical Equipment, Devices, and Supplies

To prevent supplies from becoming contaminated or compromised during storage, medical equipment, devices, and patient care items should be stored in accordance with regulatory requirements and manufacturer instructions. Key points related to storage include the following[17,18,21]:

- Storage areas should meet Facility Guidelines Institute requirements adopted by state or local building code and CMS, if applicable, and should be clean and in good repair.
- Sterile items should be stored at least 8 inches off the floor, 2 inches from outside walls, and 18 inches from ceilings.
- All items in clean storage rooms should be clean (no soiled items), and clean items should not be stored in soiled rooms.
- Expired items and items in damaged packaging (for example, torn, soiled, wet) should be discarded or reprocessed in accordance with manufacturers' instructions.
- If open shelving is used for sterile or clean storage, the bottom shelf should be solid to protect items from contamination.
- AAMI recommends using closed or covered cabinets for storage of items that are seldom used, whereas

AORN recommends that sterile items be stored in a controlled environment.

- Supplies, including those in rigid containers, should not be stored next to or under sinks, under exposed or open water or sewer pipes, or in any location where they could become wet.
- Outside shipping containers and corrugated boxes should not be used as containers in sterile storage areas.

Reprocessing Single-Use Devices

Inappropriate reprocessing of single-use devices (SUDs) can compromise patient safety. The FDA has strict requirements for reprocessing devices labeled for single use under the Federal Food, Drug, and Cosmetic Act. The FDA requires that reprocessors of these devices provide validation information that includes cleaning and sterilization and functional performance data demonstrating that each SUD will remain substantially the same after the maximum number of times the device is reprocessed. (Third-party reprocessors can be used to meet these requirements.) In other words, before a device that is intended for one use or use on a single patient during a single procedure can be reprocessed and reused, a third party or a health care facility must comply with the same requirements that apply to original equipment manufacturers.

The IP should collaborate with staff in patient care and reprocessing areas to ensure that SUDs, particularly those used in invasive procedures, are not reprocessed and reused unless the organization can meet the FDA requirements.[14] Because most health care organizations cannot meet these rigorous requirements, the majority should either use a third-party reprocessor that can meet the requirements or choose not to reprocess and reuse SUDs. The organization would benefit from a clearly written policy. The IP can be a valuable collaborator in developing the policy. Additional information about reprocessing SUDs can be found on the FDA website (http://www.fda.gov) using the search term "single-use device," and in the Resources section of this chapter.

Performance Testing and Maintenance of Sterilizers

The machinery used to sterilize medical devices and equipment supplies used for patient care must work effectively so that the organization can ensure that each item processed is safe for patient care. The importance of medical equipment maintenance and testing in IPC efforts—and specifically the maintenance and testing of sterilizers—cannot be overemphasized. An organization must have documentation that performance testing, including physical, chemical, and biological monitoring, and routine maintenance, are performed on all sterilizers in accordance with manufacturers' recommendations and standardized, accepted practices. Many IPs and accreditation compliance specialists review sterilizer performance monitoring and maintenance records to ensure that maintenance is occurring and that sterilizers are working properly. Staff members who use the sterilizers should have a clear process to follow when the sterilizer is not working properly.

Summary

Inappropriate or inadequate cleaning, disinfection, and sterilization practices have resulted in the transmission of infections to patients. These HAIs can be prevented when facilities implement appropriate infection prevention practices. Effective cleaning, disinfection, and sterilization requires meticulously detailed processes and controls. From initial evaluation of an item for intended use through implementation and quality control of reprocessing procedures, extreme care and oversight are needed. Organizations must provide facilities and equipment that promote proper procedures. IPs must be aware of current evidence-based infection prevention practices, regulations, and other requirements; new sterilization and disinfection products and technologies; and outbreaks and clusters of infection related to medical devices and equipment. These aspects affect use and reprocessing of devices and equipment at their facility. No matter where in the facility the reprocessing happens or the type of services being provided, the expectations are the same: Provide the safest possible devices and equipment for the patient.

Resources

Tools to Try

Tool 8-1. Assessment of Item for Reprocessing Form

Tool 8-2. Evaluation Steps for Medical Devices and Supplies Reprocessing

Tool 8-3. Sample Endoscope Inventory Form

Tool 8-4. Sample Endoscope Audit Form

Supplemental Resources

Devices for Which a 510(k) Should Contain Validation Data (Reprocessing Final Guidance Appendix E). This document provides a list of items that must have validation of reprocessing instruction as part of their FDA 510(k) submission. Accessed Mar 9, 2021. http://www.fda.gov/MedicalDevices/DeviceRegulationandGuidance/ReprocessingofReusableMedicalDevices/ucm436512.htm

Facility Guidelines Institute (FGI) *Guidelines for Design and Construction of Health Care Facilities*
Although the FGI *Guidelines* were updated in 2018, some states still require compliance with earlier editions of the FGI *Guidelines* or other equivalency. To ensure compliance with state requirements, organizations must identify which guidelines edition, if any, their state(s) uses. Accessed Mar 9, 2021. Adoption by state can be found at https://fgiguidelines.org/guidelines/state-adoption-fgi-guidelines/

Cleaning, Disinfection, and Sterilization Resources
US Centers for Medicare & Medicaid Services (CMS) State Operations Manual: Appendix A— Survey Protocol, Regulations and Interpretive Guidelines for Hospitals. Accessed May 26, 2021. https://www.cms.gov/Regulations-and-Guidance/Guidance/Manuals/downloads/som107ap_a_hospitals.pdf

For Deemed Organizations

CMS Infection Control Worksheet for Ambulatory Surgical Centers https://www.cms.gov/Regulations-and-Guidance/Guidance/Manuals/downloads/som107_exhibit_351.pdf

CMS Infection Control Worksheet for Hospitals

https://www.cms.gov/Medicare/Provider-Enrollment-and-Certification/SurveyCertificationGenInfo/Downloads/Survey-and-Cert-Letter-15-12-Attachment-1.pdf

US Food & Drug Administration

Reprocessing Medical Devices in Health Care Settings: Validation Methods and Labeling Guidance for Industry and FDA Staff. https://www.fda.gov/media/80265/download

Marketing Clearance of Diagnostic Ultrasound Systems and Transducers Guidance for Industry and FDA Staff. https://www.fda.gov/media/71100/download

US Food and Drug Administration

MedWatch: The FDA Safety Information and Adverse Event Reporting Program. Accessed Mar 9, 2021. http://www.fda.gov/Safety/MedWatch/. Infection preventionists should consider signing up for e-mail Safety Alerts about concerns and recalls related to medical devices and medication.

US Centers for Disease Control and Prevention Guidelines (CDC)

Disinfection and Sterilization in Healthcare Facilities, 2008 (updated 2017). https://www.cdc.gov/infectioncontrol/guidelines/disinfection/index.html

Environmental Infection Control in Health-Care Facilities, 2003 (last update July 2019). https://www.cdc.gov/infectioncontrol/guidelines/environmental/index.html

Essential Steps for Flexible Endoscope Reprocessing—Recommendations of the Healthcare Infection Control Practices Advisory Committee (HICPAC). https://www.cdc.gov/hicpac/recommendations/flexible-endoscope-reprocessing.html#Toolkit

Association for the Advancement of Medical Instrumentation (AAMI) standards

https://www.aami.org/

- ST79: Comprehensive guide to steam sterilization and sterility assurance in health care facilities (2017 with 2020 amendments)
- ST91: Comprehensive guide to flexible and semi-rigid endoscope processing in health care facilities (2015)
- ST58: Chemical sterilization and high-level disinfection in health care facilities (2018)
- ST41: Ethylene oxide sterilization in health care facilities: Safety and effectiveness (2018)

Association of periOperative Registered Nurses (AORN) Guidelines

https://www.aorn.org/guidelines

- Sterilization Packaging Systems (2019)
- Manual Chemical High-Level Disinfection (2018)
- Processing Flexible Endoscopes (2016)
- Care and Cleaning of Surgical Instruments (2020)
- Sterilization (2018)

American Academy of Ophthalmology

Guidelines for the Cleaning and Sterilization of Intraocular Surgical Instruments—2018. Accessed Mar 24, 2021. https://www.aao.org/clinical-statement/guidelines-cleaning-sterilization-intraocular

References

1. US Centers for Disease Control and Prevention (CDC). Sacred Obligation: Restoring Veteran Trust and Patient Safety. Testimony Before the Committee on Veterans Affairs U.S. House of Representatives. May 3, 2011. Accessed Apr 7, 2021. http://www.cdc.gov/washington/testimony/2011/t20110503.htm

2. Hellinger WC, et al. Outbreak of toxic anterior segment syndrome following cataract surgery associated with impurities in autoclave steam moisture. *Infect Control Hosp Epidemiol.* 2006 Mar;27(3):294–298.

3. CDC. Notes from the field: New Delhi metallo-ß-lactamase-producing *Escherichia coli* associated with endoscopic retrograde cholangiopancreatography—Illinois, 2013. *MMWR Morb Mortal Wkly Rep.* 2014 Jan 3;62(51–52):1051.

4. Alrabaa SF, et al. Early identification and control of carbapenemase-producing *Klebsiella pneumoniae*, originating from contaminated endoscopic equipment. *Am J Infect Control.* 2013 Jun;41(6):562–564.

5. Singh N, et al. Cluster of Trichosporon mucoides in children associated with a faulty bronchoscope. *Pediatr Infect Dis J.* 2003 Jul;22(7):609–612.

6. Obee PC, et al. Real-time monitoring in managing the decontamination of flexible gastrointestinal endoscopes. *Am J Infect Control.* 2005 May;33(4):202–206.

7. Orsi GB, Venditti M. Carbapenem-resistant *Klebsiella pneumoniae* transmission associated to endoscopy. *Am J Infect Control*. 2013 Sep;41(9):849–850.

8. US Food and Drug Administration. Reprocessing of Reusable Medical Devices. Updated Mar 26, 2018. Accessed Apr 7, 2021. https://www.fda.gov/medical-devices/products-and-medical-procedures/reprocessing-reusable-medical-devices

9. US Food and Drug Administration (FDA). Updated Information for Healthcare Providers Regarding Duodenoscopes. Mar 4, 2015. Accessed Apr 7, 2021. http://www.fda.gov/downloads/MedicalDevices/DeviceRegulationandGuidance/ReprocessingofReusableMedicalDevices/UCM436588.pdf

10. FDA. Infections Associated with Reprocessed Flexible Bronchoscopes: FDA Safety Communication. Sep 17, 2015. Accessed Apr 7, 2021. https://wayback.archive-it.org/7993/20170722213119/https://www.fda.gov/MedicalDevices/Safety/AlertsandNotices/ucm462949.htm

11. Kirschke DL, et al. *Pseudomonas aeruginosa* and *Serratia marcescens* contamination associated with a manufacturing defect in bronchoscopes. *N Engl J Med*. 2003 Jan;348(3):214–220.

12. Rutala WA, Weber DJ, Healthcare Infection Control Practices Advisory Committee (HICPAC). Guideline for Disinfection and Sterilization in Healthcare Facilities, 2008. Accessed Apr 7, 2021. https://www.cdc.gov/infectioncontrol/guidelines/disinfection/index.html#anchor_1555614008

13. US Centers for Medicare & Medicaid Services (CMS). Hospital Infection Control Worksheet. Accessed Apr 7, 2021. https://www.cms.gov/Medicare/Provider-Enrollment-and-Certification/SurveyCertificationGenInfo/Downloads/Survey-and-Cert-Letter-15-12-Attachment-1.pdf

14. FDA, Center for Biologics Evaluation and Research. Reprocessing Medical Devices in Health Care Settings: Validation Methods and Labeling. Guidance for Industry and Food and Drug Administration Staff. Mar 17, 2015. Accessed Mar 13, 2021. http://www.fda.gov/downloads/MedicalDevices/DeviceRegulationandGuidance/GuidanceDocuments/ucm253010.pdf

15. Society of Gastroenterology Nurses and Associates. Standards of Infection Prevention in Reprocessing Flexible Gastrointestinal Endoscopes. 2016. Accessed Apr 7, 2017. https://www.sgna.org/Practice-Resources/Position-Statements-Standards

16. ASGE Quality Assurance in Endoscopy Committee, Petersen BT, et al. Multisociety guideline on reprocessing flexible gastrointestinal endoscopes. *Gastrointest Endosc*. 2011 Jun;73(6):1075–1084.

17. Association for the Advancement of Medical Instrumentation (AAMI). Comprehensive Guide to Steam Sterilization and Sterility Assurance in Health Care Facilities. ANSI/AAMI ST79:2017. Accessed Apr 7, 2021. https://www.aami.org/detail-pages/press-release/updated-steam-sterilization-standard-for-healthcare-facilities-st79-now-available

18. Facility Guidelines Institute (FGI). 2014 Guidelines for Design and Construction of Hospitals and Outpatient Facilities. Accessed Mar 13, 2021. http://www.fgiguidelines.org/guidelines/2014-hospital-outpatient/read-only-copy/#registration_modal

19. Association of periOperative Registered Nurses (AORN). Guideline for sterilization. In Burlingame B, et al., eds. *Guidelines for Perioperative Practice*, vol. 1. Denver: AORN, 2016.

20. Hellinger WC, et al. ASCRS Ad Hoc Task Force on Cleaning and Sterilization of Intraocular Instruments: Recommended practices for cleaning and sterilizing intraocular surgical instruments. *J Cataract Refract Surg*. 2007 Jun;33(8):1095–1100.

21. Society of Gastroenterology Nurses and Associates. Standard of Infection Prevention in the Gastroenterology Setting. 2015. Accessed Apr 7, 2021. https://www.sgna.org/Practice-Resources/Position-Statements-Standards

22. Association for the Advancement of Medical Instrumentation (AAMI). Flexible and semi-rigid endoscope processing in health care facilities. ANSI/AAMI ST91:2015. http://www.healthmark.info/InstrumentRetrieval/PPE/ST91_White_Paper_2018-05-25.pdf

23. CDC. Infection Control Assessment Tool for Outpatient Settings. Accessed Mar 13, 2021. https://www.cdc.gov/infectioncontrol/pdf/ICAR/Outpatient.pdf

24. AORN. Guideline for processing flexible endoscopes. In Burlingame B, et al., eds. *Guidelines for Perioperative Practice*, vol. 1. Denver: AORN, 2016.

25. Casalegno JS, et al. High-risk HPV contamination of endocavity vaginal ultrasound probes: An underestimated route of nosocomial infection? *PLOS ONE*. 2012;7(10):e48137.

26. AORN. Guideline for care of surgical instruments. In Burlingame B, et al., eds. *Guidelines for Perioperative Practice*, vol. 1. Denver: AORN, 2016.

27. CMS. Exhibit 351: Ambulatory Surgical Center (ASC) Infection Control Surveyor Worksheet. June 26, 2015. Accessed Apr 7, 2021. https://www.cms.gov/Medicare/Provider-Enrollment-and-Certification/SurveyCertificationGenInfo/Downloads/Survey-and-Cert-Letter-15-43.pdf

Chapter 9

Communication and Education Strategies for Infection Prevention and Control Programs

By Linda R. Greene, RN, MPS, CIC, FAPIC

Disclaimer: Strategies, tools, and examples discussed in this book do not necessarily reflect Joint Commission or Joint Commission International requirements for all settings. Always refer to the most current standards applicable to your health care setting to ensure compliance.

Introduction

The ongoing and urgent need to communicate information about infections to care providers, related health care organizations, regulatory and accreditation bodies, and patients and families requires a thoughtful communication plan that is implemented and frequently reviewed, updated, and monitored. Effective and timely communication is always important. This has become increasingly clear as health care and medical communities work to manage emerging pathogens, including the spread of Novel Coronavirus 2019 (SARS-CoV-2/COVID-19) across the world. Public health concepts such as social distancing and wearing masks in public have required broad communication and education across multiple venues and by multiple organizations, such as the World Health Organization, the US Centers for Disease Control and Prevention (CDC), and state and local health departments.[1] At the organizational level, these messages need to be shared and understood by all health care workers.

For high-quality health care, communication and education are important across the entire continuum of care, not only for infection prevention and control (IPC) but also for patient safety. Effective communication is critical to meeting patient needs and providing safe, high-quality, and patient-centered care; it is also necessary for successfully managing health care delivery. To facilitate meaningful implementation and improvement, communication must take place from the top down, from the bottom up, and horizontally across the continuum of care. Lack of communication about infections can create a major barrier to implementing evidence-based practices and can result in negative outcomes for patients and a health care organization.[2]

This chapter highlights some recommended strategies for communicating with health care workers and patients, reporting infections to internal and external stakeholders, and using tools and evidence-based methods to ensure timely, accurate, and meaningful communications to influence all phases of infection prevention and control.

Communicating with and Educating Staff, Patients, and Visitors

To implement their infection prevention and control plans, organizations must be able to effectively communicate IPC practices, expectations, and responsibilities to all stakeholders. The Joint Commission elements of performance (EPs) and Joint Commission International (JCI) measurable elements (MEs) relevant to communication strategies for preventing and controlling infection are very broad, encompassing all individuals who enter the health care facility, including hospitals, nursing care centers/long term care facilities, ambulatory surgery centers or clinics, office-based surgery practices, and other outpatient care centers. The challenge is in communicating organizational expectations and patient, resident, family, and visitor responsibilities to every individual and at every point of entry into an organization. In addition, organizations are required to orient staff to the key safety content before staff provide care, treatment, and services. Key safety content may include specific processes and procedures related to the provision of care, treatment, or services; the environment of care; and IPC. Communication with health care workers regarding IPC practices is usually offered via education during orientation, when new problems arise, when practices change, and at least annually.

Educating Staff and Licensed Independent Practitioners

Orientation of all staff, including physicians, is a great opportunity to describe and stress the importance of organizational strategic goals and IPC policies and procedures. Included among these may be standard precautions and transmission-based precautions, prevention of central line–associated bloodstream infection (CLABSI), reduction of *Clostridioides/Clostridium difficile* infection, and proper use of disinfectants for cleaning the environment. An infection preventionist (IP) should work collaboratively with the medical staff office to integrate information on IPC into the orientation process for physicians and other licensed independent practitioners.

There are many approaches to providing IPC orientation. Although in-person orientation is a traditional method of education, developments during the COVID-19 pandemic have challenged organizations to identify new and creative ways to teach and learn. Examples include online, self-directed learning modules and interactive video

conferences. When in-person training is not feasible, interactive conferences provide a great opportunity to connect with the IP and have questions answered. Online-learning orientation modules may be assigned to new hires along with follow-up via video chats to discuss key points.

One challenge is orienting vendors and contractors who may enter the organization to perform work but are not officially hired and thus are excluded from the orientation program. The IP may work with the organization's legal department to identify existing and new contractors and vendors and design a plan to educate them before they enter a facility.

An organization should be able to demonstrate the success of communicating its education strategies and may do so by documenting attendance at training and continuing education programs in employee human resources records or physician credentialing files, for example. In some cases, individual employee files may be requested during on-site surveys for review of orientation and education attendance.

Once orientation to IPC practices is completed, the challenge is to provide annual updates as well as continuous education to health care workers as new practices are introduced or old practices are changed. For example, because information related to emerging infectious diseases, such as COVID-19, changes rapidly—and advice related to novel respiratory viruses and infectious diseases may also continue to evolve—IPs should actively review information for updates and guidance to evaluate the need to modify current practices and communications within their organizations. When new information becomes available, it is a good time to remind staff of routine practices that decrease the risk of transmission of any infectious agent. These routine practices should be in place regardless of any new infectious threat.[3] Some methods for educating staff about IPC practices include the following:

- Face-to-face learning: Adult learning principles should be considered. In some cases, adults are self-motivated but may also be resistant to change. Practical tools that focus on engagement and participation are useful. Starting presentations with a discussion focused on useful tools, examples, and barriers may be helpful. Online interactive platforms may substitute for actual face-to-face learning.

- Self-guided learning videos:
  - Written materials
  - Just-in-time training
  - Train-the-trainer education
  - Toolkits and infographics

Other examples of ongoing education and communication strategies include weekly newsletters, management briefs, policy change alerts, posters, and signage. Adults learn best with repeated exposures to the information. An adage for maximum effectiveness of new information is "7 times in 7 ways."[4] Often a combination of the above methods is necessary.

Figures 9-1 and 9-2, page 221, provide examples of signs that communicate messaging about COVID-19 and social distancing. Figure 9-3, page 221, illustrates how

newsletters can be an effective IPC tool for communicating with and educating staff.

The Joint Commission also has several tools that provide resources for health care workers. For example, a facility may encourage the use of The Joint Commission CLABSI toolkit, monograph, and infographic (see Figure 9-4, page 221).[5]

Toolkits provide value, as they combine evidence-based practices with practical tools for implementation. Examples are often taken from real-life experiences in actual health care settings. Many toolkits include communication tools to engage health care workers as well as data collection tools, checklists, charts to aid implementation, and evidence-based interventions. The blending of the "what" with the "how" is useful to the health care team.[6]

Figure 9-1. Evidence for Effectiveness of Face Masks

Evidence for Effectiveness of Masks

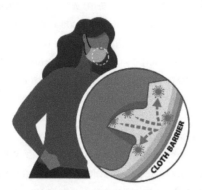

Masks are recommended as a simple barrier to help prevent respiratory droplets from traveling into the air and onto other people when the person wearing the mask coughs, sneezes, talks, or raises their voice. This is called source control. This recommendation is based on what we know about the role respiratory droplets play in the spread of the virus that causes COVID-19, paired with emerging evidence from clinical and laboratory studies that shows masks reduce the spray of droplets when worn over the nose and mouth. COVID-19 spreads mainly among people who are in close contact with one another (within about 6 feet), so the use of masks is particularly important in settings where people are close to each other or where social distancing is difficult to maintain. CDC's recommendations for masks will be updated as new scientific evidence becomes available.

Source: US Centers for Disease Control and Prevention (CDC). Guidance for Wearing Masks. Updated April 19, 2021. Accessed Jun 3, 2021. https://www.cdc.gov/coronavirus/2019-ncov/prevent-getting-sick/cloth-face-cover-guidance.html#

Figure 9-2. Messaging for Communicating Social Distancing

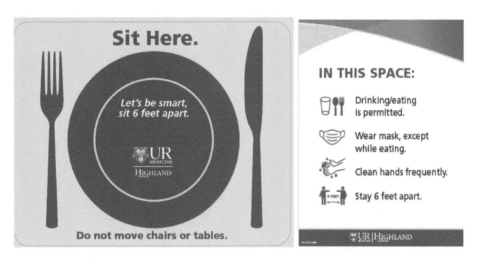

Source: University of Rochester, Highland Hospital, Rochester, NY. Used with permission.

Figure 9-3. Sample IPC Newsletter

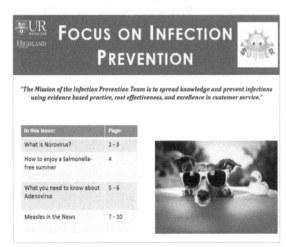

Source: University of Rochester, Highland Hospital, Rochester, NY. Used with permission.

Figure 9-4. CLABSI Prevention Infographic

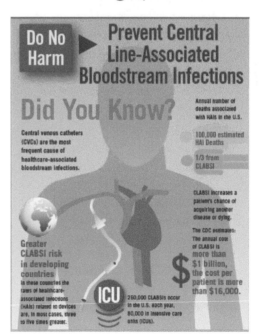

Source: The Joint Commission. *Central Line-Associated Bloodstream Infections Toolkit and Monograph.* Accessed Jun 3, 2021. https://www.jointcommission.org/resources/patient-safety-topics/infection-prevention-and-control/central-line-associated-bloodstream-infections-toolkit-and-monograph

Educating Patients, Residents, Families, and Visitors

Patients, residents, families, and visitors need to understand expectations and their responsibilities in preventing and controlling infection and how those are integrated with expected behaviors of health care workers and providers. Specific forms of IPC communication, such as newsletters, posters, electronic messages, and other printed materials, should be visible and available to individuals who enter the health care facility. This may include signage that reminds individuals to use hand hygiene and respiratory etiquette, and the organization may provide the tools to do so, such as face masks and alcohol-based hand sanitizer at entry points. Some organizations present patients with information packets upon entry to the facility; it is also important to ensure that the patient and/or patient advocate verbalizes understanding of the material. Using the teach-back method is an effective way to evaluate patient understanding. Health care workers may assess health literacy to understand the patient's ability to obtain, process, and understand basic health information. For a task that requires some psychomotor skills, such as hand hygiene, return demonstration is an important approach. The increasing popularity of telemedicine visits does not negate the need for this education. Patients can have real-time access to health care providers with opportunities to ask questions and obtain real-time feedback, and that access may be leveraged for education. Some patient education strategies that the IP can use to drive patient-centric care and engagement include the following[7]:
- Ascertaining the patient's health literacy
- Using a patient teach-back approach
- Offering educational materials in patient-preferred language and formats (such as signage, handouts, and other printed material)

The COVID-19 pandemic has heightened awareness of the importance of hand hygiene, respiratory etiquette, and masking to prevent and control the spread of infection. During the pandemic, the CDC not only stressed the importance of hand hygiene but issued guidance based on clinical and laboratory studies for wearing face masks to control transmission of the deadly virus. As part of infection prevention and control, the CDC recommends the following for patients, families, and visitors[8]:
- Wear masks with two or more layers to stop the spread of the SARS-CoV-2/COVID-19 virus.

- Wear the mask over your nose and mouth and secure it under your chin.
- Masks should be worn by people two years old and older.
- Masks should not be worn by children younger than two, people who have trouble breathing, or people who cannot remove the mask without assistance.
- It is not recommended that the general public wear masks intended for health care workers, such as, N95 respirators.

These guidelines are important in all health care settings, as other respiratory viruses, including influenza, continue to be a major concern.[9] As stated, infographics are effective tools to help educate patients, families, and visitors—particularly in ambulatory health care facilities and clinics. Figures 9-5 and 9-6 on page 223 show examples of infographics to educate patients and visitors in a variety of health care settings.

Reporting and Documenting Surveillance Within the Organization

As organizations move toward cultures of safety and high reliability, effective reporting and communication about IPC are vital.[10] This communication provides situational awareness that can help all health care providers understand the importance of IPC practices. To comply with standards on reporting infection prevention surveillance and prevention and control efforts to appropriate staff, IPs should report infection rates to leadership and care providers, according to the organization's IPC plan. This information may assist care providers in reducing or eliminating infections in ways that include, the following:
- Informing direct patient care providers about the number and identity of patient(s) who acquired particular infections, such as *Clostridioides/Clostridium difficile* infections on their units each month to track the impact of implementation strategies
- Providing information about processes and actions that protect against the spread of infection, such as hand hygiene or isolation precautions, to modify staff behaviors for improved compliance with an organization's IPC protocols

It is imperative that communication and education involve careful interpretation and analysis of data, recognition of discrepancies between policies and practices that may indicate patient or staff risk, and dissemination of

Figure 9-5. Flu Vaccine Poster

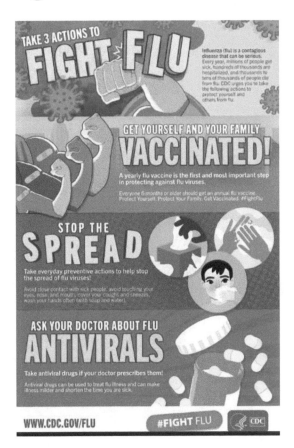

Source: US Centers for Disease Control and Prevention (CDC). Communication Resource Center. Accessed Jun 3, 2021. https://www.cdc.gov/flu/resource-center/index.htm

Figure 9-6. Clean Hands Count: Poster for Patients and Visitors

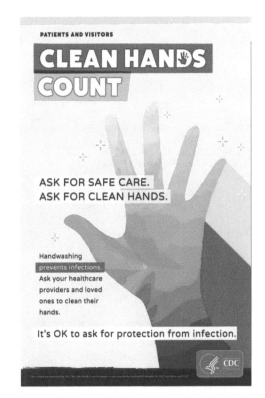

Source: US Centers for Disease Control and Prevention (CDC). Clean Hands Count Campaign. Accessed Jun 3, 2021. https://www.cdc.gov/handhygiene/campaign/index.html

information to appropriate stakeholders in an efficient, understandable, and comprehensive manner.

One of the key tasks of an IPC program is to turn data into information that can be shared with caregivers in a manner that improves practices and patient outcomes. Using data to quantify performance and reporting results is essential. Whether the objective is to improve outcomes (such as reduced catheter-associated urinary tract infections) or to improve a process of care (such as catheter insertion practices), data are central to evaluating the quality of health care. Data can help identify opportunities for improvement and can document the impact that systems-change interventions make on outcomes, such as on rates of health care–associated infections (HAIs). Measuring performance processes is critical to learning how the organization's practice

compares with best practices and how well implementation strategies are working.

When sharing data with stakeholders, it is important to display it in a meaningful manner. For example, the run chart in Figure 9-7, which shows the standardized infection ratio (SIR) for a hospital (observed/predicted), might be valuable to leadership for establishing organizational goals. The bar chart in Figure 9-8 provides surgical site infection data to monitor an outcome measure and may be helpful to the surgeon for practice improvement. The line graph in Figure 9-9 on page 225, which charts hand hygiene compliance, illustrates one way to monitor and communicate performance on key processes.

Displays of data help the infection control committee (ICC) and other stakeholders monitor outcomes and

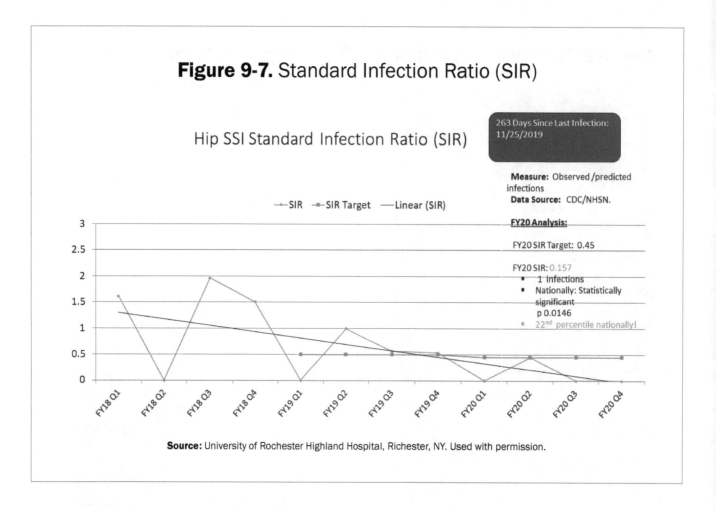

Figure 9-7. Standard Infection Ratio (SIR)

Hip SSI Standard Infection Ratio (SIR)

263 Days Since Last Infection: 11/25/2019

Measure: Observed /predicted infections
Data Source: CDC/NHSN.

FY20 Analysis:

FY20 SIR Target: 0.45

FY20 SIR: 0.157
- 1 infections
- Nationally: Statistically significant p 0.0146
- 22nd percentile nationally!

── SIR   ── SIR Target   ── Linear (SIR)

Source: University of Rochester Highland Hospital, Richester, NY. Used with permission.

Figure 9-8. Days Since Last Infection

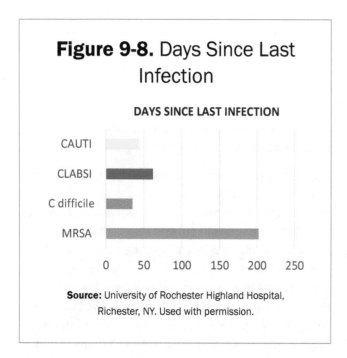

DAYS SINCE LAST INFECTION

Source: University of Rochester Highland Hospital, Richester, NY. Used with permission.

processes for improvement efforts and may drive new strategies for improvement. Tool 9-1 is a checklist that can be used to collect data on appropriate use of personal protective equipment.

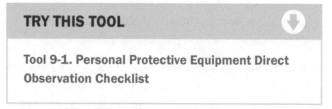

TRY THIS TOOL

Tool 9-1. Personal Protective Equipment Direct Observation Checklist

Disseminating Data

There are a variety of ways to communicate information about infection surveillance, prevention, and control to the appropriate staff. For example, in a setting that has an ICC, ICC members can communicate directly with staff. The ICC is typically composed of key leaders and staff members in the organization who are responsible for IPC program performance. These members use their expertise and experience to make recommendations for improvement. They also are responsible for sharing

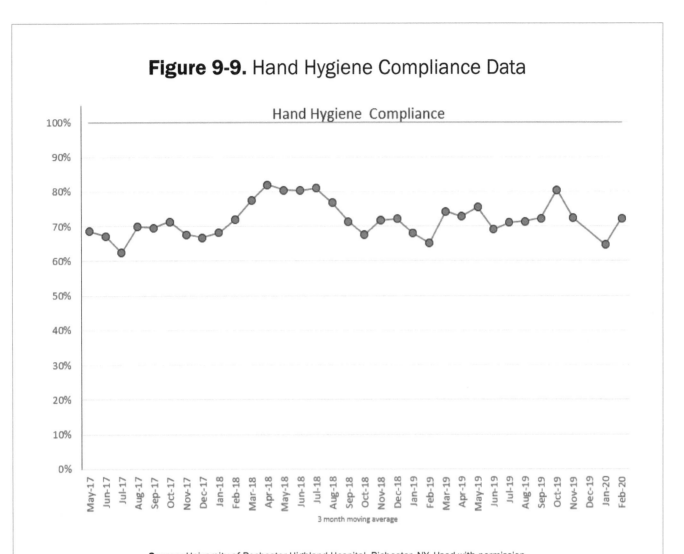

Figure 9-9. Hand Hygiene Compliance Data

Hand Hygiene Compliance

3 month moving average

Source: University of Rochester Highland Hospital, Richester, NY. Used with permission.

relevant data and information with staff in the departments they represent and with staff and physicians who provide direct patient care, where appropriate. The ICC team may actively review both process and outcome measures and may regularly request and review performance measures to directly or indirectly generate accountability. Clearly, communicating such results to senior management and throughout all levels of the organization is crucial to improvement success.

Important IPC information may be communicated both formally and informally. Table 9-1, on page 226, lists various communication types and methods and the advantages of each. Communication about the IPC program or a practice change may also be sent through a governance structure of several key committees, such as

a patient safety and quality improvement group, senior executives, or the governing body. Acute and long term care facilities—as well as specialized facilities such as dialysis centers and ambulatory surgery centers—may have specific task forces or committees dedicated to reducing specific infections (such as a CAUTI reduction task force in a hospital or a CLABSI reduction task force in a dialysis center). In the ambulatory health care setting, IPC data may be communicated through a quality group, as opposed to an ICC, which reviews overall patient safety data. Performance measures in clinics may include influenza immunization rates, communicable diseases in practices, environmental cleanliness assessments, and hand hygiene rates. Patient surveys on observations of health care worker and provider compliance are sometimes used in these settings.

Table 9-1. Communication Methods and Advantages of Each Type

Communication Types	Methods	Situations	Advantages
Direct verbal communication	1:1 verbal exchange Telephone information Meetings Unit rounds	When an important infection prevention and control–related issue needs an immediate response Unit huddles or debriefings—identified outbreak, increased incidence of rare organism Slide deck or other presentation at infection prevention, medical, or nursing staff meetings Rounding on units—device use Rounds	Ability to ask questions Opportunity to actively engage stakeholders Education in the moment Connects activities back to the patient Gives immediate feedback Promotes discussion
Policies, procedures, and guidelines	Policy or guideline development Infection prevention bundles Checklists	When a practice change or new evidence-based guideline is implemented When important information must be clearly detailed	Describes accountability Standardizes practice
Electronic communication	E-mail information Electronic reminders or alerts Internal websites with infection rates posted Screen saver messaging	When a practice change or new evidence-based guideline is implemented When important information must be clearly detailed	Describes accountability Standardizes practice Ideal for immediate messaging
Written newsletters or publications	Administrative dashboard information disseminated quickly	When information needs to be displayed	Can also be sent electronically
Educational presentations or offerings	Formal method to disseminate information in a structured manner	When new knowledge or information requires a structured approach	Structured approach

Joint Commission–accredited acute care hospitals, ambulatory surgery centers, long term care facilities, home care agencies, and other health care settings are required to collect data on a variety of HAIs and report on those data to staff and to public health authorities in accordance with law and regulation.[11] It is helpful to communicate national trends as well as local data. Valid, reliable, comparative data can be a powerful motivator for organizational change. Communication of both outcome and process measures associated with improved outcomes is an important part of a robust IPC program. Communication may be done by both formal and informal methods. Infection rates and data on compliance with evidence-based practices provide important information that can be used by staff to improve care.[12]

Providing feedback directly to physicians regarding specific outcomes, such as their own site infection rate, has been demonstrated to be effective in reducing HAIs.[13] This type of reporting can be helpful in improving compliance with recommended surgical bundles (see Tool 9-2). There are several tools available, including e-mail alerts, huddles, and debriefings. Significant events may be reviewed by a team using a tool such as the sample root cause analysis worksheet shown in Figure 9-10 on page 228. Clearly, timely communication to key stakeholders, including physicians and staff, about important IPC information is essential for identifying opportunities for improvement and a fundamental element of a well-functioning IPC program.

TRY THESE TOOLS

Tool 9-2. Root Cause Analysis Worksheet for CAUTIs

Tool 9-3. Infection Prevention Surgical Case Review (Colon Surgery)

Reporting and Communicating Outside the Organization

One of the most fundamental epidemiologic practices of an IPC program is reporting information regarding communicable diseases, such as tuberculosis (TB) or measles, to the local public health department. This reporting is essential in preventing the spread of such diseases to others in the community. Communicable disease reporting is required by law or regulation in all states and internationally. Over the past few decades,

there have been several emerging infectious diseases (EIDs) that have taken the global community by surprise and drawn new attention to EIDs, including those caused by H1N1, Ebola, Zika, and SARS-CoV-2 (COVID-19). These diseases underscore the need for timely and effective communication with local, state, and federal public health authorities.

Outbreaks that involve multidrug-resistant organisms also require prompt and thorough reporting and underscore the importance of working with local and state health care organizations. The CDC can assist in outbreak investigation, particularly if the severity in patient outcomes is significant and the source or cause of the outbreak is difficult to determine. Among its many activities, the CDC's Division of Healthcare Quality Promotion[14] investigates and responds to new and emerging infections related to adverse events among patients and health care workers. In addition, the CDC developed and maintains the National Healthcare Safety Network (NHSN), which provides health care facilities, states, regions, and the nation with data needed to progress prevention efforts to eliminate HAIs. Although local and state laws have required the reporting of communicable diseases and outbreaks for decades, what must be reported varies by state. In addition, some local regulators in international health care settings may also adopt or adapt the CDC NHSN definitions to guide surveillance methodology. IPs should become familiar with reporting requirements for their state and health care setting.

The US Centers for Medicare & Medicaid Services requires all acute care facilities to report HAIs through NHSN. A list of current or proposed reporting requirements can be found at http://www.cdc.gov/nhsn/PDFs/CMS/CMS-Reporting-Requirements.pdf.[15]

To remain compliant with local, state, and federal agency requirements, organizations should establish a methodology for continuously monitoring and identifying changes in reporting requirements so that practices are kept up-to-date. One strategy for accomplishing this is to subscribe to alerts, e-mails, newsletters, or professional societies, such as the Association for Professionals in Infection Control and Epidemiology. Reporting methods may also vary based on the location and the technological infrastructure of the organization. For example, many counties and international health care settings have electronic reporting mechanisms that include automatic reporting of communicable diseases through the

Figure 9-10. Sample Root Cause Analysis Worksheet

Topic: Catheter-Associated Urinary Tract Infections (CAUTIs) in Intensive Care Patients

What happened? (brief description)
Too many CAUTIs in the ICU (intensive care unit) in the first six months of 2020.

Why did it happen? (contributing factors)

+ factors **What prevented it from being worse?** Part of daily ICU rounds is to ask if urinary catheter in each patient was necessary.	- factors **What happened to cause the defect?** • All CAUTIs occurred when catheter was left in patient more than 6 days • Poor daily documentation of necessity • Breaking the contained system to place urimeter onto drainage system • Urine reflux (bags are not emptied when traveling off unit or mobilizing the patient) • Urine bag on floor • Inconsistent documentation regarding catheter care and securement • Not having all the supplies available on unit

What can we do to reduce the risk of it happening with a different person?

Action Plan	Responsible Person	Targeted Date	Evaluation Plan – How will we know risk is reduced?
Audit insertion procedure			
Ensure adequate catheter kits and extra catheters are available on the unit			
Standardize documentation for catheter care and securement			
Explore changing all catheters to urinometers			
Follow up with IT to understand catheter alerts and documentation expectation			

With whom shall we share our learning? (communication plan)

Who	When	How	Follow-up

Source: Adapted from https://www.ahrq.gov/professionals/education/curriculum-tools/cusptoolkit/toolkit/learndefects.html

laboratory system. These reports may be supplemented with a call or report to the local health department to provide specific patient details. Exposure tracking logs (Tool 9-4) can be used in a variety of settings to capture and report exposures to infectious diseases. Such logs can also be stored and emailed via a secure network.

TRY THIS TOOL

Tool 9-4. Infectious Disease Exposure Tracking Log

Transfer and Discharge Planning

Communicating treatment plans to prevent and control the spread of infection is required for patients and residents who require transfer to a different level of care at another facility (for example, rehabilitation, skilled nursing, or behavioral health and human services facility) or who may require hospitalization that provides comprehensive services unavailable at the transferring facility. Communicating preliminary or final laboratory test results from the transferring organization to the receiving organization, such as from blood or wound cultures including drug susceptibilities, can expedite delivery of appropriate antibiotic therapy, treatment, and barrier precautions for the patient or resident. The information communicated from the transferring agency should be directed to the internal staff at the receiving organization, who will distribute it to those who provide direct care for the patient or resident. This may include case managers, care navigators, or discharge planners who will assist with patient placement and subsequently steer the required medical care or treatment for the patient. The case manager or discharge planner is responsible for communicating any relevant information to the patient's or resident's attending physician and/or receiving health care facility. There are a number of ways to document this information; for example, an organization may document this via a note in the medical record. Some electronic medical records provide a forum for check sheets or templates that can be completed as part of the patient's medical record.

There are times when a laboratory result indicating infection in a patient is reported after the patient has been discharged from a health care facility. Generally, the laboratory is responsible for notifying the patient's provider. Communicating a positive laboratory result of a

bloodstream or wound infection to the patient's physician or receiving health care facility will expedite appropriate antibiotic treatment for the patient. This report may include information such as potential or actual infection that could require precautions to prevent and control the spread of infection (such as *Clostridioides/Clostridium difficile*) at the receiving facility. If the infectious organism is multidrug resistant, the facility may require contact precautions for the patient. In addition, the laboratory result may warrant notifying the local health department. In many localities, this information is electronically captured in a database accessed by local health departments. In these instances, the IP will also receive a copy of the information, particularly if there may have been exposure prior to discharge. It is important that these processes be identified in the organization's policies and procedures.

The IP may work with social workers and discharge planning to identify any new infections or issues. Any information communicated after discharge should be documented. Some organizations will maintain a log in the IPC department or with a case manager or other responsible party that documents the name of the receiving facility and the laboratory test or test result reported. Tool 9-5 is an example of a referral log for notifying a facility of a patient with an HAI.

TRY THIS TOOL

Tool 9-5. Referral Log of HAI Notification

Transitions and Handoff Communications

While investigating a possible HAI during routine surveillance, it sometimes becomes apparent that the infection originated at another health care organization. For example, a patient may have total hip arthroplasty at one facility but have incision and debridement of a subsequent surgical site infection at another facility. In this case, if the infection was unknown to the referring organization at the time of transfer, the referring organization would benefit from being informed of the diagnosis so it could then investigate other possible cases and interrupt further transmission of infection.

According to the NHSN rules and local and state mandatory reporting requirements, when routine surveillance identifies a surgical site infection in a patient where the initial surgery was performed at another facility, that facility should be notified of the infection. Reporting of the surgical site infection to the originating facility is important communication that assists with accurate postdischarge surveillance and accurate calculation of surgical site infection rates.

Patients and residents with a potentially communicable disease such as scabies or active TB are sometimes transferred to another facility. These infections must be communicated by the referring facility to the receiving facility. If, however, the initial assessment at a receiving facility reveals the patient has a potentially communicable condition, and the referring facility did not communicate this condition, then the receiving organization should notify the referring facility. For example, carbapenem-esistant *Enterobacteriaceae* laboratory findings from a culture collected on the day of admission from a patient who was recently transferred from another health care facility may trigger a call to the referring organization. The referring organization would benefit from being informed of the diagnosis so it could then investigate other possible cases and interrupt further transmission of this multidrug-resistant organism. The organization should identify a process to communicate such information. This communication may be by secure e-mail or phone contact. Many health care organizations keep a log of this communication, which can be made available for tracking purposes and to provide evidence of standards compliance during a survey process.

Given the constant flow of patients and residents between facilities and inpatient and outpatient settings, as well as within facilities, handoffs and transitions of care are vitally important. Transitions of care involve individual patients. They describe care when a patient moves from one level of care to another, from one institution to another, or from one system to another. One component of transitions of care is the patient handoff, which occurs outside a patient transition, such as during shift change. Handoffs refer to the interaction between health care workers when responsibility for patient care is transferred from one health care worker to another.[11] Ineffective transitions of care and poor handoff communication processes jeopardize patient safety and may result in adverse events, Thus, communication is vitally important. Every transition of care and handoff should involve steps designed to ensure that the transfer is safe, efficient, and effective. Having reciprocal arrangements with external organizations that frequently send or receive patients is important. For example, if a patient arrives at a hospital from a long term care facility with a noninfectious diagnosis and is identified on admission as having scabies, it is essential that the long term care facility be notified promptly. It is helpful to establish a communication process, particularly between the IPs or responsible parties in organizations that regularly transfer patients and residents between them. An agreement or understanding regarding a mutual reporting process to ensure consistency in practices and the flow of information will benefit the patient or resident and protect health care workers. Figure 9-11, below, is an example of medical care referral form used when a long term care resident is transferred to a hospital or an emergency department for treatment.

Figure 9-11. Medical Care Referral Form

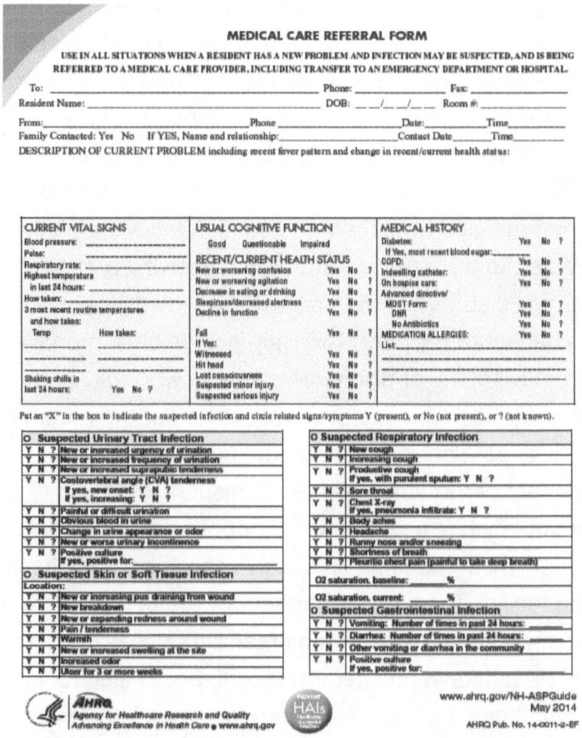

MEDICAL CARE REFERRAL FORM

USE IN ALL SITUATIONS WHEN A RESIDENT HAS A NEW PROBLEM AND INFECTION MAY BE SUSPECTED, AND IS BEING REFERRED TO A MEDICAL CARE PROVIDER, INCLUDING TRANSFER TO AN EMERGENCY DEPARTMENT OR HOSPITAL.

To: ____ Phone: ____ Fax: ____
Resident Name: ____ DOB: __/__/__ Room #: ____

From: ____ Phone ____ Date: ____ Time ____
Family Contacted: Yes No If YES, Name and relationship: ____ Contact Date ____ Time ____
DESCRIPTION OF CURRENT PROBLEM including recent fever pattern and change in recent/current health status:

CURRENT VITAL SIGNS	USUAL COGNITIVE FUNCTION	MEDICAL HISTORY
Blood pressure: ____	Good Questionable Impaired	Diabetes: Yes No ?
Pulse: ____	RECENT/CURRENT HEALTH STATUS	If Yes, most recent blood sugar: ____
Respiratory rate: ____	New or worsening confusion Yes No ?	COPD: Yes No ?
Highest temperature in last 24 hours: ____	New or worsening agitation Yes No ?	Indwelling catheter: Yes No ?
How taken: ____	Decrease in eating or drinking Yes No ?	On hospice care: Yes No ?
3 most recent routine temperatures and how taken:	Sleepiness/decreased alertness Yes No ?	Advanced directive/ MOST Form: Yes No ?
Temp / How taken:	Decline in function Yes No ?	DNR Yes No ?
	Fall Yes No ?	No Antibiotics Yes No ?
	If Yes:	MEDICATION ALLERGIES: Yes No ?
	Witnessed Yes No ?	List: ____
	Hit head Yes No ?	
Shaking chills in last 24 hours: Yes No ?	Lost consciousness Yes No ?	
	Suspected minor injury Yes No ?	
	Suspected serious injury Yes No ?	

Put an "X" in the box to indicate the suspected infection and circle related signs/symptoms Y (present), or No (not present), or ? (not known).

O Suspected Urinary Tract Infection	
Y N ?	New or increased urgency of urination
Y N ?	New or increased frequency of urination
Y N ?	New or increased suprapubic tenderness
Y N ?	Costovertebral angle (CVA) tenderness If yes, new onset: Y N ? If yes, increasing: Y N ?
Y N ?	Painful or difficult urination
Y N ?	Obvious blood in urine
Y N ?	Change in urine appearance or odor
Y N ?	New or worse urinary incontinence
Y N ?	Positive culture If yes, positive for: ____
O Suspected Skin or Soft Tissue Infection	
Location:	
Y N ?	New or increasing pus draining from wound
Y N ?	New breakdown
Y N ?	New or expanding redness around wound
Y N ?	Pain / tenderness
Y N ?	Warmth
Y N ?	New or increased swelling at the site
Y N ?	Increased odor
Y N ?	Ulcer for 3 or more weeks

O Suspected Respiratory Infection	
Y N ?	New cough
Y N ?	Increasing cough
Y N ?	Productive cough If yes, with purulent sputum: Y N ?
Y N ?	Sore throat
Y N ?	Chest X-ray If yes, pneumonia infiltrate: Y N ?
Y N ?	Body aches
Y N ?	Headache
Y N ?	Runny nose and/or sneezing
Y N ?	Shortness of breath
Y N ?	Pleuritic chest pain (painful to take deep breath)
O2 saturation, baseline: ____%	
O2 saturation, current: ____%	
O Suspected Gastrointestinal Infection	
Y N ?	Vomiting: Number of times in past 24 hours: ____
Y N ?	Diarrhea: Number of times in past 24 hours: ____
Y N ?	Other vomiting or diarrhea in the community
Y N ?	Positive culture If yes, positive for: ____

AHRQ Agency for Healthcare Research and Quality
Advancing Excellence in Health Care • www.ahrq.gov

www.ahrq.gov/NH-ASPGuide
May 2014
AHRQ Pub. No. 14-0011-2-EF

Source: Agency for Healthcare Research and Quality (AHRQ). Medical Care Referral Form. Accessed Jun 3, 2021. https://www.ahrq.gov/sites/default/files/wysiwyg/nhguide/4_TK2_T1-Medical_Care_Referral_Form.pdf

Summary

This chapter explores how communication and education continue to be significant factors affecting a health care organization's ability to detect, prevent, and mitigate infections. It discusses the need to inform and educate staff; licensed independent practitioners; and patients, residents, and their families about their roles and responsibilities in infection prevention and control. Also discussed is the increasing need to report infections, particularly those resulting in communicable diseases, HAIs, and emerging infectious disease outbreaks to appropriate authorities both internal and external to the organization. Communication about and documentation of infections are critical when transfering patients and residents from one care setting to another. Resources and downloadable tools are available to assist organizations in meeting these requirements across the continuum of care.

Resources

The following sections provide more information on this topic and can serve as a valuable reference in implementing measures to ensure a safe health care environment.

Tools to Try

Tool 9-1. Personal Protective Equipment Direct Observation Checklist

Tool 9-2. Root Cause Analysis Worksheet for CAUTIs

Tool 9-3. Infection Prevention Surgical Case Review (Colon Surgery)

Tool 9-4. Infectious Disease Exposure Tracking Log

Tool 9-5. Referral Log of HAI Notification

- Infection Prevention and Control Assessment Tool for Acute Care Hospitals. https://www.cdc.gov/infectioncontrol/pdf/icar/hospital.pdf

- Tool Kit for Reducing CAUTI in Acute Care Hospitals. https://www.ahrq.gov/hai/tools/cauti-hospitals/index.html

- The Targeted Assessment for Prevention Strategy (TAP). https://www.cdc.gov/hai/prevent/tap.html

- Billings C, et al. Advancing the profession: An updated future-oriented competency model for professional development in infection prevention and control. *Am J Infect Control.* 2019;47(6):602–614. Accessed May 20, 2021. http://www.sciencedirect.com/science/article/pii/S0196655319302317

- TeamSTEPPS. https://www.ahrq.gov/teamstepps/about-teamstepps/index.html

References

1. Centers for Disease Control and Prevention (CDC). Your Guide to Masks. Accessed Aug 10, 2020. https://www.cdc.gov/coronavirus/2019-ncov/prevent-getting-sick/about-face-coverings.html

2. Saitz R, Schwitzer G. Communicating science in the time of a pandemic. *JAMA.* 2020;324(5):443–44 4. doi:10.1001/jama.2020.12535.

3. Klompas M. Coronavirus disease 2019 (COVID-19): Protecting hospitals from the invisible. *Ann Intern Med.* 2020 May;172:619–620. https://doi.org/10.7326/M20-0751.

4. 3×3 Rule Plus 7×7 Rule to Reinforce Your Message. Accessed Dec 2, 2020. http://www.implementation-hub.com/articles/3X3_Rule_Plus_7x7_Rule.pdf

5. The Joint Commission. Central Line–Associated Bloodstream Infections Toolkit and Monograph. https://www.jointcommission.org/resources/patient-safety-topics/infection-prevention-and-control/central-line-associated-bloodstream-infections-toolkit-and-monograph

6. Barac R, et al. Scoping review of toolkits as a knowledge translation strategy in health. *BMC Med Inform Decis Mak.* 2014 Dec;14:121. https://doi.org/10.1186/s12911-014-0121-7

7. Patient Engagement Hit. 4 Patient Education Strategies That Drive Patient Activation. Accessed Jan 6, 2021. https://patientengagementhit.com/news/4-patient-education-strategies-that-drive-patient-activation

8. Centers for Disease Control and Prevention (CDC). Your Guide to Masks. Accessed Aug 10, 2020. https://www.cdc.gov/coronavirus/2019-ncov/prevent-getting-sick/about-face-coverings.html

9. Centers for Disease Control and Prevention (CDC). Frequently Asked Influenza (Flu) Questions: 2020–2021 Season. Accessed Jun 3, 2021. https://www.cdc.gov/flu/season/faq-flu-season-2020-2021.htm#anchor_1593184899499

10. Joint Commission Center for Transforming Health Care. High Reliability in Health Care Is Possible. Accessed Jun 3, 2021. https://www.centerfortransforminghealthcare.org/high-reliability-in-health-care/

11. Centers for Medicare & Medicaid Services (CMS), HHS. Medicare Program; Hospital Inpatient Prospective Payment Systems for Acute Care Hospitals and the Long-Term Care Hospital Prospective Payment System. Accessed Jun 3, 2021. https://www.govinfo.gov/content/pkg/FR-2019-05-03/pdf/2019-08330.pdf

12. Johnson JD, et al. Differences between formal and informal communication channels. *The International Journal of Business Communication* 1994;31(2):111–122. doi:10.1177/002194369403100202

13. Ko CY, et al. The American College of Surgeons National Surgical Quality Improvement Program: Achieving better and safer surgery. *Jt Comm J Qual Patient Saf*. 2015 May;41(5):199–2014.

14. Centers for Disease Control and Prevention (CDC). Division of Healthcare Quality Promotion (DHQP). Accessed Jun 3, 2021. https://www.cdc.gov/ncezid/dhqp/

15. Centers for Disease Control and Prevention (CDC). Healthcare Facility HAI Reporting Requirements to CMS via NHSN—Current or Proposed Requirements. Accessed Jun 3, 2021. http://www.cdc.gov/nhsn/PDFs/CMS/CMS-Reporting-Requirements.pdf.

Chapter 10

Occupational Health Issues

By Vicki Gillie Allen, MSN, RN, CIC, FAPIC

Disclaimer: Strategies, tools, and examples discussed in this book do not necessarily reflect Joint Commission or Joint Commission International requirements for all settings. Always refer to the most current standards applicable to your health care setting to ensure compliance.

Introduction

An occupational health program is essential to providing a safe work environment for health care workers and patients. The US Centers for Disease Control and Prevention (CDC) has identified several key elements in an effective occupational health program, including leadership and management, communication and collaboration, assessment, and education and training.[1] These elements drill down to focus on the infection prevention elements for standard precautions, staying home when ill, immunizations, and the response and management of potential infectious diseases and exposures. Collaboration among a health care organization's infection preventionist (IP), occupational health leaders, and other key stakeholders is necessary to implement and maintain a successful occupational health program.

Occupational health programs include a variety of activities designed to minimize health care workers' risk of exposure to infectious disease. These programs should work collaboratively with infection prevention and control (IPC) programs to ensure that health care workers are immune to communicable diseases that can be transmitted to patients. Protocols should be in place to promptly evaluate known or potential exposure risk to communicable diseases. An occupational health program should also have the capability to screen health care workers who may have been exposed to or who may have communicable disease(s).

The relationship between an IPC program and an organization's occupational health program varies, depending on the organization's reporting structures, patient or resident population, and services offered, as well as the prevalence of diseases in the surrounding community. In some facilities, occupational health may be assigned to the infection prevention professional. Depending on the setting, elements of an occupational health program that relate to IPC may include the following:

- Surveillance and assessments
- Immunization tracking and administration
- Education and training
- Exposure prevention and control
- Postexposure management
- Appropriate selection and use of personal protective equipment (PPE) or respirators
- Participation in outbreak investigations involving staff illness

The Joint Commission Infection Prevention and Control (IC) standards and the Joint Commission International (JCI) Staff Qualifications and Education (SQE) standards delineate what organizations must do to provide a safe work environment by preventing the transmission of infectious disease between patients and health care workers. This chapter explores some best practices, strategies, and actions health care organizations may take to help ensure compliance and patient and worker safety.

Preventing and Controlling Infectious Disease Transmission Among Patients and Staff

Joint Commission–accredited organizations are required to engage in activities that prevent the transmission of infectious disease among patients and health care workers. The following discussion describes some of the activities that IPs can use to help ensure compliance with these requirements, as they relate to occupational health.

There are two categories of infectious disease that may be targeted in meeting these standards: emerging and reemerging infectious diseases and vaccine-preventable diseases (VPDs). Occupational health is responsible for ensuring that health care workers are vaccinated against common vaccine-preventable diseases such as hepatitis B, mumps, measles, and influenza as well as screening and assessing health care workers for infections caused by emerging infectious disease, such as SARS-CoV-2 (COVID-19) and Ebola.

Emerging and Reemerging Infectious Diseases

Infectious diseases may emerge and result in outbreaks before transmissions can be controlled. Infection prevention and occupational health services professionals should stay informed of these outbreaks and evaluate the impact on their facility by assessing and screening health care workers. On January 5, 2020, the World Health Organization (WHO) provided a disease outbreak report citing cases of pneumonia—etiology unknown—in Wuhan City, Hubei Province of China, a city with a population of 19 million people.[2] The CDC followed on January 8, 2020, with recommendations for health care providers.[3] The CDC continues to provide routine updates and guidance on topics such as identification, assessment, and travel on its website and through the Health Alert Network (HAN).[4-6] By March 13, 2020, the US president declared a national emergency in response to the SARS-CoV-2 (also known as Novel Coronavirus 2019/COVID-19) pandemic.[7] State restrictions were imposed to close businesses, and shelter-in-place and stay-at-home orders were issued to limit the spread of COVID-19. All these events would have been tracked by an IP who would have appropriately screened and assessed health care workers through an occupational health program.

Developing a facility dashboard to track staff with confirmed work exposures to COVID-19 is one way to affect process outcomes. For example, while investigating a staffer exposed to COVID-19, the IP may determine if staff understand the policies and protocols related to PPE when caring for patients with known or suspected cases of SARS-CoV-2. By tracking and trending this type of data, the IP may identify the need for additional training and education when caring for these patients. Further collection and review of this data help determine the effectiveness of such an intervention. Reporting such data to the appropriate committees and stakeholders reinforces the need for data collection and interventions and validates its importance in protecting the organization's workforce.

Newly emerging pathogens, such as COVID-19, or new beliefs about adverse consequences of vaccines may affect the rate of VPDs. For example, in response to the national public health emergency and restrictions imposed by COVID-19, physician offices and medical clinics in some states were closed to routine visits. In May 2020, the CDC reported that fewer childhood vaccinations had been given.[8] Clinic closures have resulted in a decline in routine vaccinations, such as for measles, which in turn increases the risk for an outbreak of a VPD. As a preventive measure, facilities should implement processes to provide vaccines to their staff and patients. In addition, appropriate education should be given on the importance of routine vaccinations, particularly during a global pandemic.

Monitoring staff compliance, along with collecting and reporting staff VPDs, may be a component of an effective IPC plan. An example of periodic evaluation of the effectiveness of the plan for this component includes reporting staff VPD data to appropriate infection control committees in the organization, including an environment of care and safety committee, if applicable. As mentioned earlier, thorough review of such data can result in revision of protocols or additional staff education to address any trends identified.

The reemergence of VPDs, such as measles, continues to challenge clinicians. Literature from the CDC indicates that in the US in 2019, measles cases were at the highest level since 1992.[9] The CDC found that 89% of measles cases occurred in unvaccinated individuals or those who had an unknown vaccination status. The US experienced the highest number of measles cases reported since measles elimination was documented in the US (see Table 10-1 on page 236).[10]

The WHO has reported that immunizations could prevent approximately 2 to 3 million deaths annually from diseases such as diphtheria, tetanus, pertussis, influenza, and measles.[11] By maintaining a robust occupational health program, recommending or providing immunizations, and avoiding complacency about the threat of VPDs, health care organizations—both inpatient and outpatient settings—can avoid and prevent outbreaks that are becoming more of a threat in the US and internationally.[12] Also, a robust immunization program is a means to eliminate additional stress and strain on resources during a national public health emergency, such as the COVID-19 pandemic. It is important for occupational health staff and IPs to follow the most updated guidelines and best practice recommendations for VPDs applicable to the health care setting to prevent potential outbreaks and transmission of diseases such as influenza,[12] measles,[13] mumps,[14] and pertussis,[15] among others.

Some infectious diseases such as Ebola virus disease (EVD) continue with outbreaks in certain parts of the

Table 10-1. Measles Cases in the United States

Number of Measles Cases by Year Since 2010	
Year	Cases
2010	63
2011	220
2012	55
2013	187
2014	667
2015	188
2016	86
2017	120
2018	375
2019*	1,282

* Cases as of May 7, 2020. Case count is preliminary and subject to change. Data are updated monthly.

Source: US Centers for Disease Control and Prevention. Measles Cases and Outbreaks. Updated June 9, 2020. Accessed Aug 4, 2020. http:// www.cdc.gov/measles/cases-outbreaks.html

world.[16] Past outbreaks, including the 2003 Severe Acute Respiratory Syndrome (SARS) outbreak, highlight the role of health care workers in acquiring and transmitting diseases and emphasize the need for health care organizations (HCOs) to have plans to monitor, assess, and screen anyone entering the health care setting, including patients, visitors, and health care staff, to reduce potential for exposure and transmission.[16-18]

New and emerging infectious diseases, such as novel coronaviruses (SARS-CoV-1 and MERS-CV), hemorrhagic fever viruses (Lassa, Ebola), and highly pathogenic avian influenza A viruses (H5N1 and H7N9), are transmissible from person to person and carry a high mortality rate. It is important for the IP to maintain awareness of data on emerging infectious diseases and be able to verify that staff are following appropriate infection prevention and control measures to prevent exposure to and transmission of new and emerging infectious diseases. A definition of an exposure per pathogen may be approved by leadership to determine when an exposure has occurred, with implications for reporting to occupational health.

Exposure Prevention

During the 2014 Ebola outbreak, the lack of PPE and adequate health care worker training in the appropriate use of PPE placed some health care workers at higher risk for acquiring and transmitting infectious disease. And during the COVID-19 global pandemic, when nearly all hospitals have experienced the effects of COVID-19, shortages of PPE are of primary concern regarding how to best protect frontline health care workers caring for the hundreds of thousands of confirmed cases of COVID-19.[19] IPs should include emerging and reemerging infectious diseases in their facility's annual risk assessment and IPC plan and consider precautionary measures to protect health care workers. Collaboration with occupational health staff may help IPs implement processes—such as fit testing, proper donning and doffing of PPE, and compliance to VPDs—into the organization's IPC risk assessment and plan.

Health care workers and IPs must be provided with the appropriate tools and resources to prevent and control infectious diseases. The worldwide prevalence of novel diseases, such as COVID-19, should serve as a red flag to HCOs to ensure that full precautionary measures to protect health care workers are in place, including the following:

- An active immunization program that includes screening, tracking, and the need for vaccinations
- Education, training, and retraining to ensure competency on the most current guidance from professional organizations such as the CDC or WHO for specific infectious diseases, standard and transmission-based isolation precautions, and donning and doffing of PPE
- Provision of readily accessible and appropriate PPE, including appropriate use and reuse
- Contact with local and state departments of health for information. This is imperative to protect the health and well-being of all persons in the community, including patients, residents, families, and health care workers.

Local, state, and federal agencies are ideal resources for providing an IP with the tools, resources, and up-to-date evidence-based guidance necessary for managing new and emerging infectious diseases. To help mitigate risks to health care workers, an IP should understand the facility's

PPE supply chain, inventory, and usage rate and become familiar with tools and strategies made available through national, state, and professional organizations' websites to protect health care personnel.[20,21] In addition to availability and appropriate use of PPE, during the COVID-19 pandemic, health care workers also experienced physiological stress due to the long work hours, mental strain, and extended use of PPE. Organizational emergency plans should address health care worker educational needs as well as their physical and mental health needs during stressful situations to verify that appropriate protection measures are in place.[22] The involvement of IPs and frontline health care workers in a facility's emergency operations plan, drills, and exercises is one of the best ways to test that safeguards are in place and to identify gaps in facility protocols, procedures, and/or processes. (See the Resources section at the end of this chapter for CDC guidelines and resources on protecting health care personnel, as well as Chapter 5.)

Screening for Vaccine-Preventable Diseases in Health Care Organizations

Joint Commission and JCI standards are designed to help prevent transmission of VPDs from health care workers to patients/residents and vice versa. Preventing and controlling infection transmission requires proactively screening for exposure and immunity to assess facility transmission risks.

Health screenings are required for employees of Joint Commission– and JCI-accredited organizations. This requirement is located in the "Human Resources" (HR) chapter of the *Comprehensive Accreditation Manuals* and in the "Staff Qualifications and Education" chapter of the *JCI Accreditation Standards Manual*. Screenings should include general health questions, such as health history and vaccinations, and be made available to nonemployee physicians and other licensed independent practitioners. However, each organization may decide whether these screenings should be mandatory. When making this decision, organizations should consider any local or state requirements to which they must adhere. An effective occupational health program that offers vaccination is key to preventing infection among staff, patients, visitors, and others.

Screening has taken on a new meaning since the COVID-19 pandemic began. It became apparent early on that efforts to prevent and control transmission of COVID-19 within health care facilities would need to include screening of staff, visitors, and patients. Additionally, all persons who visit or have business with a health care facility, including students, volunteers, vendors, contractors, and so on, would need to be screened upon entry to prevent potential transmission of COVID-19. The CDC provides screening guidance and recommendations to health care organizations.[17]

> **TIP** Prevention and control of infection transmission between health care workers and others require proactive screening for exposure and immunity to assess facility transmission risks. Screening may need to extend beyond health care workers to patients and visitors, as demonstrated during the COVID-19 pandemic, during which active screening has consisted of one-to-one questions and temperature screening (self-reported and active checks) of all persons entering a health care facility to minimize transmission risks.

If the status of a health care worker puts others at risk of acquiring communicable diseases, the organization should provide or refer the worker for prophylaxis, treatment, counseling, or immunization to mitigate the risk. Health care workers exhibiting symptoms of infectious communicable disease should be referred to occupational health for evaluation within or outside the organization, depending on the specific communicable disease. Some communicable diseases such as COVID-19 require staff work restrictions. If quarantined, health care staff will need guidance on when it is safe to return to work. This also applies to diseases such as tuberculosis (TB), hepatitis B, varicella, pertussis, mumps, rubella, measles, and influenza.

To prevent and control the transmission of infectious diseases, an organization should document evidence of health care worker immunity to varicella, measles, mumps, and rubella. Immunization results and vaccination records should be easily accessible to organization personnel so that care staff can be appropriately assigned. In addition, having vaccine and immunity information easily accessible in the event of an exposure or an outbreak helps to efficiently implement appropriate measures to prevent and control further spread of disease and sickness.

Health care workers with the potential for blood or body fluid exposure should be immune to hepatitis B. The US Occupational Safety and Health Administration (OSHA) Bloodborne Pathogens (BBP) standard requires that employees who decline to accept the hepatitis B vaccine sign a statement of declination. Employees who decline may request and obtain the vaccination later at no cost. In addition, this vaccine should be made available after the employee has received the required OSHA BBP training and within 10 days of initial assignment.[23] Organizations should also have a process to identify and vaccinate employees whose job assignments and potential for exposure to blood or body fluids change. Most organizations take steps to ensure appropriate vaccination and immunity to these diseases as conditions of employment. In other words, if, upon testing, an employee is nonimmune, he or she is immunized as a condition of employment, unless contraindications to immunizations exist. Most organizations also allow exemptions for religious reasons.

For staff working with specific patient populations, such as neonates or children, the organization may wish to focus on screening and immunizations for staff to prevent and control infections that could jeopardize these patients. For example, because an infant younger than six months old cannot receive an influenza vaccination, a major prevention strategy for this age group is to immunize contacts, including families and health care workers. The Advisory Committee on Immunization

Practices (ACIP) recommends that health care workers receive an annual flu vaccine to protect patients and coworkers and to reduce staff absenteeism.[24]

The IP should be familiar with the screening and immunization policies and procedures for the organization and verify that they align with applicable state, local, and other government agency requirements, including the current recommendations issued by entities such as the CDC's ACIP[25] as well as other agencies. In situations such as the current COVID-19 pandemic in which a vaccine was first administered to frontline health care staff, it is important for IPs to collaborate with occupational health departments to ensure staff receive the appropriate information and education. An organization's information technology department may assist in helping to provide the data needed by IPs and occupational health teams to assess educational needs as well as appropriateness of organization policies and procedures. (See Sidebar 10-1 on page 239.)

Organizations should consider the various types of exposures that are known as well as those that can be anticipated for health care workers and have established policies, procedures, and plans to address them promptly. The organization's culture should not be punitive; it should encourage staff to report illness and not come to work when ill. These policies are an important part of an organization's infection prevention and control plan and should be developed collaboratively by infection prevention, occupational health, and human resources professionals in the organization. Assessed risks should be noted in an organization's safety analysis, which should be reviewed regularly. It is important for these plans to be in place and up to date before exposure events occur.

Consider this example: A health care worker sustains a sharps injury from a patient known to have a bloodborne pathogen. In this case, because time is of the essence (particularly if the pathogen is HIV), many facilities would use their emergency department after hours and have triage policies to ensure that exposed health care workers are assessed expeditiously.

Other facilities may have clinical staff on call who could respond immediately and provide phone counseling and assessment as well as order treatment by using established protocols and algorithms. If an organization does not have staff immediately accessible for exposure evaluation, there should be an arrangement with other facilities or the local health department to provide this

TIP Leaders and persons responsible for the IPC program should work closely with both human resources and occupational medicine departments or employee health services. These departments should set policies on the health screening and laboratory studies for both newly hired and current health care staff. In addition, these departments should work together to develop policies such as nonpunitive sick leave as well as guidelines to determine work-related versus community-related exposures, furloughs, and return-to-work policies and processes. These policies should reference the most current guidelines for infection control among health care staff.[14]

Sidebar 10-1.
Health Care Workers and Outbreak Exposure

As health care workers around the world continue to deal with Ebola and COVID-19, it has become clear that the next outbreak or pandemic is only a plane ride away.[58] However, exposures to vaccine-preventable diseases such as pertussis and measles can be avoided and controlled when organizations have surveillance and immunization response plans. When health care facilities are confronted with new or reemerging diseases, for which there may be no vaccine and much is unknown, they must rely on guidance from expert epidemiologists at organizations such as the US Centers for Disease Control and Prevention and World Health Organization to protect health care workers, patients, and the community. Current literature cites the increased risk to COVID-19 faced by health care workers as compared to the general public.[59] This risk is particularly high for health care workers who do not have access to appropriate personal protective equipment (PPE) and who must provide care to individuals with known or suspected cases of COVID-19 and Ebola. PPE availability, appropriate use, and reuse are critical to the safety and well-being of health care workers.[16,17,60] Health care organizations must prioritize procurement, education, use, and reuse of PPE for new and emerging infectious diseases in their infection prevention and control plans.

return-to-work protocols, and required documentation and reports. Communication between exposed persons and their supervisors is critical to maintain smooth operation within the organization.

When a health care worker is exposed to an infectious disease, it is important to be able to easily access immunization records to determine appropriate precautions, work restrictions, and so on. Having staff records and immunizations in an easily retrievable database can save an organization time and productivity hours.

Although some COVID-19 cases among health care workers have been linked to direct exposure at work, not all of them have been, highlighting the need for assessing, testing, immunizing, and counseling potentially infected staff during the pandemic. Until more is known about the SARS-CoV-2 virus, agencies and organizations such as the WHO,[27] CDC, and OSHA have advised and continue to advise and provide recommendations for health care staff to use standard, contact, droplet, and airborne precautions.[17,28] Despite the use of these precautions, the CDC noted in April 2020 that 9,282 COVID-19 cases in health care workers had been reported in the US. More than 90% of them were not hospitalized, but the remaining 10% were hospitalized in various stages, including intensive care, and several deaths were reported.[29] Health care workers must have access to and appropriately use PPE; this cannot be stressed enough. Recognizing that potentially highly communicable and virulent infectious diseases are only a plane ride away is an important step for organizations to be prepared on an ongoing basis. Health care works need education, training, and adequate available supplies.[30] The CDC provides guidance for donning and doffing PPE during the management of patients with EVD and COVID-19 in US hospitals.[31] Hospitals may develop their own protocols as well as training for appropriate staff.

In pandemic situations, such as COVID-19 and outbreaks such as Ebola, health care organizations should consider, at a minimum, holding daily huddles, incident command conference calls, or meetings to ensure that all departments are working together to protect and achieve patient and staff safety. In addition, organizations should have a means to identify workers who may have been exposed in pandemic and outbreak situations. IP and occupational health staff should work together, along with other organization staff, to develop policies, procedures, and plans that will be effective in identifying, handling, and reporting known and suspected exposures to

service. For those facilities where experts in exposure management are not available on site, the National Clinicians Post-Exposure Prophylaxis Hotline (PEP-Line) 888-448-4911 is available 11 a.m. to 8 p.m. Eastern Standard Time.[26]

To promptly address exposure risks, health care workers should be aware of signs, symptoms, and potential exposures that should prompt a phone call to occupational health or the IPC team.[15] Staff providing counsel to exposed health care workers should understand the organization's policies and procedures related to work restrictions, communicable illness and disease such as COVID-19. Federal, state, and local guidance and regulations should be referenced when establishing these documents. Contact tracing has been extremely important during the COVID-19 pandemic because identifying and monitoring all who may have been exposed to COVID-19 in the organization and the community is the only way to contain and prevent further transmission. Because of the complexity of contact tracing, it will likely be a shared responsibility between infection prevention teams and occupational health staff. In situations such as the current COVID-19 pandemic and community exposures, collaboration with local public health departments is essential. Staff who have been exposed should be advised and monitored for symptom development, potential quarantine, and return-to-work criteria. The IP and the organization's occupational health service should reference the CDC as well as state and local departments of health for the most up-to-date guidance for recommendations.[32]

State and Federal Agency Standards for Employee Safety

The Centers for Medicare and Medicaid Services (CMS) Condition of Participation (CoP) §482.42 for infection prevention states that a hospital must have an active hospitalwide program for the surveillance, prevention, and control of health care–associated infections and other infectious diseases.[33] Infection prevention and occupational health programs should incorporate the most up-to-date Joint Commission standards along with the CMS CoPs and appropriate state and federal laws and regulations for continuous program development. OSHA and state agencies generate regulations related to employee safety and infection transmission risk. For example, some states have requirements related to immunity for communicable diseases such as measles, mumps, and rubella.

OSHA, through its Bloodborne Pathogens standard (1910.1030),[23] requires that health care workers who have the potential for occupational exposure to blood or other potentially infectious material are offered the vaccination series against hepatitis B virus prior to engaging in activities during which they could be exposed. OSHA requires those who decline the vaccine to sign a declination form.[34] OSHA's website provides modules and tools for various health care settings that address bloodborne pathogens as well as the tuberculosis/respiratory protection standard (1910.134).[35,36] The tools outline potential hazards addressed in the standards

relative to health care settings and include model plans and programs and direct links to enforcement procedures.[36] Some states have their own occupational safety and health agency, whose requirements may differ from or be more stringent than those of OSHA.

Like OSHA, the Federal Needlestick Safety and Prevention Act (HR5178)[37] requires that frontline health care workers participate in selecting devices with engineered sharps safety protection and that all safety devices available be used, unless there is a patient or employee safety issue with the device.

The CDC also offers a comprehensive prevention workbook with tools and worksheets to assist those in occupational medicine and infection prevention in managing their entire sharps safety program.[38] In addition, the CDC provides helpful resources on its website for a comprehensive TB program.[39] This site provides guidelines, fact sheets, resource and educational materials, data, and statistics helpful for developing and maintaining a program that meets regulatory and many accreditation requirements.

In the current world of novel, communicable diseases and multidrug-resistant pathogens, it is critical for an IP to stay current and familiar with the latest evidence-based guidelines, recommendations, and requirements provided by the CDC, OSHA, the Environmental Protection Agency, and others to ensure the IPC program stays current and relevant.[40] (See the other websites listed in the Resources section at the end of this chapter.)

TIP An IPC program's annual risk assessment should include a review of occupational health experiences to identify any trends related to infection that should be addressed in the IPC plan. The annual review may include examination of occupational exposure data to VPDs as well as new and emerging diseases such as COVID-19, the facility sharps injury log, data on occupationally acquired or transmitted diseases, and information about community-acquired infections such as influenza identified in health care workers. A more in-depth discussion of risk assessment that may be incorporated into the overall IPC plan is provided in Chapter 3.

Support for Exposed Workers and Workers at Risk for Exposure

Sometimes, despite systems and practices to prevent exposures, patients or residents are exposed to infectious diseases in the health care setting. It is an organization's responsibility to provide appropriate care to a patient or resident after any exposure that may place the patient, resident, or, subsequently, his or her family or visitors at risk of acquiring an infectious disease.

Actions can be implemented to help mitigate the risk of exposure. For example, during the COVID-19 pandemic, the WHO[27] and CDC issued guidance to health care facilities for steps to provide source control and prevent acquisition and transmission of COVID-19. Some of the CDC guidance includes signage, screening, triage, and visitation restrictions.[17]

Postexposure management may include contact tracing, treatment, prophylaxis, counseling, and vaccination, as appropriate. Not only is addressing risk required when patients and residents are exposed to diseases such as TB, hepatitis B or C, varicella, pertussis, mumps, rubella, measles, and influenza, but it is also required when other transmissible infectious diseases are present for which no postexposure vaccine exists, such as blood and body fluid exposures, meningococcal meningitis, scabies, or novel and emerging pathogens, such as COVID-19 or H1N1 influenza. For example, even though there is currently no postexposure treatment for COVID-19, there are recommendations from the WHO[41] and CDC to monitor for symptom development for a period of time as well as to quarantine at home. For patients discharged following an exposure to a communicable disease and requiring home quarantine, the local or state department of public health may be involved as well. In this example, the department of health would be involved with the patient after discharge if the time period for home quarantine had not been met.[42]

> **TIP** It is a health care organization's responsibility to provide appropriate care to a patient or resident after any exposure that may place the patient, resident, or, subsequently, his or her family or visitors at risk of acquiring an infectious disease.

An IP may participate in developing and reviewing protocols for postexposure management of health care workers, patients, and residents. An IP should also collaborate with occupational health to ensure that those responsible for assessing exposed staff and other persons understand the protocols and are aware of the most current literature and recommendations surrounding postexposure management, vaccines, and prophylaxis.

To ensure consistent messaging, organizations may consider developing a script for use when counseling staff, patients, and others. Consistent messaging will ensure a standardized practice for the organization and is the best way to ensure that the right information is conveyed, laws are followed, and exposed persons have been informed of the risks from the exposure and the steps they should take to prevent an infection. For staff, patients, or residents, postexposure management should consider family members and visitors who may have been or could be at risk for secondary exposure. This is especially important during a pandemic in which no vaccine or postexposure treatment is available, and the pathogen is prevalent in the community.

An important issue for health care organizations is the accessibility of the occupational health staff or services for evaluating and caring for health care staff, patients, or residents. An organization's processes should address how evaluation and care would be identified and administered not only during occupational health office hours but after hours as well. This may occur through the emergency department, a central location off site from the organization, and through designated facility leaders. When a patient needs to be followed, the patient's primary care physician should be informed and involved in the evaluation and care.

Staff Vaccine and Immunization Programs

At minimum, health care organizations should offer vaccination against influenza to licensed independent practitioners and staff. A vaccination and immunization program not only helps to identify staff at risk for exposure to and possible transmission of VPDs but also may be integrated into an organization's overall program for quality improvement and patient safety, using measures epidemiologically important to the organization.

Annual vaccination for influenza is commonly acknowledged as a way to preserve both staff and patient or resident safety. The CDC, ACIP, and the Healthcare Infection Control Practices Advisory Committee all recommend the annual influenza vaccination for health care workers as a patient safety measure to prevent the transmission of influenza from health care workers to others.[43] During the 2018–2019 season, the CDC reports that flu vaccine coverage was highest in health care staff working in hospitals, at 95.2%, and highest in health care staff working in settings where the vaccine was required, at 97.7%.[44] Overall, during the 2018–2019 flu season, 81% of health care workers obtained the flu vaccine. Mandatory influenza vaccines were first endorsed in 2005 by professional societies and organizations, including the Society for Healthcare Epidemiology of America,[45] the Association for Professionals in Infection Control and Epidemiology,[46] and the Infectious Diseases Society of America,[47] to promote annual vaccination of health care workers as a means to improve patient safety. Since then, more than 1,000 professional organizations have come on board to promote and recognize the importance of annual flu vaccines for health care workers and patients.[48]

Annual influenza vaccination of health care workers continues to be challenging in some health care settings, including long term care, ambulatory care, and physician offices. The WHO and CDC provides toolkits that leaders can use to help increase compliance with flu vaccination in these settings.[49] International health care settings should follow their local regulations for reporting requirements.

Organizations should demonstrate that they have an annual influenza vaccination program that includes licensed independent practitioners and staff. This may be demonstrated by addressing the annual immunization program and the vaccination acceptance rates in the annual IPC plan. In addition, for some health care settings, CMS requires that influenza vaccinations be reported to CMS annually for health care workers, licensed independent practitioners, students, and volunteers. Organizations with a separate CMS certification number are required to report influenza vaccines for any paid, contract, volunteer, or student personnel having worked in the facility for one day between October 1 and March 31. Changes to reporting health care staff influenza vaccinations occurred in 2018, with reporting not required for certain health care facilities such as hospital outpatient and ambulatory surgical centers, among others.[50]

The IP has a pivotal and ongoing role in providing guidance and assistance to the occupational health service and organization leadership to develop and establish a proactive immunization program. This may involve providing literature, developing policies, developing and participating in education, and analyzing data with the occupational health service.

The IP's Role in Educating Staff

IPs should take a proactive role and collaborate with educators and occupational health staff within the organization to educate health care workers on multiple aspects of influenza, including the following:

- Diagnosis
- Transmission
- Disease impact on patients or residents, health care workers, and the community (morbidity and mortality)
- Influenza prevention measures that highlight appropriate use of PPE
- Dispelling of myths associated with influenza and the influenza vaccine (which may be the most challenging aspect of the educational effort)

Many options and tools are available for education, including posters, brochures, fact sheets, videos, webcasts, and podcasts from the CDC, local or state health departments, the WHO, and many other professional organizations (see the Resources section at the end of this chapter). In addition to external resources, internal resources such as intranet and Web-based programs can be developed. One-on-one education during rounds on units and in departments throughout the organization can also be effective. Organizations may incorporate a section on educational programs for health care workers in their IPC plan.

The IP should consider challenges and conflicts regarding influenza vaccination that may occur during an outbreak such as the COVID-19 pandemic. At the time of this writing, the CDC recommends deferring the flu vaccine for persons with suspected or confirmed COVID-19 until certain criteria have been met.[51] Information related to contingencies such as this should be considered and incorporated into the organization's IPC program, along with consent and screening forms.

If compliance with the influenza vaccine program is problematic and draws lower-than-desired rates in an organization, an IP may wish to perform a survey or convene a focus group of key staff to determine the barriers to acceptance of the vaccine. The information gained from these activities can be merged into future educational efforts or approaches to vaccine administration. Tool 10-1 provides some questions the IP may ask to assess staff immunizations in his or her facility. Answers to these questions may help inform compliance efforts.

TRY THIS TOOL

Tool 10-1. Sample Health Care Worker Influenza Vaccine Survey

> **TIP** Facility television and computer screen savers can communicate information on IPC practices such as hand hygiene, influenza vaccination, universal masking, and social distancing necessary for health care staff, patients, and visitors. IPs can work with facility marketing departments to develop appropriate methods and messaging.

Providing Access to Vaccines and Addressing Barriers

One possible barrier to immunization is staff not having access to the flu vaccine. This may occur when the vaccine is administered off-site from the primary work setting, only during occupational health office hours, which do not include evening or weekend hours, or only during certain months of the year.

One strategy for addressing this barrier is to provide the influenza vaccine at the point of care, such as by taking a cart with the vaccine and related supplies to clinical and support units or providing immunization at a convenient entry and exit point for staff, such as the employee entrance and/or time clock check-in points. Contracting with outside pharmacies is another way an organization can make the flu vaccine available to staff. It may be easier for health care workers to visit an off-site retail office or space. This eliminates the need for workers to come to the occupational health department to receive the vaccine.

Another approach is to provide the vaccine to a designated staff member on each unit, who can then

administer the vaccine to coworkers and others. Departmental and other meetings held during the influenza season can be an opportunity to vaccinate multiple staff in one convenient setting. Some organizations have expanded the weeks or months for administering the vaccine to improve vaccination rates.

> **TIP** Some organizations take advantage of the need to annually vaccinate health care workers for influenza as a way to test their mass vaccination capabilities. They choose a one- to two-day period to vaccinate as many staff as possible, thus also testing their emergency management system's ability to provide mass vaccination or prophylaxis in the event of a pandemic or bioterrorism event.

Goals and Methodology for Improving Vaccination Rates

Health care organizations' written IPC plans should incorporate goals that address prioritized risks for influenza, unprotected exposure to influenza, and methods to limit transmission of influenza in the organization. An IPC plan should also include a specific goal of improving influenza vaccination rates. The CDC provides strategies and evidence-based guidance to increase influenza vaccine acceptance, which includes hosting and resources for vaccination clinics. The benefits to the organization and the employees cannot be overlooked.[52] (See Tool 10-2 for effective approaches to increasing influenza vaccination rates.)

TRY THIS TOOL

Tool 10-2. Effective Approaches to Increasing Influenza Vaccination Rates

Tracking vaccination rates of contracted staff may occur separately from tracking of other organization health care personnel.[53] Documenting the methodology to determine influenza vaccination rates in the organization's IPC plan is one way to ensure compliance with the organization's requirements (see http://www.qualityforum.org/Home.aspx).[54]

Understanding Declination

The Joint Commission and JCI require that accredited organizations evaluate why staff do not receive the influenza vaccination. This may involve calculating vaccination rates and surveying health care workers about why they do not get vaccinated. Many organizations calculate rates of vaccine administration either overall for the organization or by various clinical or support units. Some analyze gender, profession, work shift, work setting, and other variables to get a precise picture of where there is an opportunity for improvement. It is important to note that these data may not be exact because some health care workers get their immunizations elsewhere. There should be a process to "credit" health care personnel when they get vaccines in other locations. Using sites such as Vaccine Finder allows staff to search for providers that may be more convenient and that offer seasonal influenza as well as other vaccines.[55] The Immunization Information System is a confidential, population-based computer information database that records vaccines submitted by participating providers. This system allows communities to identify populations at risk and to implement appropriate actions and interventions.[56] Information collected can then be used to target educational programs to improve vaccination acceptance. Therefore, having a method to also track health care workers immunized outside the organization can help ensure accurate vaccination rates. The National Quality Forum Measure Submission and Evaluation Worksheet 5.0 provides recommendations for the numerator and denominator.[54]

A health care organization can document reasons that staff decline the vaccine using a declination form for those who are eligible for but refuse the vaccine. This form can note receipt of the vaccine elsewhere, as many health care workers, particularly physicians, work at other facilities where they may have been immunized or are vaccinated by their personal physician or at another community site. The declination form should provide reasonable options for declining the vaccine. Download Tool 10-3 for a sample declination survey form.

TRY THIS TOOL

Tool 10-3. Declination Survey Form for Influenza Vaccination

Improving and Reporting Vaccination Rates

To improve vaccination rates according to its established goals, organizations should collect and analyze influenza immunization data and document and compare it to the goals in the annual IPC plan. Data analysis allows the organization to identify patterns and trends and to monitor its performance. The IP should provide data analysis and updates to organization leaders, committees, and councils, including recommendations for improving vaccination rates, when planning for the next influenza season.

Documentation can be reflected in the annual IPC risk assessment, plan, and evaluation. For more information, refer to Joint Commission Performance Improvement (PI) Standards PI.02.01.01 and PI.03.01.01 for compiling and analyzing data and to the Joint Commission document "Providing a Safer Environment for Health Care Personnel and Patients Through Influenza Vaccination: Strategies from Research and Practice" at https://www.jointcommission.org/-/media/tjc/documents/resources/hai/flu_monograph.pdf.[57]

There are many ways for an organization to communicate influenza vaccination data to key stakeholders. For example, an effective way is to create and use a dashboard of key infection performance indicators that is updated and provided monthly. The organization should add influenza vaccination data, including analysis, to this dashboard periodically throughout the current influenza season and at the end of the season. It should incorporate feedback and recommendations from key stakeholders into the IPC plan to guide recommendations for improvement. Organization newsletters and staff meetings are other ways to communicate influenza vaccination rate data and the effect(s) on patient or resident safety. Some recommended activities that may help an organization meet occupational health-related requirements are listed in Sidebar 10-2.

Summary

This chapter provides an overview of the infection prevention and control issues and strategies that relate to occupational health. It discusses the importance of screening and vaccinating health care workers for specific infectious diseases as well as responding to the needs of staff, patients, and residents who are infected or potentially infected. The ongoing occurrence of new and emerging infectious diseases continues to highlight the importance of protecting the health care worker and the patient/resident against infection as well as preventing and controlling subsequent transmission of infectious diseases to everyone including health care workers, patients, residents, visitors, and others. Prevention efforts, including availability, selection, and use of PPE; exposure management; and immunizations and vaccinations to prevent the spread of pathogens during infectious outbreaks are key areas of focus for IPC as it relates to occupation health and safety. Health care organizations must have plans and measures to mitigate potential harm to staff and patients. Staff and patients should be educated routinely on the importance of these prevention and control efforts. This chapter emphasizes risk assessment, planning, monitoring, and communicating to better protect patients, residents, and health care workers from infectious disease.

Resources

The following sections provide more information on this topic and can serve as a valuable reference in preserving occupational health and safety. The following tools can be accessed online:

Tools to Try
Tool 10-1. Health Care Worker Influenza Vaccine Survey

Tool 10-2. Effective Approaches to Increasing Influenza Vaccination Rates

Tool 10-3. Declination Survey Form for Influenza Vaccination

- Infection Prevention and You. PPE Do's & Don'ts. Accessed Aug 21, 2020. https://professionals.site.apic.org/infographic/ppe-dos-and-donts/

- US Centers for Disease Control and Prevention. Coronavirus 2019 (COVID-19). Optimizing Personal Protective Equipment (PPE) Supplies. Updated Jul 16, 2020. Accessed Aug 21, 2020. https://www.cdc.gov/coronavirus/2019-ncov/hcp/ppe-strategy/index.html

- US Centers for Disease Control and Prevention. The National Institute for Occupational Safety and Health (NIOSH). Emergency Response Resources. Personal Protective Equipment. Updated Nov 30, 2018. Accessed Aug 21, 2020. https://www.cdc.gov/niosh/topics/emres/ppe.html

Additional Readings

- Association for Professionals in Infection Control and Epidemiology (APIC). Accessed Aug 21, 2020. https://apic.org/

- APIC. Infection Prevention and You. Accessed Aug 21, 2020. https://professionals.site.apic.org/

- APIC. Position Paper: Influenza Vaccination Should Be a Condition of Employment for Healthcare Personnel, Unless Medically Contraindicated. Accessed Aug 21, 2020. http://www.apic.org/Resource_/TinyMceFileManager/Advocacy-PDF s/APIC_Influenza_Immunization_of_HCP_12711.PDF

- US Centers for Disease Control and Prevention (CDC). Accessed Jan 5, 2017. http://www.cdc.gov.

- CDC. Protecting Healthcare Personnel. Accessed Aug 21, 2020. https://www.cdc.gov/HAI/prevent/ppe.html

- CDC. Health care workers, occupational health, and other infection prevention guidelines. Updated October 28, 2019. Accessed Aug 21, 2020. https://www.cdc.gov/infectioncontrol/guidelines/healthcare-personnel/index.html

- CDC. Influenza. Updated Aug 21, 2020. Accessed Aug 21, 2020. https://www.cdc.gov/Flu/Index.htm

- CDC. Tuberculosis in Health Care Settings. Accessed Aug 21, 2020. https://www.cdc.gov/hai/organisms/tb.html

- Advisory Committee on Immunization Practices (ACIP). Updated Aug 20, 2020. Accessed Aug 21, 2020. http://www.cdc.gov/vaccines/acip/index.html

- CDC. Recommended Vaccines for Healthcare Workers. Accessed Aug 21, 2020. https://www.cdc.gov/vaccines/adults/rec-vac/hcw.html

- CDC. Prevention. Influenza (FLU). HCP Fight Flu Toolkit. Updated Aug 12, 2020. Accessed Aug 21, 2020. https://www.cdc.gov/flu/professionals/vaccination/prepare-practice-tools.htm

- Joint Commission Resources. Accessed Jan 5, 2017. http://www.jcrinc.com.

- The Joint Commission. Infection Prevention and Control. Accessed Aug 21, 2020. https://www.jointcommission.org/resources/patient-safety-topics/infection-prevention-and-control/

- The Joint Commission. Standards Interpretation FAQs. https://www.jointcommission.org/standards/standard-faqs/

- National Emerging Special Pathogens Training and Education Center (NETEC). NETEC Resource Library. Accessed Oct 2, 2020. https://repository.netecweb.org/

- National Federation for Infectious Diseases (NFID). Accessed Aug 21, 2020 http://www.nfid.org.

- NFID. Annual Flu Immunization Campaigns and Links to Additional Information. Accessed Aug 21, 2020. https://www.nfid.org/infectious-diseases/influenza-flu/

- Occupational Safety and Health Administration (OSHA). Accessed Aug 21, 2020. http://www.osha.gov.

- OSHA. Health Care-wide Hazards. Accessed Aug 21, 2020. https://www.osha.gov/SLTC/etools/hospital/hazards/sharps/sharps.html

- US Department of Labor. Coronavirus Resources. Accessed Aug 21, 2020. https://www.dol.gov/coronavirus

- OSHA. Tuberculosis. Accessed Aug 21, 2020. https://www.osha.gov/SLTC/etools/hospital/hazards/tb/tb.html

- Society for Healthcare Epidemiology of America (SHEA). Accessed Aug 21, 2020. http://www.shea-online.org/

- World Health Organization (WHO). Accessed Aug 21, 2020. https://www.who.int/

- WHO. Coronavirus. Accessed Aug 21, 2020. https://www.who.int/emergencies/diseases/novel-coronavirus-2019

- WHO. Influenza. Accessed Aug 21, 2020. https://www.who.int/health-topics/influenza-seasonal#tab=tab_1

References

1. US Centers for Disease Control and Prevention. Infection Control in Healthcare Personnel: Infrastructure and Routine Practices for Occupational Infection Prevention and Control Services (2019). Accessed Aug 21, 2020. https://www.cdc.gov/infectioncontrol/guidelines/healthcare-personnel/

2. World Health Organization. Pneumonia of Unknown Cause—China. Jan 5, 2020. Accessed Aug 8, 2020. https://www.who.int/csr/don/05-january-2020-pneumonia-of-unkown-cause-china/en/

3. US Centers for Disease Control and Prevention. Outbreak of Pneumonia of Unknown Etiology (PUE) in Wuhan, China. *Health Alert Network*. Jan 8, 2020. Accessed Aug 8, 2020. https://emergency.cdc.gov/han/han00424.asp

4. US Centers for Disease Control and Prevention. Update and Interim Guidance on Outbreak of 2019 Novel Coronavirus (2019-nCoV). Feb 1, 2020. Accessed Aug 8, 2020. https://emergency.cdc.gov/han/han00427.asp

5. US Centers for Disease Control and Prevention. Health Alert Network. Accessed Aug 8, 2020. https://emergency.cdc.gov/han/

6. US Centers for Disease Control and Prevention. Coronavirus (COVID-19). Accessed Aug 8, 2020. https://www.cdc.gov/coronavirus/2019-nCoV/index.html

7. Biden JR, Jr. Notice of the Continuation of the National Emergency Concerning the Coronavirus Disease 2019 (COVID-19) Pandemic. Accessed Jun 3, 2021. https://www.whitehouse.gov/briefing-room/presidential-actions/2021/02/24/notice-on-the-continuation-of-the-national-emergency-concerning-the-coronavirus-disease-2019-covid-19-pandemic/

8. US Centers for Disease Control and Prevention. Effects of the COVID-19 Pandemic on Routine Pediatric Vaccine Ordering and Administration—United States 2020. MMWR. 2020 May;69(19):591–593. Accessed Aug 4, 2020. https://www.cdc.gov/mmwr/volumes/69/wr/mm6919e2.htm?s_cid=mm6919e2_w

9. US Centers for Disease Control and Prevention. National Update on Measles Cases and Outbreaks—United States, January 1–October 1, 2019. MMWR. 2019 Oct;68(40):893–896. Accessed Aug 4, 2020. https://www.cdc.gov/mmwr/volumes/68/wr/mm6840e2.htm

10. US Centers for Disease Control and Prevention. Measles Cases and Outbreaks. Updated Jun 9, 2020. Accessed Aug 4, 2020. https://www.cdc.gov/measles/cases-outbreaks.html

11. World Health Organization (WHO). Vaccines and Immunizations. 2020. Accessed Dec 21, 2020. https://www.who.int/health-topics/vaccines-and-immunization#tab=tab_1

12. World Health Organization (WHO). Immunizations, Vaccines and Biologicals. How to Implement Seasonal Influenza Vaccination of Health Workers. Accessed Dec 21, 2020. https://www.who.int/immunization/documents/ISBN_9789241515597/en/

13. US Centers for Disease Control and Prevention. Interim Infection Prevention and Control Recommendations for Measles in Healthcare Settings. Updated Jul 19, 2019. Accessed Aug 8, 2020. https://www.cdc.gov/infectioncontrol/guidelines/measles/index.html

14. US Centers for Disease Control and Prevention. Recommendation of the Advisory Committee on Immunization Practices for Use of a Third Dose of Mumps Virus-Containing Vaccine in Persons at Increased Risk for Mumps During an Outbreak. *MMWR*. 2018 Jan;67(1):33–38. Accessed Aug 8, 2020. https://www.cdc.gov/mmwr/volumes/67/wr/mm6701a7.htm

15. US Centers for Disease Control and Prevention. Guideline for infection control in health care personnel, 1998. *Am J Infect Control*. 1998;26:289–354. Accessed Aug 8, 2020. https://www.cdc.gov/hicpac/pdf/infectcontrol98.pdf

16. US Centers for Disease Control and Prevention. Ebola (Ebola Virus Disease). 2020 Democratic Republic of the Congo Equateur Province (Ongoing). Jun 25, 2020. Accessed Aug 8, 2020. https://www.cdc.gov/vhf/ebola/outbreaks/drc/2020-june.html

17. US Centers for Disease Control and Prevention. Coronavirus Disease 2019 (COVID-19). Interim Infection Prevention and Control Recommendations for Healthcare Personnel During the Coronavirus Disease 2019 (COVID-19) Pandemic. Updated Jul 15, 2020. Accessed Aug 8, 2020. https://www.cdc.gov/coronavirus/2019-ncov/hcp/infection-control-recommendations.html

18. US Department of Health and Human Services. Office of Inspector General. Emerging Infectious Disease Preparedness & Response. Updated Mar 24, 2021. Accessed Apr 17, 2021. https://www.oig.hhs.gov/reports-and-publications/featured-topics/infectious-disease/

19. World Health Organization. WHO Coronavirus Disease (COVID-19) Dashboard. Updated on Aug 8, 2020. Accessed on Aug 8, 2020. https://covid19.who.int/

20. US Centers for Disease Control and Prevention. Coronavirus Disease 2019 (COVID-19). Summary Strategies for Optimizing the Supply of PPE during Shortages. Updated Jul 16, 2020. Accessed Aug 8, 2020. https://www.cdc.gov/coronavirus/2019-ncov/hcp/ppe-strategy/strategies-optimize-ppe-shortages.html

21. Environmental Protection Agency (EPA). Coronavirus (COVID-19) Resources for State, Local and Tribal Agencies and Associations. Updated Jul 23, 2020. Accessed Aug 8, 2020. https://www.epa.gov/coronavirus/coronavirus-covid-19-resources-state-local-and-tribal-agencies-and-associations

22. US Centers for Disease Control and Prevention. Coronavirus Disease 2019 (COVID-19). The Physiological Burden of Prolonged PPE Use on Healthcare Workers During Long Shifts. Updated Aug 7, 2020. Accessed Aug 8, 2020. https://blogs.cdc.gov/niosh-science-blog/2020/06/10/ppe-burden/

23. US Occupational Safety and Health Administration. Occupational Exposure to Bloodborne Pathogens: Final Rule: 29 CFR Part 1910. Accessed Aug 9, 2020. https://www.osha.gov/laws-regs/regulations/standardnumber/1910/1910.1030

24. US Centers for Disease Control and Prevention. Influenza Vaccination Coverage Among Health Care Personnel—United States, 2018–19 Influenza Season. Accessed Aug 9, 2020. https://www.cdc.gov/flu/fluvaxview/hcp-coverage_1819estimates.htm

25. US Centers for Disease Control and Prevention. Vaccine Recommendations and Guidelines of the ACIP. Accessed Aug 9, 2020. https://www.cdc.gov/vaccines/hcp/acip-recs/index.html

26. National Clinician's Post-Exposure Prophylaxis Hotline. Accessed Aug 15, 2020. https://aidsetc.org/aetc-program/national-clinician-consulation-center#:~:text=Post%2DExposure%20Prophylaxis%20Hotline%20(PEPline,(seven%20days%20a%20week)

27. World Health Organization (WHO). Transmission of SARS-CoV-2: Implications for Infection Prevention Precautions. Accessed Dec 21, 2020. https://www.who.int/publications/i/item/modes-of-transmission-of-virus-causing-covid-19-implications-for-ipc-precaution-recommendations

28. US Occupational Safety and Health Administration. Healthcare Workers and Employers. Accessed Aug 9, 2020. https://www.osha.gov/SLTC/covid-19/healthcare-workers.html

29. US Centers for Disease Control and Prevention. *Morbidity and Mortality Weekly Report* (MMWR) Characteristics of Healthcare Personnel with COVID-19—United States, February 12–April 9, 2020. *MMWR*. 2020 Apr;69(15):477–481. Accessed Aug 9, 2020. https://www.cdc.gov/mmwr/volumes/69/wr/mm6915e6.htm

30. Weber DJ, et al. Protecting healthcare personnel from acquiring Ebola virus disease. *Infect Control Hosp Epidemiol*. 2015 Oct;36(10):1229–1232. Accessed Aug 15, 2020. https://www.ncbi.nlm.nih.gov/pmc/articles/PMC5656048/

31. US Centers for Disease Control and Prevention. Ebola (Ebola Virus Disease). Guidance for Donning and Doffing Personal Protective Equipment (PPE) During Management of Patients with Ebola Virus Disease in U.S. Hospital. Updated Aug 30, 2018. Accessed Aug 15, 2020. https://www.cdc.gov/vhf/ebola/healthcare-us/ppe/guidance.html

32. US Centers for Disease Control and Prevention. Coronavirus Disease 2019 (COVID-19). Contact Tracing Resources. Updated Aug 13, 2020. Accessed Aug 15, 2020. https://www.cdc.gov/coronavirus/2019-ncov/php/open-america/contact-tracing-resources.html

33. State Operations Manual. Appendix A—Survey Protocol, Regulations, and Interpretive Guidelines for Hospitals. Revised Feb 21, 2020. Accessed Aug 15, 2020. https://www.cms.gov/Regulations-and-Guidance/Guidance/Manuals/downloads/som107ap_a_hospitals.pdf

34. US Occupational Safety and Health Administration. Occupational Exposure to Bloodborne Pathogens: Needlesticks and Other Sharps Injuries. Final Rule: 29CFR Part 1910. Jan18, 2001. Federal Register #: 66:5317-5325. Accessed Aug 15, 2020. https://www.osha.gov/laws-regs/federalregister/2001-01-18

35. US Occupational Safety and Health Administration. Safety and Health Topics: Tuberculosis. Respiratory Protection Standard. 1910.134. Accessed Aug 15, 2020. https://www.osha.gov/laws-regs/regulations/standardnumber/1910/1910.134

36. US Occupational Safety and Health Administration. Needlestick Sharps Injuries. Accessed Aug 15, 2020. https://www.osha.gov/SLTC/etools/hospital/hazards/sharps/sharps.html

37. US Government Information. H.R. 5178 (106th): Needlestick Safety and Prevention Act. Public Law 106-430. Nov 6, 2000. Accessed Aug 15, 2020. https://www.congress.gov/106/plaws/publ430/PLAW-106publ430.pdf

38. US Centers for Disease Control and Prevention. Sharps Safety for Healthcare Settings. Workbook for Designing, Implementing, and Evaluating a Sharps Injury Prevention Program. Updated Feb 11, 2015. Accessed Aug 15, 2020. https://www.cdc.gov/sharpssafety/resources.html

39. US Centers for Disease Control and Prevention. Tuberculosis (TB). Updated Dec 31, 2018. Accessed Aug 15, 2020. https://www.cdc.gov/tb/default.htm

40. US Occupational Safety and Health Administration. Accessed Aug 15, 2020. https://www.osha.gov/

41. World Health Organization (WHO). Considerations for Quarantine of Contacts of COVID-19 Cases. Accessed Dec 21, 2020. https://www.who.int/publications/i/item/considerations-for-quarantine-of-individuals-in-the-context-of-containment-for-coronavirus-disease-(covid-19)

42. US Centers for Disease Control and Prevention. Coronavirus Disease 2019 (COVID-19). Public Health Guidance for Community-Related Exposure. Updated Jul 31, 2020. Accessed Aug 16, 2020. https://www.cdc.gov/coronavirus/2019-ncov/php/public-health-recommendations.html

43. US Centers for Disease Control and Prevention. Influenza (Flu). Influenza Vaccination Information for Health Care Workers. Updated Dec 18, 2019. Accessed Aug 16, 2020. https://www.cdc.gov/flu/professionals/healthcareworkers.htm

44. US Centers for Disease Control and Prevention. Influenza Vaccination Coverage Among Health Care Personnel—United States, 2018–2019 Influenza Season. Sep 26, 2019. Accessed Dec 21, 2020. https://www.cdc.gov/flu/fluvaxview/hcp-coverage_1819estimates.htm

45. Talbot TR, et al. Influenza vaccination of healthcare workers and vaccine allocation for healthcare workers during vaccine shortages. *Infect Control Hosp Epidemiol.* 2005 Nov;26(11):882–890. Accessed Aug 16, 2020. https://pubmed.ncbi.nlm.nih.gov/16320984/

46. Association for Professionals in Infection Control and Epidemiology. Position Paper: APIC: Flu Vaccines Should Be Mandatory for Healthcare Personnel. Jan 27, 2011. Accessed Aug 16, 2020. https://apic.org/apic-flu-vaccines-should-be-mandatory-for-healthcare-personnel/

47. Infectious Diseases Society of America. Pandemic and Seasonal Influenza Principles for United States Action. Sep 2012. Accessed Aug 16, 2020. https://www.idsociety.org/policy--advocacy/new-page-pandemic-and-seasonal-influenza/

48. Immunization Action Coalition. Influenza Vaccination Honor Roll. Accessed Aug 16, 2020. https://www.immunize.org/honor-roll/influenza-mandates/

49. US Centers for Disease Control and Prevention. Influenza (Flu). A Toolkit for Long-Term Care Employers. Updated Oct 31, 2018. Accessed Aug 16, 2020. https://www.cdc.gov/flu/toolkit/long-term-care/index.htm

50. US Centers for Disease Control and Prevention. Healthcare Facility HAI Reporting Requirements to CMS via NHSN—Current or Proposed Requirements. Updated Jan 2019. Accessed Aug 21, 2020. https://www.cdc.gov/nhsn/pdfs/cms/cms-reporting-requirements.pdf

51. US Centers for Disease Control and Prevention. Interim Guidance for Routine and Influenza Immunization Services During the COVID-19 Pandemic. Updated Oct 20, 2020. Accessed Aug 21, 2020. https://www.cdc.gov/vaccines/pandemic-guidance/index.html

52. US Centers for Disease Control and Prevention. Influenza (Flu). Promoting Vaccination in the Workplace. Updated Aug 27, 2020. Accessed Aug 21, 2020. https://www.cdc.gov/flu/business/promoting-vaccines-workplace.htm

53. The Joint Commission. R3 Report Issue 3: Influenza Vaccination. Accessed Aug 21, 2020. https://www.jointcommission.org/standards/r3-report/r3-report-issue-3---influenza-vaccination/

54. National Quality Forum. NQF #0431 Influenza Vaccination Coverage Among Healthcare Personnel. Accessed Apr 17, 2021. https://www.qualityforum.org/Home.aspx

55. Vaccine Finder. Accessed Aug 21, 2020. https://vaccinefinder.org/

56. US Centers for Disease Control and Prevention. Immunization Information Systems (IIS). Updated June 7, 2019. Accessed Aug 21, 2020. https://www.cdc.gov/vaccines/programs/iis/index.html

57. The Joint Commission. Influenza and Other Related Diseases. Accessed Aug 21, 2020. https://www.jointcommission.org/resources/patient-safety-topics/infection-prevention-and-control/influenza-and-other-related-diseases/

58. US Centers for Disease Control and Prevention. Global Health Protection and Security. Updated May 27, 2020. Accessed Aug 23, 2020. https://www.cdc.gov/globalhealth/healthprotection/fetp/about.html

59. Nguyen LH, et al. Risk of COVID-19 among front-line health care workers and the general community: A prospective cohort study. *Lancet Public Health.* 2020 Jul 31. Accessed Aug 23, 2020. https://www.thelancet.com/journals/lanpub/article/PIIS2468-2667(20)30164-X/fulltext

60. US Centers for Disease Control and Prevention. Ebola: Personal Protective Equipment (PPE) Donning and Doffing Procedures. Updated Jul 25, 2019. Accessed Aug 23, 2020. https://www.cdc.gov/vhf/ebola/hcp/ppe-training/index.html

Chapter 11

Evaluating the Effectiveness of an Infection Prevention and Control Program

By Joan M. Ivaska, BS, MPH, CIC

Disclaimer: Strategies, tools, and examples discussed in this book do not necessarily reflect Joint Commission or Joint Commission International requirements for all settings. Always refer to the most current standards applicable to your health care setting to ensure compliance.

Introduction

Evaluation of an infection prevention and control (IPC) program is essential to determine whether the surveillance, prevention initiatives, and improvement strategies are effectively reducing risk and infections and if this improvement is based on the annual infection prevention plan. Without an intentional evaluation process, the IPC team and leaders will not know if the program is delivering value to patient safety. This chapter discusses IPC program and plan evaluation and provides tips and strategies on how to effectively evaluate the IPC program's effectiveness. The previous chapters in this book discuss how to do the following:

- Allocate resources to an IPC program
- Identify IPC risks within the program
- Create an IPC plan
- Implement interventions to reduce the likelihood and spread of infections
- Respond to infectious disease emergencies
- Communicate about IPC efforts
- Address IPC within the environment of care/facility management and safety
- Support quality and patient safety
- Support occupational health and employee safety

All these activities are critical to a successful, comprehensive IPC program, and organizations must evaluate the success of the activities and make adjustments to enhance performance as necessary. The evaluation process should include a thoughtful review of each of these components and provide direction to planning for the next year.

Evaluating the Effectiveness of Program Activities

Evaluating the effectiveness of IPC interventions and activities helps identify which activities of the IPC program are successful and which need to be changed to improve outcomes. Both The Joint Commission and Joint Commission International (JCI) address the concept of evaluation in infection prevention and control (IC) requirements. For domestic organizations, this is addressed in Standard IC.03.01.01. For international organizations, Prevention and Control of Infection (PCI) Standards PCI.5.1, PCI.14, and PCI.15 cover these concepts. These requirements encompass processes that allow IPC staff to maintain a continuous cycle of improvement. The steps in the cycle include:

- Identifying and prioritizing risks
- Developing and revising goals
- Implementing and evaluating interventions
- Sharing evaluation results organizationally
- Revising the plan

These activities, which should be reflected in the IPC plan, including the evaluation function, are similar to many of the methods used as a routine part of quality improvement (QI) efforts, such as the Institute for Healthcare Improvement (IHI) Model for Improvement Plan-Do-Study-Act (or Plan-Do-Check-Act) process, the IHI-QI, and Lean Six Sigma.[1-4]

Relevant Joint Commission Standards Addressed in This Chapter

Note: These standards were in effect at the time of publication. They refer to Joint Commission standards effective January 1, 2021. Always consult the most recent version of Joint Commission standards for the most accurate requirements for your setting.

IC.03.01.01 The [organization] evaluates the effectiveness of its infection prevention and control plan.

EP 1 The [organization] evaluates the effectiveness of its infection prevention and control plan annually and whenever risks significantly change. The evaluation includes a review of the following:
- The infection prevention and control plan's prioritized risks
- The infection prevention and control plan's goals (*See also* NPSG.07.01.01, EP 2)

- Implementation of the infection prevention and control plan's activities

EP 6 Findings from the evaluation are communicated at least annually to the individuals or interdisciplinary group that manages the patient safety program.

EP 7 The [organization] uses the findings of its evaluation of the infection prevention and control plan when revising the plan. (*See also* LD.01.02.01, EP 4)

Relevant Joint Commission International (JCI) Standards Addressed in This Chapter

Note: These standards were in effect at the time of publication. They refer to the *Joint Commission International Accreditation Standards for Hospitals, seventh edition*, ©2020. Always consult the most recent version of Joint Commission International standards for the most accurate requirements for your hospital or medical center setting.

PCI.5.1 The hospital identifies areas at high risk for infections by conducting a risk assessment, develops interventions to address these risks, and monitors the effectiveness.

ME 3 The hospital evaluates the effectiveness of the interventions and makes appropriate changes to the infection prevention and control program as needed.

PCI.14 The infection prevention and control process is integrated with the hospital's overall program for quality improvement and patient safety, using measures that are epidemiologically important to the hospital.

ME 3 The hospital uses monitoring data to evaluate and support improvements to the infection prevention and control program at least annually.

ME 5 The infection prevention and control program documents monitoring data and provides reports of data analysis to leadership on a quarterly basis.

PCI.15 The hospital provides education on infection prevention and control practices to staff, physicians, patients, families, and other caregivers when indicated by their involvement in care.

ME 4 The hospital communicates findings and trends from quality improvement activities to all staff and included as part of staff education.

An effective evaluation helps determine the extent to which the IPC program is addressing its most important risks and meeting outlined goals and objectives. Questions to answer in the evaluation process include "Is the program working?" and "Are the desired results being achieved?" The following components should be considered as part of the evaluation process:

- The program's progress toward achieving its goals and objectives
- The program's objectives and whether they should be changed, added, or removed—and why
- The previous year's successes and failures

This information may then be used in the subsequent year's risk assessment and program revision process. Part of a program's effectiveness also depends on the IPC team being a visible resource to staff and administration, demonstrating a strong commitment to infection prevention and control. It is important to demonstrate the costs and benefits of an IPC program.[5-10] This can be done by thoughtfully implementing interventions that result in decreased infections and, potentially, health care dollar savings or increased revenue. These interventions should improve patient safety and ultimately decrease costs associated with infections.

The evaluation process should be dynamic, collaborative, and multidisciplinary, taking into account all services and programs in the organization. It should evaluate risks that are facility specific, consider internal and external risks, and include thoughtful examination of the use and results of IPC activities.

> **TIP** An effective evaluation helps determine the extent to which an IPC program is addressing its most important risks and meeting outlined goals and objectives.

Joint Commission and JCI-accredited organizations are required to evaluate the effectiveness of the IPC plan at least annually and when identified and prioritized risks change. Such a review determines effectiveness, outlines activities that are still required, and indicates other issues that should be incorporated into the next year's IPC plan.

Changes in practice or services or unexpected events may result in new activities being performed during the year. Noting these changes in the annual evaluation can help IPC staff describe what actions were taken and whether they need to be incorporated into the IPC plan in the following year. When the organization adds a significant new service, such as cardiovascular surgery or neonatal intensive care, or a new site of care, such as a home health agency, these changes affect the scope of the IPC plan. The evaluation process must include a review of these changes (see Figure 11-1 on page 254). Additional information on assessing the IPC program and plan, including tools for assessing programs in a variety of health care settings, can be found in Chapter 1.

As previously mentioned, an annual risk assessment will help identify any changes that need to be made to the IPC program (see Chapter 3). The evaluation process reviews the success of the IPC program in addressing identified risks.

It may be helpful when designing IPC goals and objectives to consider a tiered approach that could indicate achievements that are minimum expectations and those that would reflect exceptional accomplishments. For example, a minimum expectation might be reducing central line–associated bloodstream infections (CLABSIs) by 20%, and an exceptional accomplishment might be achieving a rate of zero CLABSIs for a three-month period. This type of evaluation provides the organization with a more precise description of the effectiveness of the infection prevention interventions.

The intent of these requirements is to guide the organization in purposefully reviewing the activities of the infection surveillance, prevention, and control program to determine whether goals were achieved or improvement is needed. As discussed in earlier chapters, the goals are developed based on the most significant risks identified by the organization, as determined in the risk assessment, and also those functions and resources that are essential for maintaining an effective IPC program.

The IPC goals and objectives should be aligned with the organization's goals and strategies and may need to be changed as those overarching goals and strategies are changed. Many goals or objectives in one year might still be important in the next year. However, it is essential to reassess risks and review priorities for patients, residents, and staff, the environment of care, external threats, and other issues at least annually and to revise IPC goals and activities as appropriate.

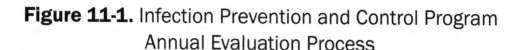

Figure 11-1. Infection Prevention and Control Program Annual Evaluation Process

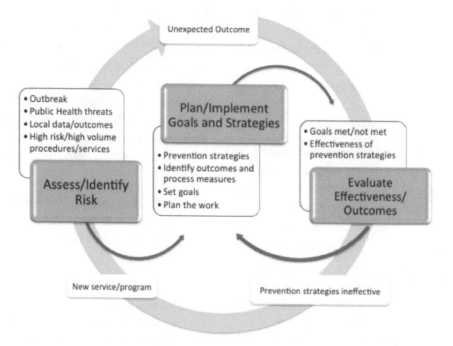

Unexpected Outcome

- Outbreak
- Public Health threats
- Local data/outcomes
- High risk/high volume procedures/services

Assess/Identify Risk

Plan/Implement Goals and Strategies

- Prevention strategies
- Identify outcomes and process measures
- Set goals
- Plan the work

- Goals met/not met
- Effectiveness of prevention strategies

Evaluate Effectiveness/ Outcomes

New service/program

Prevention strategies ineffective

This figure illustrates the ongoing evaluation process that is part of an infection prevention and control program.

The requirements for accreditation compliance also address the evaluation of activities that were carried out to achieve the IPC goals. When evaluating activities, it is important to document measurable achievements. For example, an organization could demonstrate the effectiveness of interventions in reducing the number of catheter-associated urinary tract infections by showing a reduction in the rate of such infections from the period before interventions were implemented to the period after interventions were implemented.

In the evaluation process, it is important to determine what activities added value to the IPC program and contributed to improved patient safety and what activities should perhaps be revised or replaced by others that will better help to achieve the aims of the program. For example, if an education program for appropriate cleaning of the patient's environment has not improved practices, the infection preventionist (IP) and environmental services staff may collaborate to accomplish the following:

- Identify gaps between the current and recommended best practices.
- Identify changes that can close those gaps.
- Provide education and training to increase staff compliance with proper cleaning and disinfection protocols.
- Implement a competency assessment program.
- Develop a system for routinely assessing and providing feedback on environment cleanliness to staff.

> **TIP** The Joint Commission and Joint Commission International require the following to be addressed in the IPC program evaluation:
> - Identified prioritized risks
> - The plan's measurable goals
> - Implementation of IPC activities and strategies

Communicating Findings of the Evaluation

The organization should determine the reporting structure for IPC activities, including the format and frequency of reporting. An IP should communicate to leaders and others in the organization about problems or issues throughout the year as well as successes in meeting IPC program goals and objectives. Written documentation of accomplishments based on evaluation of the IPC plan should be recorded on a scheduled, systematic basis. These reports should include barriers to meeting objectives so that new strategies may be considered in a timely fashion. Some things to consider when planning how to communicate about evaluation results include the following:

- Who are the primary audiences to receive the evaluation results? Consider individuals in leadership positions, medical staff leaders, IPC committee or safety and quality team members, and key staff, who can use the information to improve patient care.
- What kinds of information should be in the evaluation report? The report can review all IPC activities and investigations or summary data on health care–associated infections (HAIs) and goals for the next year.
- Where can that information be found, and how is it accessed? The information will be gathered from infection prevention surveillance activities, employee health, and other services or departments performing monitoring activities related to the goals and objectives.
- How can the information be effectively reported? Information can be presented verbally and also should be accompanied by some type of written report to those in the organization who are able to affect IPC practices. These may include appropriate individuals such as IPs, nurses, or groups such as a patient safety/quality improvement committee. (*See also* Chapter 9 for communication strategies.)

Each evaluation and reporting format will be somewhat different, depending on the needs and nature of the organization and its programs (see Sidebar 11-1 on page 256).

One effective way to conduct a meaningful program evaluation and to report the results is to develop a reporting template that incorporates the findings of the organizational IPC risk assessment and the subsequent results from addressing the highest-priority and ongoing risks. The risk assessment samples and tools provided in Chapter 3 of this book can serve as examples. The template could include the following columns:

- Highest-priority and continuing risks
- Goals/objectives for each risk
- Strategies developed to achieve risk reduction
- Individuals/departments responsible
- Progress toward achieving the objective or target
- Objective/goal met/not met
- Actions/recommendations for IPC program revision

The report could be taken to the IPC, quality assessment/performance improvement, and patient safety committees on a predetermined basis (for example, quarterly, biannually, annually). Such a report could also be used to keep organizational and medical staff leadership informed on the organization's progress toward reducing IPC risks. Periodic reporting helps an organiztion avoid "surprises" at the end of the year.

It is also important to communicate findings of the program evaluation, outcomes, and revisions to the IPC program goals to frontline staff. Infection prevention and control happens at the bedside, in the clinic room, in the surgical suite, and at every location and in every health care setting where patients and residents are encountered. Infection prevention and control is not a function of an office but rather is everyone's responsibility, and as such, it is essential that everyone understand the goals of the organization's IPC program and how they can contribute to its success.

Another method for describing the findings of an annual program evaluation is a summary report. An organization may already have an annual IPC committee or department report that can serve as the basis for the evaluation report. The evaluation can be performed collaboratively by individuals, a group of stakeholders, or a committee—for example, the IPC committee—and summarized in the existing report. Tool 11-1 can be used as a template for creating your own report. In addition, links to additional tools for assessing and evaluating an IPC plan are provided at the end of this chapter.

TRY THIS TOOL

Tool 11-1. Infection Prevention Annual Report and Program Evaluation

An important aspect of reporting evaluation findings is ensuring that receivers interpret the data as the sender intended. The information in the evaluation report should

Sidebar 11-1. Components of an Effective Evaluation Report

A step-by-step approach to evaluating the effectiveness of an IPC plan is to start with the previous year's plan, develop the risk assessment, and then develop the year's plan, involving a multidisciplinary team throughout the process. Because it is important to review activities and evaluate objectives, the evaluation report should consist of at least the following components:

1. A description of organizational and internal or external changes that influenced the scope of the infection surveillance, prevention, and control program/plan. This should include any significant events that altered the scope and goals of the program. Examples include public health emergencies, emerging infectious diseases, and IPC staff vacancies.

2. A review of each objective/goal of the IPC plan. This should include activities performed to meet the goals and data that show how measurable objectives are being achieved. These data may be presented in a table or a graph and may come from a variety of sources, such as from the organization's quality dashboard or from information gathered by a quality and safety team. Evaluation may include the following:
   - Quantitative data such as rate graphs and tables (for example, infection rates and compliance rates for process measures)
   - Qualitative data such as staff or patient feedback
   - Observation results using checklists that can measure hand hygiene, environmental cleaning, or isolation precaution practices. Hand hygiene observations can be reported as quantitative data by calculating the percentage of time hands are cleaned when there is an opportunity for hand hygiene or how often the technique for hand hygiene meets the criteria outlined in the organization's policies or procedures.

3. A summary of any important issue or activity that was not part of a specific goal or objective. These issues or activities may become part of the next year's objectives. Examples may include an emergency that occurred during the time frame, new construction activities, the assessment of practices at a new facility opened by the organization, or special assigned projects.

4. A summary of any special-cause investigations performed during the year (for example, cluster or outbreak investigations).

5. A description of the barriers and challenges over the year and actions implemented; this information will influence planning for the coming year.

TIP If an IPC committee exists in your organization, its members should receive a copy of the written IPC program evaluation. In addition, the chief executive officer, chief of staff, chief of nursing, patient safety leader, and other appropriate organization leaders and individuals should receive a copy.

be appropriate for the individual(s) or group. There are several ways to ensure effective communication about IPC program evaluation, including the following:
- Apply the seven Cs of effective communication: clear, correct, concise, cohesive, concrete, courteous, and complete.
- Include graphics and visual aids to enhance the written presentation.
- Document all sources, using references as appropriate.
- Maintain consistency in the presentation method(s).

Using the Findings to Revise the Plan

As the IPC program and plan are evaluated, areas for necessary future work will likely be revealed. Any problems or issues should be incorporated into the annual risk analysis; the evaluation should state whether each issue should become an IPC program objective for the following year.

> **TIP** Organizations must consider what decisions need to be made as a result of the IPC program evaluation. These might include changes to the risk assessment or priorities or changes in practice.

The IPC team may wish to incorporate the written evaluation into the IPC plan or develop it as a separate document and distribute it to appropriate leaders and medical staff (see Figure 11-2, below).

Cost Evaluation

An area to consider during the evaluation process is the cost of infections and the value of the IPC program. Measuring the cost of HAIs is difficult, and the financial impact varies among health care organizations, systems, and settings. However, there are areas on which to focus, such as length of stay, treatment costs, increased use of laboratory and other testing, and patient morbidity and mortality. In addition, there are investigation and control costs and potential legal liability. One strategy is to combine the organization's data on reducing HAI rates through its IPC efforts with estimates of benefit from well-designed studies in the health care literature, adjusting for the effects of inflation and other factors[5-11] (see Figure 11-3 on page 258). This may be presented as a cost–avoidance outcome in the program evaluation.

Figure 11-2. Sample Infection Prevention and Control Program Report for Device-Associated Infection: CLABSI

Goal	Strategies and Interventions
Reduce 20% to 0.50 per 1000 line days	• Implement daily chlorhexidine gluconate (CHG) baths. • Maintain 90% compliance with dressings dry and intact. • Maintain scrub cap compliance above 90%.
Outcome	
0.33	
Goal Met/Not Met	**Progress/Trend**
Met	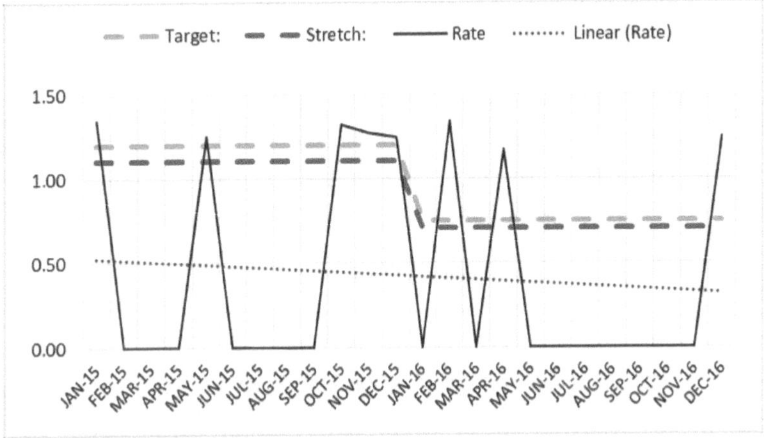
Actions and Recommendations	
• Continue to monitor next year. • Add CHG bathing to RN skills fair.	

This figure is an example of how one organization reported the evaluation of its infection prevention and control program objectives.

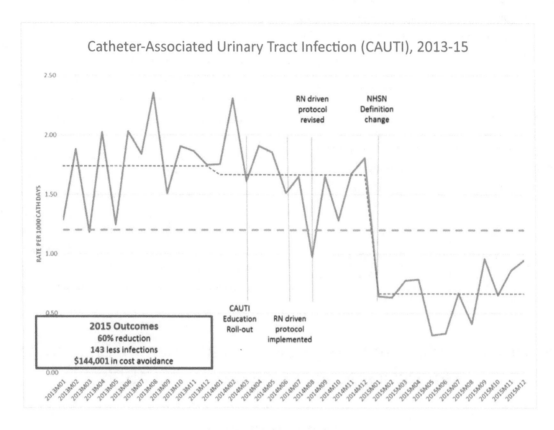

Figure 11-3. Infection Prevention Program Evaluation of HAI Costs

Catheter-Associated Urinary Tract Infection (CAUTI), 2013-15

RN driven protocol revised

NHSN Definition change

CAUTI Education Roll-out

RN driven protocol implemented

2015 Outcomes
60% reduction
143 less infections
$144,001 in cost avoidance

This figure is an example of how one organization reported the cost avoidance associated with its infection prevention and control program.

Taking a Multidisciplinary Approach to Evaluation

IPC practices are the responsibility of everyone in an organization, and having staff from throughout the facility involved in the continuous evaluation process provides a broad overview of risks and concerns associated with reducing infections in patients, residents, staff, physicians, visitors, and others.

Experience shows that promoting collaboration among individuals and departments results in broad-based solutions and can result in both individual and corporate ownership for IPC. Multidisciplinary collaboration and a systems approach increase the likelihood of a successful IPC program.[12-15]

Including others in the entire cycle, from risk assessment through evaluation, can aid in developing collaborative efforts that effectively move a specific issue from the risk column to successful and sustained resolution. The IPC staff should reinforce the importance of comprehensive organizationwide collaboration and assessment to characterize and prioritize IPC risks, identify measures for reducing those risks, and develop appropriate goals and measurable objectives.

Summary

The purpose of evaluating and analyzing the activities of an IPC program is to determine what works well and what needs to be changed. A well-designed evaluation will also provide information to leadership on the program's challenges and successes.

Resources

Refer to the following resources for helpful information on how to evaluate the effectiveness of an IPC program.

Tool to Try

Tool 11-1. Infection Prevention Annual Report and Program Evaluation

Additional Tools

- APIC. Cost Calculators. Accessed Sep 12, 2020. http://www.apic.org/Resources/Cost-calculators

- US Centers for Disease Control and Prevention. Infection Control Assessment Tools. Accessed Sep 15, 2020. https://www.cdc.gov/hai/prevent/infection-control-assessment-tools.html

- World Health Organization. Infection Prevention and Control Assessment Framework at the Facility Level. Accessed Sep 15, 2020. https://www.who.int/infection-prevention/tools/core-components/IPCAF-facility.PDF?ua=1

Additional Readings

- US Centers for Disease Control and Prevention. Framework for program evaluation in public health. *MMWR Recomm Rep.* 1999 Sep;48(RR-11):1–40. Accessed Jan 6, 2017. http://www.cdc.gov/eval/framework/index.htm

- Friedman C, et al. APIC/CHICA–Canada infection prevention control, and epidemiology: Professional and practice standards. *Am J Infect Control.* 2008 Aug;36(6):385–389.

- Bubb TN, et al. APIC professional and practice standards. *Am J Infect Control.* 2016 Jul 1;44(7):745–749. Accessed Jan 6, 2017. http://www.ajicjournal.org/article/S0196-6553(16)00155-3/pdf

- Scheckler WE, et al. Requirements for infrastructure and essential activities of infection control and epidemiology in hospitals: A consensus panel report. *Am J Infect Control.* 1998 Feb;26(1):47–60.

- Kennedy EH, Greene MT, Saint S. Estimating hospital costs of catheter-associated urinary tract infection. *J Hosp Med.* 2013 Sep;8(9):519–522.

- Stevens V, et al. Inpatient costs, mortality and 30-day re-admission in patients with central-line-associated bloodstream infections. *Clin Microbiol Infect.* 2014 May;20(5):318–324.

References

1. Bower J, Segarra-Newnham M, Tice A. Selecting change implementation strategies. In Mayhall CG, ed. *Hospital Epidemiology and Infection Control*, 3rd ed. Philadelphia: Lippincott Williams & Wilkins, 2004, 162–163.

2. Scoville R, Little K. *Comparing Lean and Quality Improvement.* IHI Innovation Series white paper. Cambridge, MA: Institute for Healthcare Improvement, 2014. Accessed Sep 12, 2020. http://www.ihi.org/resources/pages/ihiwhitepapers/comparingleanandqualityimprovement.aspx

3. Yaduvanshi D, Sharma, A. Lean Six Sigma in Health Operations: Challenges and Opportunities—"Nirvana for Operational Efficiency in Hospitals in a Resource Limited Settings." *Journal of Health Management.* 2017;19(2):203–213. https://doi.org/10.1177/0972063417699665

4. American Society for Quality. Plan-Do-Check-Act (PDCA) Cycle. Accessed Sep 12, 2020. http://asq.org/learn-about-quality/project-planning-tools/overview/pdca-cycle.html

5. Stone PW, et al. The economic impact of infection control: Making the business case for increased infection control resources. *Am J Infect Control.* 2005 Nov;33(9):542–547.

6. Arefian H, et al. Economic evaluation of interventions for prevention of hospital acquired infections: A systematic review. *PLOS ONE.* 2016;11(1):e0146381. https://doi.org/10.1371/journal.pone.0146381

7. Dick AW, et al. A decade of investment in infection prevention: A cost-effectiveness analysis. *Am J Infect Control.* 2015;43(1):4–9. https://doi.org/10.1016/j.ajic.2014.07.014

8. Raschka S, Dempster L, Bryce E. Health economic evaluation of an infection prevention and control program: Are quality and patient safety programs worth the investment? *Am J Infect Control.* 2013;41(9):773–777. https://doi.org/10.1016/j.ajic.2012.10.026

9. Rennert-May E, et al. Economic evaluations and their use in infection prevention and control: A narrative review. *Antimicrob Resist Infect Control*. 2018;7:31. https://doi.org/10.1186/s13756-018-0327-z

10. Shepard J, et al. Could the prevention of health care-associated infections increase hospital cost? The financial impact of health care-associated infections from a hospital management perspective. *Am J Infect Control*. 2020;48(3):255–260. https://doi.org/10.1016/j.ajic.2019.08.035

11. Scott RD, US Centers for Disease Control and Prevention. The Direct Medical Costs of Healthcare-Associated Infections in U.S. Hospitals and the Benefits of Prevention. Mar 2009. Accessed Apr 6, 2021. https://www.cdc.gov/HAI/pdfs/hai/Scott_CostPaper.pdf

12. Waters HR, et al. The business case for quality: Economic analysis of the Michigan Keystone Patient Safety Program in ICUs. *Am J Med Qual*. 2011 Sep–Oct;26(5):333–339.

13. Perencevich EN, et al. Society for Healthcare Epidemiology of America. Raising standards while watching the bottom line: Making a business case for infection control. *Infect Control Hosp Epidemiol*. 2007 Oct;28(10):1121–1133.

14. Jain M, et al. Decline in ICU adverse events, nosocomial infections and cost through a quality improvement initiative focusing on teamwork and culture change. *Qual Saf Health Care*. 2006 Aug;15(4):235–239.

15. Cima R, et al. Colorectal surgery surgical site infection reduction program: A national surgical quality improvement program–driven multidisciplinary single-institution experience. *J Am Coll Surg*. 2013 Jan;216(1):23–33.

Chapter 12

Integrating Infection Prevention and Control into Patient Safety and Performance Improvement

By Kathleen A. Gase, MBA, MPH, CIC, FAPIC

Disclaimer: Strategies, tools, and examples discussed in this book do not necessarily reflect Joint Commission or Joint Commission International requirements for all settings. Always refer to the most current standards applicable to your health care setting to ensure compliance.

Introduction

As discussed in Chapter 11 of this book, one of the most important reasons for evaluating the effectiveness of an organization's infection prevention and control (IPC) plan is to determine if the actions and interventions in the plan decreased infections and improved patient safety.

Infection prevention and control are integral to an organization's patient safety, quality of care, and performance improvement (PI) programs. As such, The Joint Commission National Patient Safety Goal® (NPSG) NPSG.7 for domestic health care organizations and International Patient Safety Goal® (IPSG) IPSG. 5 for international health care settings address reducing the risk of health care–associated infections (HAIs). These goals promote specific improvements in patient safety by focusing on hand hygiene, preventing specific HAIs, and responding to incidents that involve infections.

The purpose of this chapter is to explore strategies and best practices related to hand hygiene and reducing HAIs and to discuss how to help ensure compliance by using some basic PI tools. These tools do not represent an exhaustive list and may also be applied to other IPC issues.

Despite having long been recognized as causing significant morbidity and mortality, HAIs continue to be troublesome.[1,2] Although progress has been made in preventing some HAIs, they are among the most common adverse events in health care. They can happen in any health care facility, including hospitals, ambulatory surgery centers, hemodialysis, and long-term care

facilities to name a few. Approximately 1 in 25 currently hospitalized patients has at least one HAI; an estimated 687,000 HAIs and 72,000 deaths occurred in US acute care hospitals in 2015.[3]

From the outset, NPSG.7 and IPSG.5 have focused on reducing the risk of HAIs by encouraging health care organizations to implement evidence-based guidelines for hand hygiene. The US Department of Health and Human Services has identified reduction of HAIs as an agency priority and provides the National Action Plan to eliminate HAIs in specific health care settings. *See* Resources section at the end of this chapter for more information.

Organizations accredited by The Joint Commission and Joint Commission International (JCI) are expected to improve performance based on their stated goals. Evidence-based practices must be implemented and monitored to prevent and control infections. As discussed in Chapter 11, an organization must measure the effectiveness of its IPC program as a *routine* part of its PI and evaluation activities.

The risk of adverse events—including those that involve infections—in the health care environment is related to the type of care, treatment, and services provided by an organization. All IPC requirements are program specific, and organizations accredited by The Joint Commission and JCI must be aware of which requirements pertain to their setting and the care, treatment, and services they provide. The following sections address some strategies and recommendations to help organizations eliminate HAIs.

TIP

With current knowledge and available technology, health care organizations that aggressively target specific HAIs have sustained decreases, with some reporting infection rates close to zero—a target previously thought to be unattainable.[4,5]

Relevant Joint Commission Standards Addressed in This Chapter

Note: These standards were in effect at the time of publication. They refer to Joint Commission standards effective January 1, 2021. Always consult the most recent version of Joint Commission standards for the most accurate requirements for your setting.

NPSG.07.01.01 Comply with either the current Centers for Disease Control and Prevention (CDC) hand hygiene guidelines and/or the current World Health Organization (WHO) hand hygiene guidelines.

IC.02.05.01 Implement evidence-based practices to prevent health care–associated infections due to the following:

- Multidrug-resistant organisms (MDROs)
- Central line–associated bloodstream infections (CLABSI)
- Catheter-associated urinary tract infections (CAUTI)
- Surgical site infections (SSI)

PI.02.01.01 The [organization] compiles and analyzes data.

Relevant Joint Commission International (JCI) Standards Addressed in This Chapter

Note: These standards were in effect at the time of publication. They refer to the *Joint Commission International Accreditation Standards for Hospitals, seventh edition,* ©2020. Always consult the most recent version of Joint Commission International standards for the most accurate requirements for your hospital or medical center setting.

IPSG.5 The hospital adopts and implements evidence-based hand-hygiene guidelines to reduce the risk of health care–associated infections.

IPSG.5.1 Hospital leaders identify care processes that need improvement and adopt and implement evidence-based interventions to improve patient outcomes and reduce the risk of hospital-associated infections.

PCI.14 The infection prevention and control process is integrated with the hospital's overall program for quality improvement and patient safety, using measures that are epidemiologically important to the hospital.

PCI.15 The hospital provides education on infection prevention and control practices to staff, physicians, patients, families, and other caregivers when indicated by their involvement in care.

Using Evidence-Based Guidelines to Set Goals for Improvement

Although proper hand hygiene is a widely accepted IPC intervention, many studies show that hand hygiene by health care staff is poor.[6,7] By consistently ensuring that all staff follow the Centers for Disease Control and Prevention[8] or World Health Organization[9] hand hygiene guidelines, health care organizations may successfully reduce the risk of infectious agents and HAIs.

Although hand hygiene is accepted as a cornerstone of IPC, it nevertheless remains difficult to improve compliance and sustain these improvements over time. The Joint Commission Center for Transforming Healthcare offers a number of resources designed to improve patient safety and compliance with hand hygiene practices. See Sidebar 12-1 for details on the Center's *Hand Hygiene Targeted Solutions Tool® (TST®)*. Organizations that have successfully improved hand hygiene compliance have used multimodal, multidisciplinary approaches that include strategies such as the following[10-14]:

- Ensuring management and leadership support of hand hygiene programs
- Educating health care staff, patients, residents, and visitors about the importance of hand hygiene and how to properly clean hands
- Providing appropriate hand hygiene facilities and products in convenient locations
- Hanging posters and other reminders to clean hands near sinks, in restrooms, and at other strategic locations

---

Sidebar 12-1. The Hand Hygiene Targeted Solutions Tool® (TST®)

To help increase hand hygiene compliance, Joint Commission Center for Transforming Health Care (the Center) offers a systematic and data-driven problem-solving based tool that guides health care organizations through step-by-step processes to measure actual performance, identify barriers to success, and establish solutions that are customized to address targeted needs.

The Hand Hygiene TST is a Web-based application designed to use evidence-based solutions to help health care organizations reduce the frequency of HAIs. Key features of the online application include the following:

- Strategies to define and measure hand hygiene issues that are specific to an organization
- Video scenarios to train observers on how to collect data
- Real-time data analysis
- Ways to improve the compliance rate with tailored solutions
- Completion in 12 to 16 weeks
- A control plan to sustain success

Hospitals that participated in the hand hygiene improvement initiative cited dramatic improvements in hand hygiene compliance within their organizations. For example, a typical 200-bed hospital that used the Hand Hygiene TST reported the following results:

- Prevented 130–140 health care–associated infections
- Prevented eight deaths
- Avoided annual medical costs estimated between $2.3 and $2.8 million

In addition to the Hand Hygiene TST, the Center offers similar modules for improving patient safety, which address topics such as hand-off communications, falls prevention, and reducing surgical site infections. Resources on these topics include videos, fact sheets, brochures, and implementation guides designed to assist organizations with their patient safety and performance improvement efforts.

Source: Joint Commission Center for Transforming Healthcare. Hand Hygiene Targeted Solutions Tool. Accessed Apr 6, 2021. https://www.centerfortransforminghealthcare.org/products-and-services/targeted-solutions-tool/hand-hygiene-tst/

- Encouraging patients, residents, and families to speak up and ask health care staff to clean their hands
- Creating and implementing incentive programs and competitions
- Measuring compliance with hand hygiene procedures and providing feedback to health care staff on their performance
- Engaging champions of hand hygiene to lead campaigns
- Using staff role models
- Instituting a culture of patient safety and leadership and health care staff accountability

Organizations should be able to show that they have implemented policies and procedures based on IA, IB, and IC recommendations of the required guideline(s) (incorporated by reference into state regulation) and chosen guideline(s), in the absence of a required guideline. In addition, health care worker adherence to recommended hand hygiene practices should be monitored, and workers should be provided with feedback on their performance. As part of this effort, organizations may set a specific quantitative goal to improve hand hygiene compliance. Failure mode and effects analysis— a step-by-step approach to identifying all possible failures—is one PI tool that can be used to identify issues and possible improvement goals. Regardless of the monitoring method, health care staff should receive feedback on organizational goals for improvement.[15]

Targeting HAIs for Elimination

To comply with Joint Commission and Joint Commission International requirements, accredited organizations should implement evidence-based policies and practices to reduce the risk of the following health care–associated infections:

- Multidrug-resistant organisms (MDROs)
- Central line–associated bloodstream infections (CLABSIs)
- Catheter-associated urinary tract infections (CAUTIs)
- Surgical site infections (SSIs)

Domestic organizations also should measure and monitor their IPC processes, outcomes, and compliance for these HAIs by using evidence-based guidelines or best practices. International organizations also are required under JCI Standard IPSG.5.1 to improve patient outcomes and reduce the risk of HAIs by identifying care processes and adopting and implementing evidence-based interventions. Such interventions may include infection prevention bundles for CLABSI, ventilator-associated pneumonia, CAUTI, SSI, and severe sepsis.

Infection prevention bundles are sets of evidence-based practices that, when implemented collectively, can improve patient outcomes. Care bundles can potentially enhance compliance with evidence-based process measures and may help to create reliability and consistency when they are simple, clear, and concise. Using bundled interventions is an effective way to implement change and improve the culture of safety in health care by promoting teamwork, measuring compliance, and providing feedback and accountability to frontline staff and leaders to improve care. See Chapter 6 for clinical strategies for using infection prevention bundles.

To improve patient outcomes, health care organizations should focus on improving the safety and quality of the care, treatment, and services they provide. The best way to achieve this is by measuring performance of processes that support care and then using the data collected to drive improvement. Analyze data from internal sources to identify patterns and trends and monitor performance. Health care organizations also are encouraged to use external databases to compare their performance with that of other similar organizations and care settings on specific topics and share incidence data with stakeholders.

Multidrug-Resistant Organisms

The presence of MDROs that can cause infections is on the rise not only in health care organizations but also in communities. Joint Commission standards require that organizations implement evidence-based practices to prevent HAIs, but these requirements do not prescribe which evidence-based guidelines to use unless required by law and or government regulations, such as the US Centers for Medicare & Medicaid Services Conditions of Participation/Conditions for Coverage. The following are recommended strategies and evidence-based guidelines to prevent infections due to MDROs[16-18]:

- Conduct a risk assessment.
  - Periodically assess the prevalence or incidence of MDROs in patients, health care staff, and the community.
  - Identify epidemiologically important MDROs.
  - Integrate MDRO risk assessment into the overall IPC risk assessment or create a standalone document.
  - Document findings in the IPC plan (as discussed in Chapter 3).

- Educate health care staff.
  - Develop and implement education activities about HAIs, MDROs, and IPC strategies based on the risk assessment and surveillance findings.[18]
  - Provide education at the time of hire and annually thereafter, or more frequently as needed, based on risk assessment, turnover, or changes in the patient population.
  - Evaluate the effectiveness of education by monitoring compliance with IPC practices and the occurrence of MDROs.
- Educate patients.
  - Provide education about HAIs, MDROs, and IPC strategies to patients infected or colonized with an MDRO; educate family members as needed.
  - Include educational pamphlets, videos, scripted discussions, or a combination of techniques, depending on the learning levels of the patient and family.
- Conduct surveillance.
  - Based on the risk assessment, monitor laboratory reports for MDROs.
  - Conduct surveillance for MDROs in accordance with local, state, and federal regulatory requirements. Consider evidence-based recommendations and guidelines when developing surveillance plans.[19]
  - Use recognized surveillance methodology and criteria to identify patients infected and colonized with an MDRO.[19]
  - Use PI or patient safety tools to identify MDRO issues or opportunities for improvement (for example, cause-and-effect diagrams, brainstorming, process flow maps).
- Provide surveillance data to key stakeholders.
  - Provide incidence MDRO surveillance data (prevention processes and/or outcomes) to health care staff involved in IPC activities and key stakeholders, including leaders, licensed independent practitioners, nursing staff, and other clinicians.
  - Provide information as part of the infection prevention or quality and safety committee meetings or send direct communications to stakeholders.
  - Present information graphically with short written explanations.
  - Leaders may need to provide additional support or assistance with removing barriers. Leaders should recognize and reward health care staff working to prevent and control MDROs.

- Create policies and practices.
  - Develop and implement IPC policies and practices for MDRO prevention that meet applicable regulatory requirements and that are aligned with evidence-based standards, professional organization guidelines, and best practices.

Central Line–Associated Bloodstream Infections

In 2018, approximately 20,000 CLABSIs were reported by US acute care hospitals, leading to increased morbidity and mortality, as well as extended hospital stays.[3] As noted earlier in this chapter, The Joint Commission does not prescribe which evidence-based guidelines should be used to prevent HAIs unless required by law and/or government regulations. Tools 12-1 and 12-2 can help evaluate organizational activities related to CLABSI prevention and adherence to central line insertion practices.

TRY THESE TOOLS
Tool 12-1. Central Line–Associated Bloodstream Infection (CLABSI) Assessment **Tool 12-2. Central Line Insertion Practices Adherence Monitoring**

The following strategies and guidelines may be used to help prevent CLABSI and to support compliance with the relevant standards discussed in this chapter[20,21]:

- Educate health care staff.
  - Develop and implement educational activities on HAIs and CLABSIs, as well as IPC strategies and activities based on the risk assessment and surveillance findings.
  - Educate and train all health care staff involved in central venous catheter (CVC) insertion and maintenance care.
  - Educate at the time of hire, annually thereafter, and when CVC insertion or maintenance care activities are added to staff job responsibilities.
  - Evaluate the effectiveness of education by monitoring compliance with IPC protocols and the occurrence of CLABSI.
- Educate patients.
  - Prior to insertion of a CVC, health care staff should educate the patient and family as needed about CLABSI prevention strategies.

- Include educational pamphlets, videos, scripted discussions, or a combination of techniques, depending on the learning levels of the patient and family.
- Create policies and practices.
  - Develop and implement IPC policies and practices for CLABSI prevention that meet applicable regulatory requirements and are aligned with evidence-based standards, professional organization guidelines, and best practices.
- Conduct a risk assessment.
  - Periodically assess the incidence of CLABSI to identify at-risk populations.
  - Integrate CLABSI risk assessment into the overall IPC risk assessment or create a standalone document (see Chapter 3).
  - Document findings in the IPC plan (as discussed in Chapter 3).
- Conduct surveillance.
  - Based on the risk assessment, monitor the occurrence of CLABSI in specific patient populations.
  - Ensure compliance with local, state, and federal surveillance and reporting requirements.
  - Use recognized surveillance methodology and criteria to identify CLABSI.[19]
  - Evaluate the effectiveness of CLABSI prevention activities and education efforts by monitoring prevention process and outcome measures.
- Provide surveillance data to key stakeholders.
  - Provide CLABSI surveillance data (outcomes and processes) to health care staff involved in CVC insertion and maintenance and key stakeholders, such as clinical and executive leaders.
  - Encourage posting and discussion of CLABSI rates in clinical areas.
  - Leaders may need to provide additional support or assistance with removing barriers. Leaders should recognize and reward health care staff working to prevent CLABSI.
- Implement standardized CVC insertion and care protocols, including the following:
  - CVC insertion checklist[4]
  - Hand hygiene prior to insertion or manipulation
  - Optimal catheter site selection
  - Restricted femoral vein use
  - Standardized cart or kit with all supplies needed for CVC insertion
  - Maximal sterile barrier precautions for central line

insertion (sterile gloves, sterile gown, large sterile drape, mask/face shield, and cap)
  - Appropriate antiseptic for skin prep
  - Disinfected catheter hubs and injection ports before every access.
  - CVC dressing change kit and checklist
- Remove nonessential CVC.
  - Establish a mechanism for routinely evaluating all patients with a CVC to assess for continued need.
  - Incorporate a follow-up mechanism to ensure prompt CVC removal when no longer needed.

Surgical Site Infections

Despite national prevention efforts and continued public reporting of data, SSIs remain a common and costly HAI; approximately 160,000–300,000 SSIs occur each year in the US, and there was no significant change in incidence between 2017 and 2018.[3,22-24] The consequences of these infections can be devastating. As stated in previous sections, Joint Commission requirements are not prescriptive unless required by law or government regulations. Tool 12-3 offers a checklist for developing and evaluating SSI prevention activities.

TRY THIS TOOL

Tool 12-3. Surgical Site Infection (SSI) Prevention

The following strategies may be used to prevent SSIs and support compliance with the standards addressed in this chapter[25]:

- Educate health care staff, including physicians.
  - Develop and implement education activities about HAIs, SSIs, and IPC strategies based on the risk assessment and surveillance findings.
  - Educate all health care staff involved in surgical procedures.
  - Educate staff at the time of hire, annually thereafter, and when involvement in surgical procedures is added to staff job responsibilities.
  - Evaluate the effectiveness of education by monitoring compliance with IPC protocols and the occurrence of SSIs.
- Educate patients.
  - Prior to surgical procedures, health care staff should educate the patient, and his or her family, as needed, about SSI prevention strategies.

- ◦ Include educational pamphlets, videos, scripted discussions, or a combination of techniques, depending on the learning levels of the patient and family.
- • Create policies and practices.
  - ◦ Develop and implement IPC policies and practices for SSI prevention that meet applicable regulatory requirements and are aligned with evidence-based standards, professional organization guidelines, and best practices.[25]
  - ◦ Evaluate multidisciplinary bundles with key stakeholders and consider procedure-specific interventions when applicable.[26]
- • Conduct a risk assessment.
  - ◦ Periodically assess the health care organization's patient population, types of surgical procedures performed, and regulatory and reporting requirements for your state or territory. Assess the occurrence of SSIs to identify at-risk populations.
  - ◦ Integrate SSI risk assessment into the overall IPC risk assessment or create a standalone document.
  - ◦ Document findings in the IPC plan (as discussed in Chapter 3).
- • Conduct surveillance.
  - ◦ Based on the risk assessment, monitor the occurrence of SSIs in specific surgical populations.
  - ◦ Ensure compliance with local, state, and federal surveillance and reporting requirements.
  - ◦ Use recognized surveillance methodology and criteria to identify SSIs.[19]
  - ◦ Evaluate the effectiveness of SSI prevention activities and education efforts by monitoring prevention process and outcome measures.
- • Provide surveillance data to key stakeholders.
  - ◦ Provide SSI surveillance data (outcomes and processes) to health care staff involved in surgical procedures and key stakeholders such as clinical and executive leaders.
  - ◦ Leaders may need to provide additional support or assistance with removing barriers. Leaders should recognize and reward health care staff working to prevent SSI.

Catheter-Associated Urinary Tract Infections

CAUTI is the leading cause of HAIs related to indwelling urinary devices. Morbidity attributable to CAUTI is limited, but due to the high frequency of events, the burden is substantial.[27,28] Many prevention and reduction efforts

have been focused on CAUTI with varying success; a decrease of 8% was seen in the US between 2017 and 2018.[3] Tool 12-4 provides a checklist for evaluating CAUTI practices and activities.

TRY THIS TOOL

Tool 12-4. Catheter-Associated Urinary Tract Infection (CAUTI) Assessment

The following strategies may be used to prevent CAUTI and support compliance with the standards addressed in this chapter[27-29]:

- • Educate health care staff.
  - ◦ Develop and implement educational activities about HAIs, CAUTIs, and IPC strategies based on the risk assessment and surveillance findings.
  - ◦ Include all health care staff involved with indwelling urinary catheter insertion and care.
  - ◦ Ensure all indwelling urinary catheters have an appropriate indication for use; assess daily.[30]
  - ◦ Educate staff at the time of hire, annually thereafter, and when indwelling urinary catheter insertion or care activities are added to staff job responsibilities.
  - ◦ Evaluate the effectiveness of education by monitoring compliance with IPC protocols and the occurrence of CAUTI.
- • Educate patients.
  - ◦ Prior to insertion of an indwelling urinary catheter, health care staff should educate the patient and family as needed about CAUTI prevention strategies.
  - ◦ Education may include pamphlets, videos, scripted discussions, or a combination of techniques, depending on the learning levels of the patient and family.
- • Create policies and practices.
  - ◦ Develop and implement IPC policies and practices for CAUTI prevention that meet applicable regulatory requirements and are aligned with evidence-based standards, professional organization guidelines, and best practices.
- • Conduct a risk assessment.
  - ◦ Periodically assess the occurrence of CAUTI to identify at-risk populations.
  - ◦ Integrate CAUTI risk assessment into the overall IPC risk assessment or create a standalone document.

- Document findings in the IPC plan (as discussed in Chapter 3).
- Conduct surveillance.
  - Based on the risk assessment, monitor the occurrence of CAUTI in specific patient populations.
  - Ensure compliance with local, state, and federal surveillance and reporting requirements.
  - Use recognized surveillance methodology and criteria to identify CAUTI.[19]
  - Evaluate the effectiveness of CAUTI prevention activities and education efforts by monitoring prevention process and outcome measures.
- Provide surveillance data to key stakeholders.
  - Provide CAUTI surveillance data (outcomes and prevention processes) to health care staff involved with indwelling urinary catheter insertion and care and key stakeholders such as clinical and executive leaders.
  - Leaders may need to provide additional support or assist with removing barriers. Leaders should recognize and reward health care staff working to prevent CAUTI.
- Ensure that standardized indwelling urinary catheter insertion and maintenance care protocols are implemented.
- Ensure that catheters are inserted based on appropriate indication.
- Remove nonessential indwelling urinary catheters.
  - Establish a mechanism for routinely evaluating all patients with an indwelling urinary catheter to assess for continued need.
  - Incorporate a follow-up mechanism to ensure prompt indwelling urinary catheter removal as soon as possible and/or when no longer needed.

Managing Sentinel Events Related to Health Care–Associated Infections

As noted throughout this chapter, HAIs continue to be a significant contributor to patient morbidity and mortality. An HAI may be classified as a sentinel event. A sentinel event is a patient safety event (not primarily related to the natural course of the patient's illness or underlying condition) that reaches a patient and results in any of the following:

- Death
- Permanent harm
- Severe temporary harm

> **TIP** **Appropriate Indications for Indwelling Urinary Catheter Placement[30]**
>
> - Patient has acute urinary retention or bladder outlet obstruction
> - Need for accurate measurements of urinary output in critically ill patients
> - Perioperative use for selected surgical procedures:
>   - Patients undergoing urologic surgery or other surgery on contiguous structures of the genitourinary tract
>   - Anticipated prolonged duration of surgery (catheters inserted for this reason should be removed in post-anesthesia care unit)
>   - Patients anticipated to receive large-volume infusions or diuretics during surgery
>   - Need for intraoperative monitoring of urinary output
> - To assist in healing of open sacral or perineal wounds in incontinent patients
> - Patient requires prolonged immobilization (for example, potentially unstable thoracic or lumbar spine, multiple traumatic injuries such as pelvic fractures)
> - To improve comfort for end-of-life care if needed

In the above definition, severe temporary harm is defined as critical, potentially life-threatening harm lasting for a limited time with no permanent residual effect but requires the following: transfer to a higher level of care/monitoring for a prolonged period of time, transfer to a higher level of care for a life-threatening condition, or additional major surgery, procedure, or treatment to resolve the condition, according to The Joint Commission's Sentinel Event Policy.

The Joint Commission and JCI adopted a formal Sentinel Event Policy in 1996 to help health care organizations that experience serious adverse events improve safety and learn from those sentinel events. Careful investigation and analysis of patient safety events, and strong corrective actions that provide effective and sustained system improvement, are essential to reduce risk and prevent patient harm. The Sentinel Event Policy explains how The Joint Commission partners with organizations that have experienced a serious patient safety event to protect the patient, improve systems, and prevent further harm. The policy is found in the "Sentinel Events" chapter of each *Comprehensive Accreditation Manual* or its *E-dition®* counterpart. Per the Sentinel Event Policy, an appropriate response includes all the following:

- A formalized team response that stabilizes the patient, discloses the event to the patient and family, and provides support for the family as well as staff involved in the event
- Notification of organization leadership
- Immediate investigation
- Completion of a comprehensive systematic analysis for identifying the causal and contributory factors
- Strong corrective actions derived from the identified causal and contributing factors that eliminate or control system hazards or vulnerabilities and result in sustainable improvement over time
- Timeline for implementation of corrective actions
- Systemic improvement

Joint Commission Leadership (LD) Standard LD.03.09.01, Element of Performance (EP) 5 and JCI Quality Improvement and Patient Safety (QPS) Standard QPS.7, Measurable Element (ME) 2 require accredited organizations to conduct thorough and credible comprehensive systematic analyses (for example, root cause analyses) in response to sentinel events. Leaders should disseminate the results of these analyses to all staff who provide services related to the patient safety event being investigated. Organizations should inform the patient or surrogate decision maker about unanticipated outcomes of care, treatment, or services that relate to sentinel events according to Rights and Responsibilities of the Individual (RI) Standard RI.01.02.01, EP 20 and JCI Patient-Centered Care (PCC) Standard PCC.3.1, ME 4.

Infection Prevention and Control, Patient Safety, and Performance Improvement

Protecting patients while providing more complex health care is challenging. With every advancement in the medical field—new equipment and tools, new procedures, and new techniques—providers must do everything possible to ensure that patients have the best opportunity to emerge from the health care system without an avoidable complication. Collaboration among IPC, patient safety,

and PI departments has never been more important.

By working together, these groups can more effectively and efficiently affect patient care. PI professionals can accelerate change and transition by partnering with other experts—such as infection preventionists (IPs), patient safety staff, and others—to appropriately develop and implement interventions. Often the patient safety team can assist in measuring the success of those interventions. IPs should develop collaborative relationships with quality and safety professionals and may serve on committees and teams that address strategies for performance improvement.

The structure of how the three departments join forces will undoubtedly look different at each facility and in various health care settings. The key to success is that the relationship and communication exist to facilitate the joining of forces. It is much more difficult to positively affect patient care if IPC teams are working separately from patient safety and performance improvement teams. By working together, interventions can be built on the momentum of previous successes and can move forward more quickly and more efficiently.

Summary

IPC is an integral component of an organization's patient safety and PI programs. The interventions discussed in this chapter focus on evidence-based practices shown to reduce the risk of infection, thus improving patient safety.

IPC plays an essential role in improving performance. By collaborating with others in the organization to rigorously and accurately measure outcomes and processes of care, providing surveillance data, and implementing and promoting feasible and effective IPC interventions, a culture of safety can be achieved.

Resources

Tools to Try

Tool 12-1. Central Line–Associated Bloodstream Infection (CLABSI) Assessment

Tool 12-2. Central Line Insertion Practices Adherence Monitoring

Tool 12-3. Surgical Site Infection (SSI) Prevention

Tool 12-4. Catheter-Associated Urinary Tract Infection (CAUTI) Assessment

Hand Hygiene

- Association for Professionals in Infection Control and Epidemiology. Implementation Guides, Hand Hygiene. Accessed Jan 6, 2017. http://www.apic.org/Professional-Practice/Implementation-guides

- Centers for Disease Control and Prevention. Hand Hygiene in Healthcare Settings. Accessed Jan 6, 2017. http://www.cdc.gov/handhygiene/

- Infection Prevention and Control Canada. Information About Hand Hygiene. Accessed Jan 6, 2017. https://ipac-canada.org/hand-hygiene.php

- Institute for Healthcare Improvement. How-to Guide: Improving Hand Hygiene. Accessed Jan 6, 2017. http:// www.ihi.org/resources/pages/tools/howtoguideimprovinghandhygiene.aspx

- Joint Commission Center for Transforming Healthcare. Hand Hygiene Targeted Solutions Tool. Accessed Apr 6, 2021. https://www.centerfortransforminghealthcare.org/products-and-services/targeted-solutions-tool/hand-hygiene-tst/

- The Joint Commission. Hand Hygiene. Accessed Jun 4, 2021. http://www.jointcommission.org/topics/hai_hand_hygiene.aspx

- World Health Organization. Hand Hygiene. Accessed Jun 4, 2021. http://www.who.int/gpsc/5may/Hand_Hygiene_Why_How_and_When_Brochure.pdf

- The Joint Commission, Speak Up: Five Things You Can Do to Prevent Infection. Accessed Jun 4, 2021. http://www.jointcommission.org/assets/1/6/Infection_Control_brochure.pdf

Health Care–Associated Infections

- US Department of health and Human Services. Office of Disease Prevention and Health Promotion. National HAI Action Plan to Prevent Health Care–Associated Infections: Road Map to Elimination. Accessed January 28, 2021. https://health.gov/our-work/health-care-quality/health-care-associated-infections/national-hai-action-plan

Multidrug-Resistant Organisms

- Association for Professionals in Infection Control and Epidemiology. Implementation Guides, *Clostridium difficile* Infections. Accessed Aug 24, 2020. http://www.apic.org/Professional-Practice/Implementation-guides

- Strategies to Prevent *Clostridium difficile* Infections in Acute Care Hospitals: 2014 Update. Accessed Aug 24, 2020. https://www.cambridge.org/core/journals/infection-control-and-hospital-epidemiology/article/strategies-to-prevent-clostridium-difficile-infections-in-acute-care-hospitals-2014-update/D5ADD87BD88203703AF85707CE799F6E

- Strategies to Prevent Methicillin-Resistant *Staphylococcus aureus* Transmission and Infection in Acute Care Hospitals: 2014 Update. Accessed Aug 24, 2020. https://www.cambridge.org/core/journals/infection-control-and-hospital-epidemiology/article/strategies-to-prevent-methicillinresistant-staphylococcus-aureus-transmission-and-infection-in-acute-care-hospitals-2014-update/E4CB8361054B5FA8588CFB04C445682A

- Association for Professionals in Infection Control and Epidemiology. Implementation Guides, Methicillin-Resistant *Staphylococcus aureus* (MRSA). Accessed Aug 24, 2020. http://www.apic.org/Professional-Practice/Implementation-guides

- Association for Professionals in Infection Control and Epidemiology. Implementation Guides, *Acinetobacter*. Accessed Aug 24, 2020. http://www.apic.org/Professional-Practice/Implementation-guides

- US Centers for Disease Control and Prevention. Be Antibiotics Aware. Accessed Apr 26, 2021. https://www.cdc.gov/antibiotic-use/index.html

- US Centers for Disease Control and Prevention. Methicillin-Resistant *Staphylococcus aureus* (MRSA). Accessed Aug 24, 2020. http://www.cdc.gov/mrsa/

Central Line–Associated Infections

- Association for Professionals in Infection Control and Epidemiology. Implementation Guides. Central Line–Associated Bloodstream Infection. Accessed Aug 24, 2020. http://www.apic.org/Professional-Practice/Implementation-guides

- Institute for Healthcare Improvement. Central Line–Associated Bloodstream Infection. Accessed Aug 24, 2020. http://www.ihi.org/resources/Pages/Tools/HowtoGuidePreventCentralLineAssociatedBloodstreamInfection.aspx

- The Joint Commission. Central Line–Associated Bloodstream Infection. Accessed Aug 24, 2020. http://www.jointcommission.org/topics/hai_clabsi.aspx

Surgical Site Infections

- Association for Professionals in Infection Control and Epidemiology. Implementation Guides, Orthopedic Surgical Site Infections. Accessed Aug 24, 2020. http://www.apic.org/Professional-Practice/Implementation-guides

- Association for Professionals in Infection Control and Epidemiology. Implementation Guides, Guide for the Prevention of Mediastinitis Surgical Site Infections Following Cardiac Surgery. Accessed Aug 24, 2020. http://www.apic.org /Professional-Practice/Implementation-guides

- American College of Surgeons. Surgical Patient Education Program. Accessed Aug 24, 2020. https://www.facs.org/education/patient-education

- Institute for Healthcare Improvement. How-to Guide: Prevent Surgical Site Infections. Accessed Aug 24, 2020. http://www.ihi.org/resources/pages/tools/howtoguidepreventsurgicalsiteinfection.aspx

Catheter-Associated Urinary Tract Infections

- Association for Professionals in Infection Control and Epidemiology. Implementation Guides, Catheter-Associated Urinary Tract Infections. Accessed Aug 24, 2020. http://www.apic.org/Professional-Practice/Implementation-guides

- Centers for Disease Control and Prevention. Catheter-Associated Urinary Tract Infections (CAUTI). Accessed Aug 24, 2020. http://www.cdc.gov/HAI/ca_uti/uti.html

- Institute for Healthcare Improvement. Catheter-Associated Urinary Tract Infection (CAUTI). Accessed Aug 24, 2020. http://www.ihi.org/topics/cauti/Pages/default.aspx

- The Joint Commission. Catheter-Associated Urinary Tract Infections (CAUTI). Accessed Aug 24, 2020. https://www.jointcommission.org/resources/patient-safety-topics/infection-prevention-and-control/catheter-associated-urinary-tract-infections-cauti/

Sentinel Events

- The Joint Commission. Sentinel Event Policy and Procedures. Accessed Aug 24, 2020. https://www.jointcommission.org/resources/patient-safety-topics/sentinel-event/sentinel-event-policy-and-procedures/

- The Joint Commission: Root Cause Analysis in Health Care: Tools and Techniques. Accessed August 24, 2020. https://www.jcrinc.com/-/media/deprecated-unorganized/imported-assets/jcr/default-folders/items/ebrca15samplepdf.pdf?db=web&hash=D9A527F917C81876009A950394FE8D69

Patient Safety and Performance Measurement and Improvement

- Agency for Healthcare Research and Quality. Quality and Patient Safety Resourcs. Accessed Aug 24, 2020. https://www.ahrq.gov/patient-safety/resources/index.html

- US Centers for Medicare & Medicaid Services. Quality of Care Center. Accessed Aug 24, 2020. https://www.cms.gov/Center/Special-Topic/Quality-of-Care-Center.html

- Institute for Healthcare Improvement. Accessed Aug 24, 2020. http://www.ihi.org

- National Quality Forum. Accessed Aug 24, 2020. http://www.qualityforum.org

References

1. Burke JP. Infection control—A problem for patient safety. *N Engl J Med*. 2003 Feb;348:651–656.

2. Leape LL, et al. The nature of adverse events in hospitalized patients—Results of the Harvard Medical Practice Study II. *N Engl J Med*. 1991 Feb;324(6):377–384.

3. US Centers for Disease Control and Prevention. Healthcare-Associated Infections. HAI Data. Accessed Aug 24, 2020. https://www.cdc.gov/hai/data/index.html

4. Bell T, O'Grady, N. Prevention of central line–associated bloodstream infections. *Infec Dis Clin North Am*. 2017 Sep;31(3):551–559.

5. Infection Control Today. Getting to Zero: Implications for Infection Prevention. Oct 15, 2009. Accessed Aug 24, 2020. https://www.infectioncontroltoday.com/view/getting-zero-implications-infection-prevention

6. Ellingson K, et al. Strategies to prevent healthcare-associated infections through hand hygiene. *Infect Control Hosp Epidemiol*. 2014 Aug;35(8):937–960.

7. Lambe KA, et al. Hand Hygiene Compliance in the ICU: A Systematic Review. *Crit Care Med*. 2019 Sep;47(9):1251–1257.

8. US Centers for Disease Control and Prevention: Guideline for hand hygiene in health-care settings. Recommendations of the Healthcare Infection Control Practices Advisory Committee and the HICPAC/SHEA/APIC/IDSA Hand Hygiene Task Force. *MMWR Recomm Rep*. 2002 Oct;51(RR-16):1–45. Accessed Aug 24, 2020. http://www.cdc.gov/mmwr/PDF/rr/rr5116.pdf.

9. World Health Organization. WHO Guidelines on Hand Hygiene in Health Care. 2009. Accessed Aug 24, 2020. https://apps.who.int/iris/bitstream/handle/10665/44102/9789241597906_eng.pdf.

10. Lydon S, et al. Interventions to improve hand hygiene compliance in the ICU: A systematic review. *Crit Care Med*. 2017 Nov;45(11):1165–1172.

11. Caris MG, et al. Nudging to improve hand hygiene. *J Hosp Infect*. 2018 Apr;98(4):352–358.

12. Lankford MG, et al. Influence of role models and hospital design on the hand hygiene of healthcare workers. *Emerg Infect Dis*. 2003 Feb;9(2):217–223.

13. Pittet D. Improving adherence to hand hygiene practice: A multidisciplinary approach. *Emerg Infect Dis*. 2001 Mar–Apr;7(2):234–240.

14. Schweizer ML, et al. Searching for an optimal hand hygiene bundle: A meta-analysis. *Clin Infect Dis*. 2014 Jan;58(2):248–259.

15. American Society for Quality. Failure Mode and Effects Analysis (FMEA). Accessed Aug 24, 2020. https://asq.org/quality-resources/fmea

16. Siegel JD, et al. Healthcare Infection Control Practices Advisory Committee. Management of Multidrug-Resistant Organisms in Healthcare Settings, 2006. Accessed Aug 24, 2020. https://www.cdc.gov/infectioncontrol/pdf/guidelines/mdro-guidelines.pdf

17. Cohen AL, et al. Recommendations for metrics for multidrug-resistant organisms in healthcare settings: SHEA/HICPAC position paper. *Infect Control Hosp Epidemiol*. 2008 Oct;29(10):901–913.

18. The Society for Healthcare Epidemiology of America. Compendium of Strategies to Prevent HAIs. Accessed Jan 28, 2021. https://www.shea-online.org/index.php/practice-resources/priority-topics/compendium-of-strategies-to-prevent-hais

19. US Centers for Disease Control and Prevention. National Healthcare Safety Network (NHSN). Updated Jan 2021. Accessed Jan 28, 2021. https://www.cdc.gov/nhsn/pdfs/pscmanual/12pscmdro_cdadcurrent.pdf

20. Marschall J, et al. Strategies to prevent central line-associated bloodstream infections in acute care hospitals: 2014 update. *Infect Control Hosp Epidemiol*. 2014 Jul;35(7):753–771.

21. O'Grady NP, et al., and Healthcare Infection Control Practices Advisory Committee (HICPAC). Guidelines for the Prevention of Intravascular Catheter-Related Infections. US Centers for Disease Control and Prevention, 2011. Accessed Aug 24, 2020. https://www.cdc.gov/infectioncontrol/pdf/guidelines/bsi-guidelines-H.pdf

22. US Agency for Healthcare Research and Quality. Healthcare Cost and Utilization Project: Statistics on Hospital Stays. 2013. Accessed Apr 2016. http://hcupnet.ahrq.gov/.

23. Scott RD, US Centers for Disease Control and Prevention. The Direct Medical Costs of Healthcare-Associated Infections in U.S. Hospitals and the Benefits of Prevention. Mar 2009. Accessed Dec 30, 2016. http://www.cdc.gov/HAI/pdfs/hai/Scott_CostPaper.pdf

24. Zimlichman E, et al. Health care-associated infections: A meta-analysis of costs and financial impact on the US health care system. *JAMA Intern Med*. 2013 Dec;173(22):2039–2046.

25. Anderson DJ, et al. Strategies to prevent surgical site infections in acute care hospitals: 2014 Update. *Infect Control Hosp Epidemiol.* 2014 Jun;35 (6):605–627.

26. Berrios-Torres SI, et al. Centers for Disease Control and Prevention guideline for the prevention of surgical site infection, 2017. *JAMA Surg.* 2017 Aug;152(8):784–791. Accessed Aug 24, 2020. https://jamanetwork.com/journals/jamasurgery/fullarticle/2623725

27. Saint S, et al. A program to prevent catheter-associated urinary tract infection in acute care. *N Engl J Med.* 2016;374:2111–2119.

28. Magill SS, et al. Changes in prevalence of health care-associated infections in U.S. hospitals. *N Engl J Med.* 2018;379:1732–1744.

29. Lo E, et al. Strategies to prevent catheter-associated urinary tract infections in acute care hospitals: 2014 update. *Infect Control Hosp Epidemiol.* 2014 May;35(5):464–479.

30. Gould CV, et al. Guideline for the Prevention of Catheter-Associated Urinary Tract Infections 2009. Updated Feb 2017. Accessed Aug 24, 2020. https://www.cdc.gov/infectioncontrol/pdf/guidelines/cauti-guidelines-H.pdf

Index

oversight of, 12, 14, 15, 25

prevention of HAIs as goal of, 11, 27

reporting and communicating finding of evaluation of, 255–256, 257

resources for, 259

resources to support, 13, 14, 16, 34, 36, 44–45, 46–47, 126

revision and updating of, 251, 252, 257

standards related to, 11–13, 25–26, 27, 38, 125–127, 251, 252

strategies and resources for development and implementation of, 2–5

work processes for, priority and efficiency of, 21–22

zero preventable infections goal of, 2

Infection Prevention and Control Canada (IPAC Canada)/ Community and Hospital Infection Control Association of Canada (CHICA-Canada), 22

Infection preventionist (IP)

authority and responsibility of, 11–12, 13, 14, 15–17, 20, 25, 27

authority to institute control measures in response to infection risk, 16, 17

communication and collaboration for multidisciplinary approach to IPC activities, 23, 26

competencies and professional practice standards for, 22–25, 27–28, 45–46

competency assessments of, 16

duties of, 12, 25

job description for, 17, 18–20, 25, 27, 28

leadership and influence of, 45–46

planning activities role of, 44

qualifications of, 13, 25–26

staffing ratio recommendations, 21

Infection Prevention Society, 22

Infectious diseases, 126. *See also* Epidemics and pandemics

capabilities to identify and investigate, 16

changes in the environment and challenges from, 44, 47

exposure prevention, 236–237

globalization and global disease threats, 1

growth in exposure to, 1

high-consequence infectious diseases (HCIDs), 39, 57, 59

isolation of patients with, 126

leadership responsibility for resources for preparedness efforts for, 39

mitigation and management of emerging, re-emerging, and evolving diseases, 1, 44, 111, 235–236

outbreak investigations, 90, 92, 101–103, 126, 139–141

planning and preparing for threats from, 1, 44, 107–108

prevention of transmission of, 234–241

reporting emerging, reemerging, and evolving diseases, 227, 229

reporting of data and control of outbreaks of, 100, 239–240

risk assessment process for highly infectious diseases, methodology and construct for, 57, 59

risk assessment protocol for patients from other countries, 111

risk-based data-driven approach to reduction in (PCI.5), 53, 91

risks related to, 51

social and economic effects of, 1

surveillance of events and performance measures related to, 96

survey on preparedness for, 44

symptoms and syndromes associated with, 114, 117

vaccine-preventable diseases (VPDs), 234, 235, 236, 237–240

Infectious Disease Society of America (IDSA)

clinical strategies resources, 158

evidence-based practice guidance from, 151

influenza vaccination guidance and resources, 242

risk assessment for policies and procedures and guidance from, 55

risks assessment and review of data and guidelines from, 61

Influenza and influenza vaccination program

access to vaccines, 243

barriers to acceptance of the vaccine, 242–243

declination reporting, 244

influenza vaccinations for staff (IC.02.04.01), 90, 234

mandatory vaccination recommendations, 242

rate of vaccination, 242

resources for, 246–247

sample tracer questions for, 70

screening and immunization of staff, 238

staff education on, 242, 245

staff vaccination programs, 241–245

surveillance of events and performance measures related to, 96

vaccination rate data reporting, 101, 243, 244

vaccination reporting requirements, 242

Influx of infectious patients

airborne infection isolation requirements, planning and preparing for, 118–119

communication related to, internal and external, 120

planning for and organizational capabilities to deliver care, treatment, and services, 108–110, 111–114, 115, 116

policies, procedures, and plans for response to, 111

PPE supply management and optimizing use of PPE during an, 130

process to manage patients with contagious diseases, 91

protection and care for health care workers during, 120

recognition of infectious disease emergency, 114–117

recognizing potential for, 110–111, 121–122

recovery and mitigation, 121

and reprioritization of risks, 56–57

response to, 110–111, 117–120

standards related to, 107–108, 109, 110–111, 123

surge capacity for, 118–119

Information technology (IT) and health informatics. *See also* Data and information

computer workstations and networking to support IPC, 43

electronic communication security, 43

electronic health records (EHRs), 43

IPC program support with, 43

surveillance program use of, 101

Injection safety

One & Only Campaign (CDC), 128, 129

protocols and practices in non-hospital settings related to, 14

resources for, 161

standard precautions and safe injection practices, 127, 128, 129

Injuries to patients (EC.04.01.01), 170

Injuries to staff (EC.04.01.01), 170

Institute for Healthcare Improvement (IHI)

clinical strategies resources, 159

HAI-prevention resources from, 270–271

practice bundles and strategies from, 151–152

quality improvement methods and guidance from, 251

International Association of Healthcare Central Service Materiel Management (IAHCSMM)

expertise as clinical resource for IPC, 17

International Patient Safety Goals (IPSG)

care processes improvement through evidence-based interventions (IPSG.5.1), 262, 264

hand-hygiene guidelines, adoption and implementation of evidence-based (IPSG.5), 53, 261, 262

Isolation strategies, 131

J

The Joint Commission

clinical strategies resources, 158–159

as deeming authority to survey on behalf of CMS, 190

mission and vision statement, 39, 40

requirements versus recommendations, 190, 193

risks assessment and review of data from, 61

Joint Commission Center for Transforming Healthcare, 263–264

Joint Commission International (JCI)

IPC requirements of, 2

mission and vision statement, 39, 40

requirements versus recommendations, 190, 193

risks assessment and review of data from, 61

Joint Commission Resources (JCR)

collaboration with APIC, 3–5

mission and vision statement, 39, 40

mission of, 3

K

Klebsiella pneumoniae carbapenemase (KPC), 71

L

Laboratory and laboratory resources

reference laboratories, 47

resources to support infection prevention and control program and activities, 34, 47

response to infection risks with cultures and testing, 16, 17

Laws, regulations, and guidelines

compliance with and an effective IPC program, 16

Leadership

change to improve performance, management of, 34, 44–45

characteristics of successful, engaged leaders, 37

clinical resources, responsibility for identification of and decisions about, 17, 20–22, 26, 27

collaboration and success of, 46

communication and success of, 45

culture of safety and quality, support for, 33, 37, 47

governing body, 39

importance for effective IPC program, 4

IP role in, 44

planning activities for safe, quality care
(LD.03.03.01), 34

planning and preparing for infectious disease
emergencies, 1, 44, 107–108, 111–114

Pneumonia. *See also* Ventilator-associated pneumonia
and infections

community-acquired pneumonia (CAP) protocol for TB
risk identification, 115–116

impact on patients, 1

locations for acquisition of, 1

Population-specific risks

care setting–specific risk assessments to identify,
57–58, 60

evaluation with risk assessment process, 71, 74

monitoring of, 54

stratification method for risk assessment, 54

Practice bundles and strategies, 151–153

Preconstruction risk assessment (PCRA), 70, 170, 172,
180

Prevention and Control of Infections (PCI) standards

cleaning and disinfecting environment and
environmental surfaces (PCI.7), 171

construction and renovation, management of risks
during (PCI.11), 171–172

data collection and analysis to reduce infection rates
(PCI.5), 126

emergency preparedness program

development, implementation, and evaluation of
(PCI.12.2), 13

global communicable diseases, focus on
response to (PCI.12.2), 13

emergency preparedness program development,
implementation, and evaluation (PCI.12.2),
107–108, 109, 123

infection prevention and control (IPC) program

resources to support infection prevention and
control program (PCI.3), 13, 36, 46–47

risk-based data-driven approach to health care–
associated infection prevention and control
program (PCI.5), 53, 91, 97

risk identification, management, and reduction
as part of design and implementation of
(PCI.4), 53, 92, 101

infection prevention and control activities, data
collection and analysis on (PCI.14), 126, 218

infection prevention and control process integration
into quality improvement and patient safety
program (PCI.14), 91, 97, 234, 252, 262

infection prevention and control program, reporting
results of (PCI.1), 218

infectious waste, disposal of (PCI.8), 171

IPC requirements and measurable elements (MEs),
2, 125

isolation of patients with infectious diseases
(PCI.12), 126

medical equipment and devices

infection risk reduction activities related to
(PCI.6), 192

single-use devices (PCI.6.1), 192

patients with contagious diseases, process to
manage influx of (PCI.12.1), 91

personal protective equipment requirements
(PCI.13), 126

processes associated with infection risks,
identification of (PCI.4), 126

resources allocation approval by leadership for IPC
(PCI.3), 126

responsibility to manage infection prevention and
control activities (PCI.1), 13, 91, 97

risk assessment and management–related
standards, 51, 53

risk assessment of areas of high risk for infection
(PCI.5.1), 53, 91, 252

risk-based data-driven approach to health care–
associated infection prevention and control
program (PCI.5), 53

staff education on IPC practices (PCI.15), 91–92, 97,
218, 252

staff roles and responsibilities for preventing
infections (PCI.2), 27

transmission-based precautions (PCI.12), 126

Procedures

practice bundles and strategies for infection
prevention, 151–153

risk assessment process for evaluation of infections
risks related to, 72, 74, 78

surveillance of events and performance measures
related to, 93

Processes and systems

best-practices approach embedded in routine
practice, 116

change to improve performance, leadership
management of, 34, 44–45

identification of processes associated with infection
risks, 126

importance to safe, quality care, 37–38

IPC work processes, priority and efficiency of, 21–22

planning to establish processes for safe, quality care, 34, 44

risk assessment for policies and procedures related to, 54–55, 56

risks assessment and review of, 61

standards related to reduction in infection risks, 125–127

Process measures and data, 55, 93, 94, 95

Program management

IP competency in, 46

Pseudomonas aeruginosa, 8, 173

Public health departments

collaboration with, 16

communication with and reporting IPC information to, 218, 227, 229

communication in response to infection risks, 17, 110–111

e-mail alerts from, 54

emergency response process and communication with, 120

expertise as clinical resource for IPC, 17

health and illness monitoring by, 54

information sharing and communicating trends to recognize potential influx of infectious patients, 110–111, 121–122

reporting infection and surveillance data to, 100, 239–240

risk assessment process role of, 54

risks assessment and review of data and information from, 61

Q

Qualitative risk assessment method, 63–64

gap analysis, 63–64, 65–66

SWOT (strengths, weaknesses, opportunities, and threats) analysis, 64, 67

Quality assurance activities

importance for effective IPC program, 15, 16

surveillance data use in, 16

Quality Improvement and Patient Safety (QPS)

IPC–related requirements and measurable elements (MEs), 2

risk management program to identify and reduce safety risks (QPS.10), 52

Quality improvement and patient safety program

approval and oversight of (GLD.1.2), 35

communication of information about (GLD.4.1), 35

development and implementation of (GLD.4), 35

integration of infection prevention and control

process into (PCI.14), 91, 97, 234, 252, 262

Quality of care and patient safety

barriers and challenges in non-hospital settings, 14

change to improve, leadership management of, 44–45

implementation of changes to improve, 44–45

infection-related risks to, 1

IPC importance for, 3, 4, 15, 16, 261, 269

leadership influence and responsibility for, 37–45

leadership support for culture of safety and quality, 33, 37

planning activities for safe, quality care, 34, 44

resources to support, 44–45, 271

staffing and resources to support, 34

staffing for, 12

staff role in, 12

staff roles and responsibilities for, 34

successful implementation of patient safety and IPC initiatives, 153–156

systems critical to, 37–45

Quantitative risk assessment method, 62–63

R

Reference laboratories, 47

Reprocessing. *See* Cleaning, disinfection, and sterilization processes and program

Resources. *See* Equipment, space, supplies, and resources; Staffing and personnel resources

Respiratory hygiene and cough etiquette, 113, 127, 128–129

Respiratory infections and diseases. *See also* COVID-19/ SARS-CoV-2 coronavirus pandemic

CDC poster on stopping the spread of, 138

risk-based data-driven approach to reduction in (PCI.5), 53, 91

surveillance of events and performance measures related to, 95

Risk assessment and management

annual risk assessment for IPC program, 240

areas of high risk for infection, risk assessment of (PCI.5.1), 53, 91, 252

continuous process of and written risk assessment as living document, 56, 57, 77

control measures in response to infection risk

authority statement example, 17

authority to institute, 16, 17

examples of measures, 16, 17

data-driven risk-based approach to health care– associated infection prevention and control program (PCI.5), 53

resources for comparing surveillance data, 76

responsibility for planning, managing, and implementing, 92, 97

risks identification through surveillance activities and analysis of data, 55, 60–61, 92–97, 127

scope and methods for surveillance, 81

staffing for, 17

standards related to, 89, 90–92, 125–127

surveillance plan, 81, 92

elements of a written plan, 94–96

work processes for, priority and efficiency of, 21–22

written surveillance reports, 97, 100

Survey Analysis for Evaluating Risk® (SAFER®) Matrix, 67, 68–69

SWOT (strengths, weaknesses, opportunities, and threats) analysis, 64, 67

T

Teams and teamwork. *See* Collaboration and teams

TeamSTEPPS® (AHRQ), 152–153

Temporary closing a unit or ward of in response to infection risks with, 16

Time study for IPC activities, 22, 27

Tracer activities and methodologies

assessment and evaluation of internal risks with, 67

influenza vaccination program, sample questions for, 70

risk assessment policies and procedures through, 55

Tracer methodology

assessment and evaluation of internal risks with, 70

Training. *See* Staff education, training, and orientation

Transfer and discharge of patients

communication and planning for, 229

handoff communications, 229–230

medical care referral form, 230

transfer of a patient/resident who has an infection that needs monitoring, treatment, and/or isolation, 90, 96, 100, 218, 229–230

Transmission-based precautions, 16, 17

CDC guidelines on, 130–131

focus and scope of, 130

implementation of, 125

isolation strategies, 131

PPE use during, 131–132

standards related to, 125, 126

surveillance of events and performance measures related to staff compliance with protocols, 95

Try This Tool resources, 9

Tuberculosis (TB)

case example, 115–116

transfer of patient with, 230

U

Urinary catheters and urinary tract infections (UTIs). *See also* Catheter-associated urinary tract infections (CAUTIs)

evidence-based practices implementation and reduction in, 2

impact on patients, 1

locations for acquisition of, 1

risk-based data-driven approach to reduction in (PCI.5), 53, 91

surveillance of events and performance measures related to staff compliance with protocols, 95

Utility system, management of risks associated with, 169, 171, 174–177, 184

V

Vaccine-preventable diseases (VPDs), 234, 235, 236, 237–240

Vaccines and vaccination programs. *See also* Influenza and influenza vaccination program

COVID-19 and emergence of vaccine-preventable diseases, 235

evaluation of vaccine-preventable diseases with risk assessment process, 71

faster development of vaccines, 1

screening for vaccine-preventable diseases, 237–240

staff vaccination and immunization program, 234, 241–244

surveillance of events and performance measures related to, 96

Vancomycin-resistant *Enterococci* (VRE), 71, 95, 130–131, 173

Ventilator-associated pneumonia and infections

costs related to, 2

nurse-physician collaboration for reduction in, 45

practice bundles and strategies for prevention of, 151, 152

surveillance of events and performance measures related to, 93

Vision of organization. *See* Mission, vision, and goals of organization

Visitors

communication processes and systems to communicate IPC information with, 44

restrictions on in response to infection risks, 16, 17

W

Water supply and system, 173, 174–176, 184

World Health Organization (WHO)

    clinical strategies resources, 161–162

    environment of care resources, 185

    evidence-based practices based on guidance from, 15

    hand hygiene guidelines, compliance with, 52, 262, 263, 270

    infection reports from, 61

    infectious disease exposure prevention guidance, 239, 241

    influenza vaccination guidance and resources, 242

    IPC program and IP professional practice assessment tools, 28, 259

    mask and social distancing guidance, 135, 217

    multidisciplinary approach to IPC activities, support for, 45

    occupational health resources, 246–247

    risk assessment and infection prevention and control (IPC) plan plan resources, 84

    risks assessment and review of data and guidelines from, 61

    standard precautions practices, 193

    surveillance resources, 104

    vaccine-preventable diseases (VPDs) guidance from, 235

Z

Zika virus, 1